Basic Science for the Clinical Electrophysiologist

Guest Editor

CHARLES ANTZELEVITCH, PhD, FHRS, FACC, FAHA

CARDIAC ELECTROPHYSIOLOGY CLINICS

www.cardiacEP.theclinics.com

Consulting Editors

RANJAN K. THAKUR, MD, MPH, MBA, FHRS
ANDREA NATALE, MD, FACC, FHRS

March 2011 • Volume 3 • Number 1

SAUNDERS an imprint of ELSEVIER, Inc.

W.B. SAUNDERS COMPANY
A Division of Elsevier Inc.

1600 John F. Kennedy Boulevard • Suite 1800 • Philadelphia, Pennsylvania 19103-2899

http://www.theclinics.com

CARDIAC ELECTROPHYSIOLOGY CLINICS Volume 3, Number 1
March 2011 ISSN 1877-9182, ISBN-13: 978-1-4557-0423-1

Editor: Barbara Cohen-Kligerman
Developmental Editor: Donald Mumford

Cardiac Electrophysiology Clinics (ISSN 1877-9182) is published quarterly by Elsevier Inc., 360 Park Avenue South, New York, NY 10010-1710. Months of issue are March, June, September, and December. Subscription prices are $167.00 per year for US individuals, $250.00 per year for US institutions, $88.00 per year for US students and residents, $187.00 per year for Canadian individuals, $279.00 per year for Canadian institutions, $239.00 per year for international individuals, $299.00 per year for international institutions and $126.00 per year for Canadian and foreign students/residents. To receive student/resident rate, orders must be accompanied by name of affilliated institution, date of term, and the signature of program/residency coordinator on institution letterhead. Orders will be billed at individual rate until proof of status is received. Foreign air speed delivery is included in all Clinics subscription prices. All prices are subject to change without notice. **POSTMASTER:** Send address changes to Cardiac Electrophysiology Clinics, Elsevier Health Sciences Division, Subscription Customer Service, 3251 Riverport Lane, Maryland Heights, MO 63043. **Customer Service: 1-800-654-2452 (US and Canada). From outside of the US and Canada, call 314-477-8871. Fax: 314-447-8029. E-mail: JournalsCustomerService-usa@elsevier.com (for print support); JournalsOnlineSupport-usa@elsevier.com (for online support).**

Reprints. For copies of 100 or more of articles in this publication, please contact the Commercial Reprints Department, Elsevier Inc., 360 Park Avenue South, New York, NY 10010-1710. Tel.: 212-633-3812; Fax: 212-462-1935; E-mail: reprints@elsevier.com.

Printed and bound by CPI Group (UK) Ltd, Croydon, CR0 4YY

Transferred to Digital Print 2011

Cover illustration: Representation of a rotor and its properties. (*Left*) Computational simulation of spiral waves originated by a rotor in a 2D structure. (*Center*) Progressive decrease of the conduction velocity (CV) due to the steeper convex curvature towards the tip of the wave front. (*Right*) Progressive decrease of the wavelength (WL) towards the center of rotation (core). The shortest wavelength is localized near the core.

Contributors

CONSULTING EDITORS

RANJAN K. THAKUR, MD, MPH, MBA, FHRS
Professor of Medicine, and Director,
Arrhythmia Service, Thoracic and
Cardiovascular Institute, Sparrow Health
System, Michigan State University,
Lansing, Michigan

ANDREA NATALE, MD, FACC, FHRS
Executive Medical Director, Texas Cardiac
Arrhythmia Institute at St David's Medical
Center, Austin, Texas; Consulting Professor,
Division of Cardiology, Stanford University,
Palo Alto, California; Clinical Associate
Professor of Medicine, Case Western
Reserve University, Cleveland, Ohio;
Senior Clinical Director, EP Services,
California Pacific Medical Center, San
Francisco, California; Department of
Biomedical Engineering, University of Texas,
Austin, Texas

GUEST EDITOR

**CHARLES ANTZELEVITCH, PhD, FHRS,
FACC, FAHA**
Gordon K. Moe Scholar; Executive Director
and Director of Research, Professor of
Pharmacology, Masonic Medical Research
Laboratory, Utica; Upstate Medical University,
Syracuse, New York

AUTHORS

FADI G. AKAR, PhD
Mount Sinai School of Medicine, New York,
New York

**CHARLES ANTZELEVITCH, PhD, FHRS,
FACC, FAHA**
Gordon K. Moe Scholar; Executive Director
and Director of Research, Professor of
Pharmacology, Masonic Medical Research
Laboratory, Utica; Upstate Medical University,
Syracuse, New York

ANDREAS S. BARTH, MD
Department of Medicine, The Johns Hopkins
Bayview Hospital, Baltimore,
Maryland

CONNIE R. BEZZINA, PhD
Associate Professor, Heart Failure
Research Center, Department of Clinical
and Experimental Cardiology, Academic
Medical Center, Amsterdam,
The Netherlands

ALEXANDER BURASHNIKOV, PhD, FHRS
Research Scientist, Masonic Medical
Research Laboratory, Utica, New York

IRA S. COHEN, MD, PhD
Leading Professor of Physiology and
Biophysics, Department of Physiology and
Biophysics, Health Sciences Center; Director,
Institute for Molecular Cardiology, Stony Brook
University, Stony Brook, New York

LIA CROTTI, MD, PhD
Section of Cardiology, Department of Lung,
Blood and Heart, University of Pavia;
Department of Cardiology, Fondazione
IRCCS Policlinico San Matteo, Pavia, Italy

DAVID N. EDWARDS, MD, PhD
Division of Cardiology, The Johns Hopkins
University, Baltimore, Maryland

SUSAN P. ETHERIDGE, MD
Division of Pediatric Cardiology and the Nora
Eccles Harrison Cardiovascular Research
and Training Institute, University of Utah
School of Medicine, Salt Lake City, Utah

HARRY A. FOZZARD, MD
Otho S.A. Sprague Distinguished Service
Professor of Medical Sciences, Emeritus,
Cardiac Electrophysiology Laboratories,
Department of Medicine, The University
of Chicago, Chicago, Illinois

LIOR GEPSTEIN, MD, PhD
Professor of Physiology and Cardiology,
The Sohnis Family Research Laboratory for
Cardiac Electrophysiology and Regenerative
Medicine, The Bruce Rappaport Faculty of
Medicine, Technion-Israel Institute of
Technology, Haifa, Israel

ROBERTO INSOLIA, PhD
Section of Cardiology, Department of Lung,
Blood and Heart, University of Pavia;
Department of Cardiology, Fondazione
IRCCS Policlinico San Matteo, Pavia, Italy

JOSÉ JALIFE, MD
Professor of Internal Medicine and The Cyrus
and Jane Farrehi Professor of Cardiovascular
Research; Professor of Molecular and
Integrative Physiology; Director, Department
of Internal Medicine, Center for Arrhythmia
Research, University of Michigan, Ann Arbor,
Michigan

DARWIN JEYARAJ, MD
Instructor of Medicine, Heart and Vascular
Center, MetroHealth Campus of Case Western
Reserve University, Cleveland, Ohio

JOHN C. LOPSHIRE, MD, PhD
Assistant Professor of Medicine and Cellular
and Integrative Physiology, Division of

Cardiology, Department of Medicine, Krannert
Institute of Cardiology, Indiana University
School of Medicine, Indianapolis, Indiana

ROOS F.J. MARSMAN, MSc, PhD
Student, Heart Failure Research Center,
Department of Clinical and Experimental
Cardiology, Academic Medical Center,
Amsterdam, The Netherlands

DAVID FILGUEIRAS RAMA, MD
Visiting Fellow in Basic Cardiac
Electrophysiology, Department of Internal
Medicine, Center for Arrhythmia Research,
University of Michigan, Ann Arbor, Michigan

DAVID S. ROSENBAUM, MD
Professor of Medicine, Biomedical
Engineering, Physiology and Biophysics;
Chief of Cardiology, Heart and Vascular
Center, MetroHealth Campus of Case
Western Reserve University, Cleveland,
Ohio

MICHAEL R. ROSEN, MD
Gustavus A. Pfeiffer Professor of
Pharmacology and Professor of Pediatrics;
Director, Center for Molecular Therapeutics,
Columbia University Medical Center,
New York, New York

GUY SALAMA, PhD
University of Pittsburgh, School of Medicine,
The Cardiovascular Institute, Pittsburgh,
Pennsylvania

**PETER J. SCHWARTZ, MD, FAHA,
FACC, FESC**
Section of Cardiology, Department of Lung,
Blood and Heart, University of Pavia;
Department of Cardiology, Fondazione IRCCS
Policlinico San Matteo, Pavia; Laboratory
of Cardiovascular Genetics, IRCCS Istituto
Auxologico Italiano, Milan, Italy; Department
of Medicine, University of Stellenbosch,
Cape Town; Department of Medicine,
Cardiovascular Genetics Laboratory, Hatter
Institute for Cardiology Research, Cape Heart
Centre, Faculty of Health Sciences, University
of Cape Town, Observatory, South Africa;
Chair of Sudden Death, Department of Family
and Community Medicine, College of
Medicine, King Saud University, Riyadh,
Saudi Arabia

JOHN C. SHRYOCK, PhD
Senior Director, Biology, Cardiovascular
Therapeutic Area, Gilead Sciences, Inc,
Palo Alto, California

GORDON F. TOMASELLI, MD
Michel Mirowski MD Professor of Cardiology,
Chief of Cardiology, The Johns Hopkins
University, Baltimore, Maryland

MARTIN TRISTANI-FIROUZI, MD
Division of Pediatric Cardiology and the Nora
Eccles Harrison Cardiovascular Research
and Training Institute, University of Utah
School of Medicine, Salt Lake City, Utah

DONGQI WANG, MD, PhD
Professor, The First Affiliated Hospital, Medical
School of Xi'an Jiaotong University, Xi'an,
China

ARTHUR A.M. WILDE, MD, PhD
Professor of Cardiology, Heart Failure
Research Center, Department of Clinical and
Experimental Cardiology, Academic Medical
Center, Amsterdam, The Netherlands

GAN-XIN YAN, MD, PhD
Professor, The First Affiliated Hospital, Medical
School of Xi'an Jiaotong University, Xi'an,
China; Professor, Lankenau Institute for
Medical Research and Main Line Health
Heart Center, Wynnewood, Pennsylvania

DOUGLAS P. ZIPES, MD
Distinguished Professor of Medicine and
Pharmacology and Toxicology, Division of
Cardiology, Department of Medicine,
Krannert Institute of Cardiology, Indiana
University School of Medicine, Indianapolis,
Indiana

Contents

Basic cardiac EP was a rich field before midcentury, but it was revolutionized by the development of the micropipette and the voltage clamp, and subsequently by molecular biology. A small number of talented scientists have built the field, but it now is large and relates to all parts of the biomedical enterprise. Although progress has been propelled by membrane biophysicists, major contributions have been made by scientists with primarily clinical cardiac questions. The field has grown in size and content to where direct focus on cardiac therapy, both drugs and devices, is possible.

Pathophysiological remodeling of cardiac function occurs at multiple levels, spanning the spectrum from molecular and subcellular changes to those occurring at the organ-system level. Of key importance to arrhythmias are changes in electrophysiological and calcium handling properties at the tissue level. This review discusses how high-resolution optical mapping of action potential and calcium transients has advanced our understanding of basic arrhythmia mechanisms associated with multiple cardiovascular disorders, including the long QT syndrome, heart failure, and ischemia-reperfusion injury. The article focuses on the role of repolarization gradients and calcium-mediated triggers in the initiation and maintenance of complex arrhythmias in these settings.

A cardiac arrhythmia simply defined is a variation from the normal heart rate and/or rhythm that is not physiologically justified. Recent years have witnessed important advances in our understanding of the electrophysiologic mechanisms underlying the development of a variety of cardiac arrhythmias. This article discusses the mechanisms responsible for cardiac arrhythmias, which are generally divided into 2 major categories: (1) enhanced or abnormal impulse formation (ie, focal activity) and (2) conduction disturbances (ie, reentry).

Advances in modern laboratory technologies and techniques over the past decade, including electrophysiologic and genetic analyses, have uncovered many novel mechanisms underlying sudden cardiac death, the J wave being one example. J wave syndromes include a spectrum of disorders that involve accentuation of the I_{to}-mediated epicardial action potential notch in different regions of the heart, leading to the development of prominent J waves, early repolarization, and ST segment elevation on the ECG. Phase 2 reentry has been identified as the trigger in J wave syndromes, and enhanced dispersion of repolarization as the substrate, giving rise to polymorphic ventricular tachycardia and fibrillation and sudden death. This article summarizes current knowledge about J wave syndromes, linking bench work with the bedside.

The hallmark of electrophysiologic remodeling in heart failure is arrhythmogenic prolongation of the action potential. Downregulation of repolarizing K^+ currents and bioenergetic pathways are hallmarks of electrophysiological remodeling. Ion transport and mitochondrial bioenergetic transcripts are tightly co-regulated, with a predicted increase in electrical instability in the failing myocardium. Cardiac resynchronization therapy (CRT) significantly shortens the action potential particularly in myocytes isolated from the lateral wall of the left ventricle during dyssynchronous contraction. This partial normalization of the electrical phenotype may provide an explanation for the reduced risk for arrhythmias and better prognosis after CRT.

Electronic pacemakers are the standard of care for certain cardiac disorders of rate and rhythm. This article discusses future alternative biologic pacemakers. The advantages that biologic pacing might offer are discussed as are current approaches to implementation. This article concludes that proof of principle has been demonstrated but that several hurdles remain before this new improved technology can become the standard of care.

This article describes the electrophysiologic basis for ventricular electrical remodeling, often manifest clinically as cardiac memory. The initiating mechanisms, signaling pathways, and transcription factors that participate in cardiac memory are reviewed. The evidence highlights the considerable plasticity of cardiac muscle in response to various pathophysiological insults. Insights into the highly regional nature of ventricular remodeling are provided. Elucidation of the ionic, molecular, and signaling pathways operative in specific regions will enhance development of pharmacologic, biologic, and device therapies to ameliorate cardiac remodeling or possibly induce reverse remodeling where therapeutically beneficial.

Timothy syndrome (TS) is a rare primarily sporadic disorder that affects the development of many organ systems. The first case of TS was reported in 1992 in a German report describing an infant with 2:1 atrioventricular block, prolonged QT interval, syndactyly, and subsequent sudden death. L-type calcium channels are critical for normal excitation-contraction coupling by providing the initial calcium influx that triggers a secondary release of calcium from the sarcoplasmic reticulum. The differential expression of the L-type calcium channels has implications for the severity of TS symptoms.

Mutations in the cardiac voltage-gated sodium channel encoded by the SCN5A gene have been linked to multiple cardiac arrhythmia syndromes, including the long QT syndrome, the Brugada syndrome, and cardiac conduction disease. The clinical severity of these disorders ranges from mild or even quiescent disease to life-threatening conditions. This article reviews insight gained on mutant sodium channels associated with these disorders, how these lead to disease, and the impact that this knowledge has had on the management of patients with these disorders.

Potassium channels are key players in the control of cardiac action potential, and their dysfunction can lead to atrial and ventricular arrhythmias. Mutations in genes encoding voltage-gated potassium channels, leading to their loss of function, cause long QT syndrome and Andersen-Tawil syndrome. Mutations in potassium-channel genes, leading to their gain of function, cause short QT syndrome and familial atrial fibrillation. Recently, the potassium-channel K_{ATP} has been implicated in early repolarization syndrome and in Brugada syndrome.

Enhanced late sodium channel current (I_{Na}) in the heart is arrhythmogenic. Although normally small and without a demonstrable physiologic role, late I_{Na} is enhanced in many pathologic conditions, including ischemia and heart failure. An enhanced late I_{Na} provides significant additional depolarizing current and Na^+ influx throughout the plateau of the action potential and contributes to reduction of repolarization reserve and Na^+-induced Ca^{2+} loading of myocytes. Arrhythmic activity associated with enhanced late I_{Na} includes diastolic depolarization, early and late afterdepolarizations, triggered activity, alternans, and torsades de pointes tachyarrhythmias. Inhibition of late I_{Na} has been demonstrated to reduce arrhythmogenesis.

Atrial fibrillation (AF) is an epidemiologic problem, that has a huge impact on hospitalization costs and on overall health care. Only a profound and complete understanding of the mechanisms involved in the initiation and maintenance of AF will allow the generation of more specific prevention and/or treatment of new episodes. Insights into AF mechanisms derived from the use of appropriate experimental and numerical models have crucial relevance in attempts to improve patient care and to develop new and more specific therapies. This article focuses on current knowledge about such mechanisms and their translation to real clinical situations.

Atrial fibrillation (AF) is a growing clinical problem associated with increased morbidity and mortality. Although rhythm control strategies are preferable to those of rate control, pharmacologic therapy capable of widely applicable, safe, and effective AF suppression is not available. Recent studies have uncovered significant differences in the characteristics of atrial and ventricular sodium channels, leading to identification of drugs capable of atrial-selective inhibition of sodium channel current (I_{Na}). These agents are capable of atrial-selective depression of I_{Na}-dependent parameters and thus effective and safe suppression of AF. This review describes this and other strategies under development for the pharmacologic management of AF.

In the field of clinical cardiac electrophysiology, many of the commonly utilized diagnostic and therapeutic tools employed by the practicing clinician derive their origin from basic science discoveries. This trend continues in this rapidly evolving field. It is incumbent upon practicing clinicians in this field to acquire and maintain an understanding of basic science cardiac electrophysiology principles to aid in clinical practice. This will allow them to practice clinical care of their patients with a solid foundation built upon these principles, to independently assess the utility and efficacy of newly introduced diagnostic and therapeutic tools, and to actively participate in the acquisition of new basic science knowledge related to arrhythmias and conduction system disease.

Cardiac Electrophysiology Clinics

READ THE CLINICS ONLINE!

Access your subscription at:
www.theclinics.com

Such a Long Journey – From Phenotype to Molecular Mechanisms

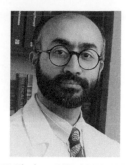 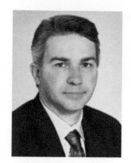

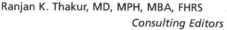

Ranjan K. Thakur, MD, MPH, MBA, FHRS   Andrea Natale, MD, FHRS
Consulting Editors

"Life can only be understood backwards; but it must be lived forwards."

    Soren Kierkegaard (Danish Philosopher, 1813–1855)

While genes may be involved in causing various arrhythmias by effects on one or more molecular mechanisms (such as ion channels), the final common pathway to arrhythmogenesis is still re-entry, after depolarizations or altered automaticity. In cardiac electrophysiology, our understanding often progresses "backwards" from defining the clinical spectrum, to the immediate arrhythmia mechanism, to the genetic and molecular under-pinnings. A deeper understanding of clinical arr-hythmias requires going on this journey, though it may be backwards. The reward of these efforts is not only a deeper understanding but also the potential to discover therapies to improve our patients' lives.

Briefly, a case in point is that of the Brugada syndrome. In Southeast Asia, the problem of sudden death in young men during sleep has been recognized for quite some time (Lai Tai in Thailand, Bangungut in the Phillipines and Pokkuri in Japan). The first clinical description of this phenomenon appeared in the early 1990s, followed by the recognition of ST elevation in the right pre-cordial leads and ventricular ectopy causing reen-trant ventricular arrhythmias, leading to sudden death. Then, the sodium channel was implicated along with the SCN5A gene. Although our understanding is not yet complete, this case demonstrates how human understanding prog-resses ever deeper.

This issue of the *Cardiac Electrophysiology Clinics* focuses on "Basic Science for the Clinical Electrophysiologist." It is imperative that as our understanding of arrhythmias deepens, the clinician is able to make sense of the new knowledge. This requires periodic reinforcement of the fundamentals. Dr Antzelevitch is a renowned basic scientist and he has assembled a panel of internationally respected experts to elucidate basic science concepts as they relate to a modern understanding of arrhythmogenesis. The subject may appear hard and somewhat removed from day-to-day clinical care, but it is truly fundamental knowledge and clinicians should be well acquainted with it. We hope that readers will give the articles in this issue the care that Dr Antzelevitch and his colleagues have expended in preparing them.

Ranjan K. Thakur, MD, MPH, MBA, FHRS
Thoracic and Cardiovascular Institute
Sparrow Health System
Michigan State University
405 West Greenlawn, Suite 400
Lansing, MI 48910, USA

Andrea Natale, MD, FHRS
Texas Cardiac Arrhythmia Institute
Center for Atrial Fibrillation at
St David's Medical Center
1015 East 32nd Street, Suite 516
Austin, TX 78705, USA

E-mail addresses:
thakur@msu.edu (R.K. Thakur)
andrea.natale@stdavids.com (A. Natale)

cardiacEP.theclinics.com

Preface
Basic Science for the Clinical Electrophysiologist

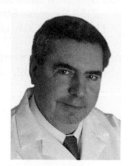

Charles Antzelevitch, PhD, FHRS
Guest Editor

It has been a distinct pleasure and privilege to serve as editor of this issue of the *Cardiac Electrophysiology Clinics* focused on "Basic Science for the Clinical Electrophysiologist." Cardiac electrophysiology has witnessed remarkable progress in recent years with major advances in our understanding of the genetic, molecular, biophysical, and cellular mechanisms underlying the development of cardiac arrhythmias. We have invited reviews by leading experts who have contributed prominently to their respective fields and have remained at the cutting edge of scientific discovery.

Dr Fozzard leads off the series with a historical accounting of the gradual transition from clinical to cellular, biophysical, and molecular aspects of cardiac electrophysiology over the past century. Drs Salama and Akar then discuss how state-of-the-art tools have advanced our understanding of basic arrhythmia mechanisms associated with multiple cardiovascular disorders, with particular focus on high-resolution optical action potential and calcium transient imaging.

In the next two articles, Drs Burashnikov, Yan, and I provide an overview of the genetic, molecular, and cellular mechanisms underlying arrhythmogenesis, in particular, the J wave syndromes.

These include Brugada and early repolarization syndromes, the latter being the subject of intense investigation in recent months. Drs Edwards, Barth, and Tomaselli focus their attention on arrhythmias associated with heart failure, whose prognosis remains poor despite remarkable improvements in medical therapy.

Drs Cohen and Gepstein provide us a fascinating tour of the world of biological pacemakers, describing the diverse and creative strategies being developed. Drs Rosenbaum, Jeyaraj, and Rosen discuss the physiological and pathophysiological factors underlying cardiac memory and its clinical implications. Drs Tristani-Firouzi, Etheridge, Marsman, Bezzina, Wilde, Crotti, Insolia, and Schwartz review the incredible progress made in our understanding of channelopathies involving defects in genes encoding various subunits of the calcium, sodium, and potassium channels. Dr Shryock explores the mounting evidence linking late sodium channel current activity to cardiac arrhythmogenesis and the development of drugs that selectively target this current.

Drs Rama and Jalife focus on the intricate mechanisms underlying the development of atrial fibrillation (AF), and Dr Burashnikov and I discuss

Card Electrophysiol Clin 3 (2011) xv–xvi
doi:10.1016/j.ccep.2010.12.001

pharmacological management of AF, the most common arrhythmia encountered in clinical practice and one that is creating a very significant epidemiologic problem. Finally, Drs Lopshire and Zipes close the series with a discussion of how commonplace therapies born at the basic science bench top find their way to the bedside practice of medicine.

The articles presented in this issue are designed to highlight how basic science discoveries in cardiac electrophysiology have been and continue to be made, how they are translated into clinical therapy, and how they are ultimately refined to become part of evidence-based clinical practice.

Charles Antzelevitch, PhD, FHRS
Masonic Medical Research Laboratory
2150 Bleecker Street
Utica, NY 13501, USA

Upstate Medical University
Syracuse, NY 13202, USA

E-mail address:
ca@mmrl.edu

History of Basic Science in Cardiac Electrophysiology

Harry A. Fozzard, MD

KEYWORDS

- Heart • Micropipettes • Voltage clamp • Ion channels
- Mechanisms of arrhythmias

PREFACE

Basic cardiac electrophysiology (EP) has been inspired by 2 disciplines, clinical cardiology and membrane/cellular biophysics. Early in the twentieth century, the field was clinically oriented, seeking to understand the relation between disease and cardiac electrograms. Other scientists, motivated by a desire to understand natural systems, were studying the general origin of cellular electric properties. Although communication between the 2 areas has sometimes been suboptimal, they merged to form our modern basic cardiac EP. Modern electronics and digital computers have also been critical to both basic and clinical EPs, providing essential tools for both basic insights and clinical applications of cardiac EP. The field has flourished with good ideas.

Understanding the origin of ideas is fraught with difficulty. Ideas typically derive from interaction, combined with contemplation and study. However, scientific creative processes are rarely explained in a form accessible to a historian. The scientific literature has developed a publishing format that is focused on how to reproduce the reported results, not on how the ideas were developed. Hodgkin[1] describes the problem thus: scientists tend to publish how the experiments should have been conceived and performed rather than how the investigators actually stumbled on their answers. Consequently, the important creative process is often obscured in the otherwise voluminous scientific literature.

It is a pleasure to try to tell the story of basic cardiac EP. I have organized it around the work of the major scientific forebearers, chosen from those whom I knew first- or secondhand. Many have contributed greatly to EP in general, but I have mentioned only those who seem to me to have had a particularly large effect on the cardiac branch of the field. In contrast to the typical scientific article, this article references old articles, which often contain insights we are in danger of losing. This exposition necessarily reflects my personal experiences; I ask forbearance for this. Morton Arnsdorf intended to coauthor this article with me. I have been influenced by his thoughts, and miss greatly the contribution he would have made to this effort.

THE BIOPHYSICAL ERA
Microelectrodes for Transmembrane Potential Recording

The major technical breakthrough that transformed basic cardiac EP was development of the fine-tipped glass micropipette that could record transmembrane potentials without injuring the cell. For decades, glass pipettes had been used for bioelectric studies recording localized surface potentials or transmembrane potentials from large cells.[2,3] The giant axon of the squid (giant because of fusion of multiple smaller axons) could be studied with pipettes, but they were too large for cardiac cells. Negative intracellular potentials were not in doubt, but values were uncertain and description of the action potential was qualitative. A common method

Supported by NIH, NHLBI grant HL065661.
Cardiac Electrophysiology Laboratories, Department of Medicine, The University of Chicago, 5841 South Maryland Avenue, Chicago, IL 60637, USA
E-mail address: hafozzar@uchicago.edu

Card Electrophysiol Clin 3 (2011) 1–10
doi:10.1016/j.ccep.2010.10.010

for study of the heart was recording of injury potentials, the difference between a distal outside electrode and one close to a freshly damaged region, but the cardiac injury current was short lived because the muscle healed over.[4]

It was Ling,[5] working with skeletal muscle in Gerard's Chicago laboratory, who first successfully made microelectrodes that could record transmembrane potentials accurately. His pipettes were less than 1 μm in outer diameter, pulled by hand from capillary tubing over a small gas-oxygen flame, and filled by boiling with isotonic potassium chloride (KCl) solution. The recording system had a high resistance and poor frequency response, so only steady potentials could be recorded correctly. Electrophysiologists either came to the Chicago laboratory to learn the Ling-Gerard method or, in some cases, successfully reproduced the method independently. A genealogy of how the micropipette method spread between 1950 and 1970 from Chicago, Illinois to cardiac electrophysiologists was compiled by Weidmann.[6] Key individuals in the early spread of micropipette use were Alan Hodgkin, Ichiji Tasaki, Brian Hoffman, and the Woodbury brothers.

For European electrophysiologists, it was Alan Hodgkin's visit to Chicago in 1949 that enabled him to bring the method back to Cambridge, England. With William Nastuk, his visitor from New York, he used a cathode follower system that recorded the skeletal muscle action potential. This system showed a significantly positive overshoot that depended on the concentration of outside sodium.[7] They also used 3 M KCl to fill the pipettes, increasing their conductivity and reducing the junction potential, resulting in a frequency response adequate for recording the action potential. Nastuk, tiring of the hand method, designed the first automatic pipette puller. Hodgkin taught Silvio Weidmann, who was in his Cambridge laboratory, and Edouard Coraboeuf, who was visiting the laboratory from Paris, France. They used the Hodgkin-Nastuk cathode follower system to record the first cardiac action potentials from dog cardiac Purkinje fibers.[8] Meanwhile, in Salt Lake City, Utah, Lowell and Walter Woodbury along with Hans Hecht, the chief of Cardiology, recorded the frog ventricular action potential using a string galvanometer.[9] My direct questioning of Silvio Weidmann and Walter Woodbury failed to determine which laboratory was exactly the first to record cardiac action potentials; both insisted that the honor was shared, although we can say that Hans Hecht was the definitely first clinician. This response characterizes to me the collegial noncompetitive spirit of electrophysiologists in the early years after World War (WW) II.

The Physiology department at SUNY Downstate, Brooklyn, New York was already a center for cardiac EP under its chairman Chandler Brooks when young Brian Hoffman quickly applied the intracellular microelectrode method. Hoffman and Cranefield[10] (recently from the laboratory of Eyster and Meek[11] at the University of Wisconsin) thoroughly explored cardiac EP. The monumental Hoffman achievement was no doubt in part stimulated by the year that Silvio Weidmann spent there before he returned to Bern, Switzerland. A host of cardiac electrophysiologists, both basic and clinical, were mentored by Brian Hoffman and Paul Cranefield in Brooklyn and subsequently at the Columbia University College of Physicians and Surgeons and the Rockefeller Institute.

Ichiji Tasaki was an exceedingly creative electrophysiologist developing the gap method of recording action potentials, although his early work in Japan was missed by much of the field because during WWII, his publications were in Germany, sent via German U-boats. Subsequently, he worked in Cambridge and Bern, and then in St Louis, Missouri, introducing the microelectrode technique to electrophysiologists at Washington University, who then taught me.

The Voltage Clamp

In 1952, Hodgkin and Huxley[12] published their extraordinary series of articles on voltage clamp studies of the squid's giant axon, describing Na^+ and K^+ currents as functions of membrane voltage and time, earning them the Nobel Prize in 1963. This thorough description of membrane excitability and the proposal for membrane sodium and potassium transport structures (ie, channels) stunned the electrophysiology community, and it was a decade before this huge step in understanding excitability could be incorporated into general understanding. What led to their great leap forward?

The discussion leads to Cole[3] who was a physicist studying the passive and active properties of membranes. After WWII, Cole worked at the University of Chicago in the Institute for Radiobiology and Biophysics (an outgrowth of the Manhattan Project to develop biologic applications of nuclear physics). A statistics colleague, L. J. Savage, had suggested to him that the best way to study active membrane properties was to control the transmembrane voltage and measure the current required. During the summer of 1947, Cole shared a laboratory at the Woods Hole Marine Biological Laboratory with Marmont,[13] who was developing a method to insert a wire axially into the giant axon of the squid. With guard chambers around a central chamber, he was able to control the voltage uniformly across the axon membrane in the central chamber and record the feedback current required. During off hours of that summer, Cole used this first voltage clamp to record the currents from a set of voltage steps, showing an early inward current and a delayed outward current. He inferred that the delayed outward current was carried by K^+ but did not understand the transient inward current.

Meanwhile, Hodgkin and Huxley were released from their wartime work in England on radar and military electronics and resumed their collaboration in Cambridge, demonstrating the likely role of sodium (Na^+) as the carrier of excitatory current and also trying to develop a voltage control method.[1] While Hodgkin was in the United States with a Rockefeller Fellowship, he had worked with Cole at Woods Hole in 1938 and maintained a correspondence with him. Cole wrote of his first voltage clamp experiments, and Hodgkin arranged to visit Cole in Chicago in March 1948, during a trip to New York to visit his wife's parents. It must have been an exciting visit in Chicago, and both researchers give considerable credit to each other in inferring the ionic basis of excitability from the preliminary recordings.[3] Upon return to Cambridge, Hodgkin built the voltage clamp apparatus that he, Huxley, and Bernard Katz would begin to use that fall at the Marine Laboratory in Plymouth, England. In the next few years, Hodgkin and Huxley[12] completed their analysis of the voltage and time dependencies of Na^+ and K^+ conductances, described them with partial differential equations, and solved the equations to show that they could indeed reproduce the squid action potential and conduction. Huxley integrated the equations with a mechanical calculator because digital computers were not available. Electrophysiologists were stunned by the beauty of the result. Over the next decade, Cole, Tasaki, Woodbury, and only a few others were able to comprehend the power of this achievement and build on the concepts. How did these ideas influence cardiac EP?

Silvio Weidmann was a Swiss neurophysiologist who was sent to Hodgkin's laboratory in 1948 by Torsten Teorell, his mentor in Uppsala, Sweden. Weidmann[14] learned the microelectrode method from Hodgkin, and on July 16, 1949, he was offered the chance to record from the heart of a dog that had been killed after being used to demonstrate Starling's Law of the heart. Hodgkin pointed out that Weidmann now had the opportunity "to rediscover the whole of cardiac electrophysiology." Weidmann understood thoroughly the revolutionary work of Hodgkin and Huxley on the squid axon. Upon return to Bern, Switzerland,

he devised a method to control the membrane potential at a point in a cardiac Purkinje fiber using 2 micropipettes and the plate amplifiers of an oscilloscope. Using this arrangement, he demonstrated that the Hodgkin-Huxley model of voltage and time dependency of Na^+ and K^+ conductances explained qualitatively the cardiac action potential,[15,16] the effects of local anesthetic drugs,[17] and many other cardiac electrical phenomena.

At University College, London, where Andrew Huxley became the Chairman in 1960, Otto Hutter had a graduate student named Denis Noble. Noble,[18] intrigued by the Hodgkin-Huxley concepts, used an early digital computer to show that reasonable extrapolation of available cardiac experimental data could lead to the calculation of a cardiac Purkinje fiber action potential and associated pacemaker potential. This work highlighted numerous critical issues in cardiac electrogenesis, which only quantitative study could resolve. For example, the upstroke velocity would require a density of Na^+ channels that exceeded even the density of the Na^+ channels of nerves. The reduced conductance contributing to the plateau was modeled as an instantaneous function of membrane potential,[19] although membrane conductance appeared to decrease progressively during the plateau. Of course, no calcium (Ca^{2+}) current was included because it had not yet been demonstrated. This pioneering work reviewed all critical data to that point and set the agenda for the next decade of basic cardiac EP.

In Bern, Carmeliet[20] had demonstrated that cardiac Purkinje fibers could be shortened to a few millimeters and yet retain their normal resting and action potential characteristics as a result of healing over at the ties or cut ends. Deck and colleagues[21] in Heidelberg, Germany used this shortened Purkinje strand for voltage clamp study of K^+ currents. Hecht and colleagues[22] also exploited the short Purkinje strand for voltage clamp. I learned of the method at a meeting in Milan, Italy in 1963 and quickly built the clamp apparatus to resolve the problem of excess membrane capacity relative to the number of Na^+ channels.[23] Noble (who had moved to Oxford) and his graduate student Tsien[24] soon showed that there are several different types of delayed rectifier K^+ currents in addition to the inward rectifier current, presaging the plethora of cardiac K^+ currents that are now known.

Calcium Current

The critical role of calcium in influencing and generating muscle contraction was well known by this time, but how the action potential triggered an increase in intracellular Ca^{2+} was unknown. The most uncertain part of the ionic mechanism of the cardiac action potential was the plateau and eventual repolarization, and a Ca^{2+} current could contribute to it. Several early reports supported the idea of such a Ca^{2+} current in crustacean muscle.[25,26] Among many interested in the question was Reuter,[27] who was studying the mechanism of effect of catecholamines on cardiac contraction. In 1964, he moved to Bern and at his suggestion we tried some pilot experiments that clearly demonstrated that cardiac muscle has a Ca^{2+} current during the plateau.[27] He also demonstrated the critical Na^+-Ca^{2+} countertransport system in cardiac muscle,[28,29] which because of its electrogenicity (more than 2 Na^+ exchanged for each Ca^{2+}) also affects repolarization. Subsequently, several types of Ca channels have been found in the heart, and even more types in the central nervous system.

Catechols have a dramatic effect on cardiac function, and it was important to understand how this was achieved. Exploring the mechanism of catecholamine effect on breakdown of glycogen, Earl Sutherland pioneered the field of second messenger modulation via phosphorylation (Nobel Prize in 1974). The role of Ca current in catecholamine enhancement of contraction was resolved by Tsien and Weingart[30] Tsien moved to Yale when he left Denis Noble's laboratory), partly by showing an effect of phosphorylation on the Ca^{2+} channel to increase Ca^{2+} current. The cascade of G protein involvement, cyclic AMP production, and channel phosphorylation was explored by Trautwein and Hescheler,[31] which was important because the cardiac Ca^{2+} channel was the first ion channel to be shown to have second messenger modulation. Now it is clear that most or all channels in the heart and other excitable tissues are modulated in multiple ways under both physiologic and pathologic conditions, including drug mechanisms for therapeutic and toxic effects.

The voltage clamp also made it possible to study the expected dependence of cardiac contraction on membrane voltage and the associated Ca^{2+} current.[32–34] Ca^{2+} current was not sufficient to activate the contractile proteins directly, but it triggered the release of Ca^{2+} from the sarcoplasmic reticulum[35,36] via its action on its ryanodine receptor release channel (CICR). The CICR experiments were first done by Duane Hellam in Podolsky's National Institute of Health laboratory using the skinned fiber preparation of Natori, and then by Lincoln Ford, who after working with Andrew Huxley came to Chicago. CICR is particularly important for the heart.[37] The spectacular success of intracellular optical indicators developed by Richard Tsien's brother Roger (Nobel Prize in 2008) was initiated in part by the latter's interest in monitoring levels of cardiac cell Ca^{2+}.[38]

Single Channel Recordings

At a conference at the New York Academy of Sciences I attended in 1961, some of the last holdouts finally accepted the idea that cells were bounded by a discrete impermeant membrane rather than simply by a sol-gel transition with different ion exchange properties. Hodgkin and Huxley[12] were careful not to refer to channels but to ion transport molecules. Proof of existence of these channels as gated pores with ion selectivity in biologic membranes was elusive. Bimolecular lipid membranes could be constructed, which when doped with various proteins showed discrete steplike changes in conductance,[39] suggesting gated channels. The mathematical predictions of the behavior of randomly opening channels, called membrane noise, was developed by Katz and Miledi[40] for the analysis of acetylcholine-activated motor end plate currents (Katz received the Nobel Prize in 1970 for his work on synaptic transmission). Anderson and Stevens[41] predicted that the single channel conductances of those channels would be about 32 picosiemens, a reasonable number, but outside the recording range of conventional methods. Suction pipettes had been long used in EP to record potentials from small patches of membrane. The Nobel Prize in 1991 was awarded to Erwin Neher and Bert Sakmann for perfecting the method and recording accurately the gating behavior of single channels.[42] Now the stochastic behavior of one molecule (or complex of a few molecules) composing a single channel could be monitored directly, demonstrating categorically the existence of gated channels. Strong suction would also rupture the membrane beneath the patch pipette, providing open electric and solution access to the cell interior and allowing high-quality voltage clamp of single cells, a boon for investigators studying the small cardiac cells that were becoming available through cell isolation and culture. Recording of the first single cardiac channels was done in Bern.[43]

The membrane's role in electrogenesis was also demonstrated by methods that allowed perfusion of the interior of cells, first applied for the giant axon of squid.[44] The first controlled intracellular perfusion of single cardiac cells[45] used a method developed in Kiev, Ukraine by Kostyuk[46] for single snail neurons. This method has the advantage of allowing direct application and withdrawal of ions, metabolites, and drugs to and from the inner side of the membrane. Another major step in clarifying the properties of ion channels was the successful recording of gating currents at the University of Pennsylvania by Cole's former student Armstrong and his collaborator Bezanilla.[47] Hodgkin and Huxley[12] had speculated that for channels in the membrane to respond to changes in membrane voltage, they must be charged, and that the membrane field caused or permitted conformational changes that could open or shut the pore. Small outward currents preceded the inward Na^+ currents, but proper study had to await better clamps and computer-based data acquisition. These gating currents have been used in the heart to investigate the molecular mechanism of action of local anesthetics,[48] building on Weidmann's[17] original experiments. Indeed, the development of fast programmable digital computers that could be dedicated to experimental control has made modern cardiac EP possible. One milestone in their application to the field was the LINC computer developed at the Lincoln Laboratories, Massachusetts Institute of Technology, and in 1963 the parts were distributed to 24 electrophysiologists by the NIH, including one to Woodbury, who introduced computer systems to a generation of cardiac scientists. For example, the LINC was used for the first real-time monitoring of cardiac rhythm in newly developed coronary care units.[49]

Gap Junctions and Spread of Current

The electrocardiogram is the extracellular representation of the complex spread of depolarization and subsequent repolarization of the atria and ventricles, and the sequence of this electrical process is critical to the mechanical function of the heart.[50] This electrical continuity of heart muscle has led to its being called a syncytium, yet it has long been clear from anatomic studies that the heart is composed of separate independent cells.[51] Furthermore, if the heart is damaged, the injured borders seal themselves electrically and continue to function in contrast to skeletal muscle cells[4]; otherwise, surgery on the heart would be nearly impossible and myocardial infarction would have a universal lethality. Electric coupling between cells is almost as if the cell membrane barriers were nonexistent.[52] Cell coupling could be from chemical synaptic transmission (although conduction is sufficiently fast to make this implausible), from fast electric coupling by depolarization of the narrow intercalated disk space (conceptually valid, but also slow), or from direct cytoplasmic connection via

channels. There was a vigorous argument for some time that direct cytoplasmic contact did not exist.[53] However, conduction in heart muscle is achieved via electrotonic spread of current.[54] Weidmann[55] showed intracellular diffusion of radioactive K^+ along a strand of ventricular muscle composed of many cells in series and that the effective resistance between cells was about the same as that along the length of a 125 micron single cell. The ability of cardiac muscle to heal over at the site of injury was shown by Délèze[56] in Bern to depend on the presence of Ca^{2+} in the outside medium and that it occurred 1 to 3 cell lengths back from the injury, as if the intercalated disk at that site, formerly having low resistance, had developed high resistance. Thus the existence of special low-resistance junctions between cells was gradually established for many tissues, including the heart and nerves.[57] Eventually, the functional study of gap junctions could be done by electric recordings from the cardiac cell pairs[58] and by inserting the purified junctional channels in artificial membrane bilayers.

JOINING WITH MOLECULAR BIOLOGY

Proof of the existence of ion channels and insight into their molecular function required determination of their molecular structure. This knowledge was also needed to resolve the question if the heart channels were the same as those in the nerve/brain or were unique structures with their own special functions. The rapidly developing field of molecular biology intersected EP in the early 80s. The first step was to purify the channel protein of interest and obtain some partial sequence, from which to make probes to locate the messenger RNA. The problem is that ion channels are found only in trace quantities in membranes, but the eel electric organ has a very high concentration of acetylcholine receptor (AChR) channels and Na channels. The AChRs were purified and partially sequenced[59] and then successfully cloned by Noda and colleagues.[60] Using tagged tetrodotoxin as marker, Agnew and colleagues[61] succeeded in purifying enough of the Na^+ channel to allow Noda and colleagues[62] to determine the coding DNA sequence for it. Shortly thereafter, Numa's laboratory in Kyoto, Japan reported 3 mammalian brain Na^+ channel sequences. Thus began a new era for cardiac EP.

The cardiac Na^+ channel was cloned by 2 laboratories, more or less simultaneously, using information about the sequences of brain channels. A consortium of investigators found 2 isoforms of Na^+ channels in skeletal muscle,[63] of which one was prominent in denervated or embryonic skeletal muscle (and resistant to tetrodotoxin). The same isoform was independently cloned from cardiac muscle.[64] We discovered this identity when Bob Barchi came to Chicago to help Rogart and me prepare for a Program Project grant proposal, and by calling back to his laboratory, he confirmed that the 2 clones were identical. As always, it is critical that the clone express the functional protein in order for one to be certain that it is correct.[65] So far there is only one isoform unique to the heart, with a one–amino acid residue difference that confers its resistance to tetrodotoxin,[66,67] although some brain isoforms have been identified in the heart and the cardiac isoform has been found in brain.

Cloning of the first K$^+$ channel required a different approach. Many drosophila mutants had been characterized by geneticists during the years.[68] One mutant called Shaker was characterized as having a skeletal muscle defect probably related to action potential repolarization. By locating the chromosomal region with the genetic defect and sequencing large regions, the gene was found.[69] The Shaker clone provided probes that have resulted in cloning of many different K$^+$-selective channels from a variety of species, benefiting from the signature sequence that endowed the channels with K$^+$ selectivity.[70]

Mark Keating was a cardiology fellow in San Francisco who decided to look for a mechanism of lethal arrhythmia by finding the mutations that caused the long QT (LQT) syndrome. He reasoned, as did others, that K currents controlled repolarization, and that LQT syndromes resulted from an abnormality in a K channel. He joined the faculty in Salt Lake City, which had both a strong cardiac EP group and an outstanding genetics program, taking advantage of the special opportunity of working with Mormon populations. The first success of this approach was the report of a mutation in a K$^+$ new channel KCNQ1 and in a human version of the drosophila ERG channel (HERG).[71] These 2 molecules, along with their accessory subunits, probably constitute the 2 K$^+$ currents originally described by Noble and Tsien[24] that are responsible for cardiac repolarization. Now it is clear that LQT syndrome is associated with mutations in either K$^+$ or Na$^+$ channels or modulation of these channels.

A channel of particular importance to cardiac cells is the gap junction channel. The first gap junction subunit was cloned in 1984,[72] followed shortly by cloning of the main ventricular muscle isoform, connexin 43.[73] Purkinje fibers and atrial muscle mainly express a different isoform, connexin 40. More than 25 different isoforms have been cloned. Expression of gap junctional channels may be crucial for any effort to rebuild cardiac muscle from stem cells.

The ability to clone and express ion channels has provided information about their molecular function, including identifying the structures responsible for the key properties of permeation; selectivity; voltage-sensitivity; gating; and modification by second messengers, toxins, and drugs. This is gradually leading to new approaches to cardiac arrhythmia control. A major advance in ion channel science and in the search for therapeutic approaches was the successful X-ray analysis of the 3-dimensional structure of a bacterial K$^+$ channel (KcsA),[74] and then Shaker and other K$^+$ channels, recognized by award of the 2003 Nobel Prize to Rod MacKinnon (shared with Peter Agre who determined the structure of the water channel).

PURSUING THE ELECTROPHYSIOLOGIC BASIS OF ARRHYTHMIAS
Delayed Afterpotentials

For more than a century, it has been known that high stimulation rates suppress intrinsic physiologic pacemakers[75] as anyone who has used direct current shock to convert fast atrial rhythms can attest. However, cardiac glycosides could enhance the intrinsic rate of sinus node cells,[76] and in the presence of the drug, stimulation often provoked ectopic rapid rhythms.[77] As antiarrhythmic drugs were being developed, animal models were needed for testing, and ouabain-induced ventricular tachycardia/fibrillation was popular. The mechanism of this arrhythmia interested Lederer and Tsien[78] at Yale, who showed that digitalis induced an oscillatory change in membrane potential that could reach threshold for repetitive firing (also see[79]). Digitalis blocked the Na$^+$ pump, loading the cell with Na$^+$, which in turn loaded the cell with Ca^{2+} via Na-Ca exchange, setting in motion the further periodic release of Ca^{2+} from the sarcoplasmic reticulum (the CICR process). The elevated levels of intracellular Ca^{2+} generated an inward current, causing cyclic depolarization.[80] The only arrhythmias definitely caused by this mechanism are digitalis toxicity and inherited exercise-induced ventricular tachycardia, because of a mutation in the sarcoplasmic reticulum Ca release channel (ryanodine receptor) that sensitizes the channel to CICR. However, elevated levels of cellular Ca^{2+} occur in many pathologic conditions associated with lethal arrhythmias, such as heart failure, these arrhythmias may also depend on the delayed afterpotential mechanism.

Fibrillation

Fibrillation is a major cardiac problem, including both atrial fibrillation and lethal ventricular fibrillation. The concepts of excitatory loops because of unidirectional block and reentry have long been appreciated, as well as the need for a critical mass of tissue to sustain the rhythm. Transmembrane recordings first showed that the action potentials at a single point during ventricular fibrillation were relatively normal, with short durations related to firing frequency and occasional reduced amplitude responses.[81] A major step to understand fibrillation was the computer simulation by Moe and colleagues[82] incorporating the concept of excitation with dispersion of recovery intervals. The conflicting ideas for fibrillation have been a protected ectopic pacemaker with disorganized spread of excitation, circular excitation around an unexcitable barrier (eg, an infarcted area), or reentry by slow conduction of excitation unidirectionally through damaged, but living tissue. The conditions for conduction to be slow enough to allow excitation to emerge after recovery of the adjacent tissue seemed to be explained by the kinetics of Ca^{2+} channels, but not Na^+ channels. Allessie and colleagues[83] showed clearly that fibrillation could be maintained without a physical barrier because the excitability process could create a (nonstationary) functional area of inexcitable tissue. A crucial feature in the onset and maintenance of fibrillation is heterogeneity of action potential duration, which depends in part on intrinsically different expression of repolarizing currents.[84] Although some fibrillation resulted from general quasi-uniform changes in excitability (eg, afterpotentials produced by digitalis), more often the rhythm is triggered by one mechanism and sustained by another. Removal of the trigger region was the logical approach to prevention, and this was especially feasible if the trigger was a region of slow precarious conduction, such as injured cells adjacent to a myocardial infarct. This logic provided the rationale for ablation therapy, in which the small region composed of offending living cells is destroyed.

LQT Insights

Two valuable insights have come from the cloning of LQT mutants. First, a common Na channel mutant (deltaKPQ) associated with LQT interferes with repolarization by increasing the occurrence of bursting of the channel, adding a slowly decaying component to the Na^+ current.[85] This bursting prolongs the plateau of the action potential by the mechanism suggested by Noble[18] and is reminiscent of the mode 2 behavior of Ca^{2+} channels provoked by phosphorylation.[86] The delayed phase of Na^+ channel inactivation can also be seen under some circumstances in cloned normal Na channels.[87] This mechanism has also been suggested for arrhythmia in heart failure, and drugs that preferentially block this slowly decaying component are being sought.

The second valuable insight is the mechanism of drug-induced LQT. The Cardiac Arhythmia Suppression Trial report emphasized that antiarrhythmic drugs can also be proarrhythmic, a fact well known to older clinicians. One major mechanism of this proarrhythmic effect is blocking HERG,[88] allowing the development of a simple laboratory test to determine if a newly developed drug is likely to cause LQT syndrome.

CREATIVE CENTERS

Midcentury, the number of investigators in basic cellular EP was sufficiently small; hence, communication was informal. Rockefeller Fellowships, such as the one that brought Alan Hodgkin to the United States, contributed significantly to the development of the field internationally. WWII brought most electrophysiologic research to a halt, but its exploitation of radar, gunnery, and nuclear sciences provided invaluable experience in electronics for some key investigators, such as Hodgkin, Huxley, Woodbury, Katz, and Cole. During these times most university scientists devoted most of their school year to teaching, but during the summer they were free to experiment. Woods Hole and Plymouth Marine Biological Laboratories not only provided access to squid giant axons but also encouraged intimate collaboration and exchange of ideas. Gordon Research Conferences in New Hampshire were especially important for the fledgling basic cellular cardiac EP community. Established scientific societies (eg, the American Heart Association and the [British] Physiological Society, the newly founded Biophysical Society, and subsequently the Heart Rhythm Societies) were crucial, and the small Cardiac Electrophysiology Society grew from a forum for discussing interesting electrocardiograms to a valuable venue for exchanging ideas. The Physiological Laboratories in Cambridge (and its closely associated group at University College, London), the Physiology and Biophysics programs at the University of Chicago, and the Rockefeller Institute played particularly important roles in developing the modern cellular EP that galvanized the cardiac field.

Although individual laboratories have always been potent sources of ideas and major work, some programs have been developed for training of the increasing number of young people entering the field of basic cardiac EP. A typical pattern of training was to obtain one's basic training in one group, additional training in another, and take sabbaticals in a third group, so any listing is inevitably partial and incomplete. Nevertheless, these clusters were important in the development of cardiac electrophysiologists. Some of these electrophysiologists include Weidmann and Reuter in Bern, Switzerland; Noble in Oxford, England; Woodbury in Salt Lake City, Utah and Seattle, Washington; Hoffman in New York; Fozzard in Chicago; Tsien at Yale, Connecticut; Moe in Utica, New York; Zipes in Indianapolis, Indiana; Sano and Irisawa in Japan; Trautwein in Heidelberg and Homberg, Germany; Carmeliet in Leuven, Belgium, and Coraboeuf in Paris, France. The number of cardiac electrophysiologists is now legion.

SUMMARY

Basic cardiac EP was a rich field before midcentury, but it was revolutionized by the development of the micropipette and the voltage clamp, and subsequently by molecular biology. A small number of talented scientists have built the field, but it now is large and relates to all parts of the biomedical enterprise. Although progress has been propelled by membrane biophysicists, major contributions have been made by scientists with primarily clinical cardiac questions. The field has grown in size and content to where direct focus on cardiac therapy, both drugs and devices, is possible. It will be important to remember the physiologic and biophysical roots and not lose the multidisciplinary exchange that has made this field so creative.

REFERENCES

1. Hodgkin AL. Chance and design. Cambridge (UK): Cambridge University Press; 1992.
2. Blinks LR. The relation of bioelectric phenomena to ionic permeability and to metabolism in large plant cells. Cold Spring Harbor Symposia 1940;8:204–14.
3. Cole KS. Membranes, ions, and impulses. Berkley (CA): University of California Press; 1968.
4. Engelmann TW. Ueber the Leitung der Erregung im Herzmuskel. Pflugers Arch Physiol 1875;11:465–80.
5. Ling G, Gerard RW. The normal membrane potential of frog Sartorius fibers. J Cell Comp Physiol 1950;34: 383–96.
6. Weidmann S. The microelectrode and the heart. In: Kao FF, Koizumi K, Vassalle M, editors. Research in physiology. Bologna (Italy): Aulo Gaggi Publisher; 1971. p. 3–25.
7. Nastuk WL, Hodgkin AL. The electrical activity of single muscle fibers. J Cell Comp Physiol 1950;35: 39–73.
8. Coraboeuf E, Weidmann S. Potential de repos et potentials d'action du muscle cardiaque. CR Soc Biol Paris 1949;143:1329–31.
9. Woodbury LA, Woodbury JW, Hecht HH. Membrane resting and action potentials from single cardiac muscle fibers. Circulation 1950;1:264–6.
10. Hoffman BF, Cranefield PF. Electrophysiology of the heart. New York: McGraw-Hill; 1950.
11. Eyster JAE, Meek WJ. The origin and conduction of the heart beat. Physiol Rev 1921;1:1–43.
12. Hodgkin AL, Huxley AF. A quantitative description of membrane current and its application to conduction and excitation in nerve. J Physiol 1952;117:500–44.
13. Marmont G. Studies on the axon membrane. I A new method. J Cell Comp Physiol 1949;34:351–82.
14. Weidmann S. Membrane excitation in cardiac muscle. Circulation 1961;24:499–505.
15. Weidmann S. Effect of current flow on the membrane potential of cardiac muscle. J Physiol 1951;115: 227–36.
16. Weidmann S. The effect of the cardiac membrane potential on the rapid availability of the sodium-carrying system. J Physiol 1955;127:213–24.
17. Weidmann S. Effects of calcium ions and local anesthetics on the electrical properties of Purkinje fibres. J Physiol 1955;129:568–82.
18. Noble D. A modification of the Hodgkin-Huxley equations applicable to Purkinje fibre action and pacemaker potentials. J Physiol 1962;160:317–52.
19. Katz B. Les constants electriques de la membrane du muscle. Arch Sci Physiol 1949;2:285–99.
20. Carmeliet E. Chloride ions and the membrane potential of Purkinje fibres. J Physiol 1961;156: 375–88.
21. Deck KA, Kern R, Trautwein W. Voltage clamp technique in mammalian cardiac fibres. Pflugers Arch 1964;280:50–62.
22. Hecht HH, Hutter OF, Lywood DW. Voltage-current relation of short Purkinje fibres in sodium deficient solution. J Physiol 1964;170:5P.
23. Fozzard HA. Membrane capacity of the cardiac Purkinje fibre. J Physiol 1966;182:255–67.
24. Noble D, Tsien RW. Outward membrane currents activated in the plateau range of potentials in cardiac Purkinje fibres. J Physiol 1969;200:205–31.
25. Fatt P, Ginsborg BL. The ionic requirements for the production of action potentials in crustacean muscle fibres. J Physiol 1958;142:516–32.
26. Hagiwara S, Chichibu S, Naka KI. Effects of various ions on the resting and spike potentials of barnacle muscle. J Gen Physiol 1964;48:163–79.
27. Reuter H. Divalent cations as charge carriers in excitable membranes. Prog Biophys Mol Biol 1973; 26:1–43.
28. Reuter H, Seitz N. Dependence of calcium flux from cardiac muscle on temperature and external ion composition. J Physiol 1968;195:451–507.

29. Baker PF, Blaustein MP, Hodgkin AL, et al. The influence of calcium on sodium efflux in squid axons. J Physiol 1969;200:431—58.

30. Tsien RW, Weingart R. Inotropic effect of cyclic AMP in calf ventricular muscle studied by a cut end method. J Physiol 1976;260:117—41.

31. Trautwein W, Hescheler J. Regulation of cardiac L-type calcium current by phosphorylation and G-proteins. Annu Rev Physiol 1990;52:257—74.

32. Fozzard HA, Hellam DC. Relationship between membrane voltage and tension in voltage-clamped cardiac Purkinje fibres. Nature 1968;218:588—9.

33. Morad M, Trautwein W. The effect of the duration of the action potential on contraction in the mammalian heart muscle. Pflugers Arch 1968;299:66—84.

34. Beeler GW Jr, Reuter H. The relation between membrane potential, membrane currents, and activation of contraction in ventricular myocardial fibres. J Physiol 1970;207:211—29.

35. Ford LE, Podolsky RJ. Regerative calcium release within muscle cells. Science 1970;167:58—9.

36. Endo M, Tanaka M, Ogawa Y. Calcium-induced release of calcium from the sarcoplasmic reticulum of skinned skeletal muscle. Nature 1970;228:34—6.

37. Fabiato A, Fabiato F. Contractions induced by a calcium-triggered release of calcium from the sarcoplasmic reticulum. J Physiol 1975;249:469—96.

38. Marban E, Rink TJ, Tsien RW, et al. Free calcium in heart muscle at rest and during contraction measured with Ca-sensitive microelectrodes. Nature 1980;286:845—50.

39. Hladky SB, Hayden DA. Discreteness of conductance change in bimolecular lipid membranes in the presence of certain antibiotics. Nature 1970;225:451—3.

40. Katz B, Miledi R. The statistical nature of the acetylcholine potential and its molecular components. J Physiol 1972;224:665—700.

41. Anderson CR, Stevens CF. Voltage clamp analysis of acetylcholine produced end-plate current fluctuations at frog neuromuscular junctions. J Physiol 1973;235:655—91.

42. Hamill OP, Marty A, Neher E, et al. Improved patch clamp techniques for high resolution current recording from cells and cell-free membrane patches. Pflugers Arch 1981;391:85—100.

43. Reuter H, Stevens CF, Tsien RW, et al. Properties of single calcium channels in cardiac cell culture. Nature 1982;297:501—4.

44. Baker PF, Hodgkin AL, Shaw TI. Replacement of the axoplasm of giant nerve fibres with artificial solution. J Physiol 1962;164:330—54.

45. Makielski JC, Sheets MF, Hanck DA, et al. Sodium current in voltage clamped internally perfused canine cardiac Purkinje cells. Biophys J 1987;52:1—11.

46. Kostyuk PG. Intracellular perfusion of nerve cells and its effects on membrane current. Physiol Rev 1984;64:435—54.

47. Armstrong CM, Bezanilla F. Currents related to movements of gating particles of the sodium channels. Proc Natl Acad Sci U S A 1973;96:4158—63.

48. Hanck DA, Makielski JC, Sheets MF. Kinetic effects of quarternary lidocaine block of cardiac sodium channels: a gating current study. J Gen Physiol 1994;103:19—43.

49. Fozzard HA. Computer handling of coronary care unit data. Med Clin North Am 1973;57:143—54.

50. Scher AM, Spach MS. Cardiac depolarization and repolarization and the electrocardiogram. In: Berne RM, Sperelakis N, editors. Handbook of physiology, the cardiovascular system, vol. 1. Baltimore (MD): American Physiological Society; 1979. p. 357—92.

51. Sjostrand FS, Andersson E. Electron microscopy of the intercalated discs of cardiac muscle tissue. Experientia 1954;9:369—71.

52. Weidmann S. The electrical constants of Purkinje fibres. J Physiol 1952;118:348—60.

53. Sperelakis N. Additional evidence for high resistance intercalated discs in the myocardium. Circ Res 1963;12:676—83.

54. Barr L, Dewey MM, Berger W. Propagation of action potentials and the structure of the nexus in cardiac muscle. J Gen Physiol 1965;48:797—823.

55. Weidmann S. The diffusion of radiopotassium across intercalated disks of mammalian cardiac muscle. J Physiol 1966;187:323—42.

56. Délèze J. The recovery of resting potential and input resistance in sheep heart injured by knife or laser. J Physiol 1970;208:547—62.

57. Loewenstein WR. Junctional intercellular communication: the cell-to-cell membrane channel. Physiol Rev 1981;61:829—913.

58. Maurer P, Weingart R. Cell pairs isolated from adult guinea pig and rat hearts: effects of $[Ca^{2+}]$ ion nexal membrane resistance. Pflugers Arch 1987;409: 394—402.

59. Raftery MA, Hunkapillar MW, Strader NB, et al. Acetylcholine receptor: complex of homologous subunits. Science 1980;208:1454—7.

60. Noda M, Furatani Y, Takahashi H, et al. Cloning and sequence analysis of calf DNA and human genomic DNA encoding a-subunit precursor of muscle acetylcholine receptor. Nature 1983;305:818—23.

61. Agnew WS, Levinson SR, Brabson JS, et al. Purification of the tetrodotoxin-binding component associated with the voltage-sensitive sodium channel from *Electrophorus electricus* electroplax membranes. Proc Natl Acad Sci U S A 1978;75:2606—10.

62. Noda M, Shimizu S, Tanabe T, et al. Primary structure of *Electrophorus electricus* sodium channel deduced from cDNA sequence. Nature 1984;312: 121—7.

63. Kallen RG, Sheng Z-H, Yang J, et al. Primary structure and expression of a sodium channel

characteristic of denervated and immature rat skeletal muscle. Neuron 1990;4:233—42.

64. Rogart RB, Cribbs LL, Muglia LK, et al. Molecular cloning of a putative tetrodotoxin-resistant rat heart Na channel isoform. Proc Natl Acad Sci U S A 1989;86:8170—4.

65. Cribbs LL, Satin J, Fozzard HA, et al. Functional expression of the rat heart I Na channel isoform. FEBS Lett 1990;275:195—200.

66. Satin J, Kyle JW, Chen, et al. A mutant of TTX-resistant cardiac sodium channels with TTX-sensitive properties. Science 1992;256:1202—5.

67. Backx PH, Yue DT, Lawrence JH, et al. Molecular localization of an ion-binding site within the pore of mammalian sodium channels. Science 1992;257:248—51.

68. Ganetsky B. Genetic analysis of ion channel dysfunction in *Drosophila*. Kidney Int 2000;57:766—71.

69. Tempel BL, Papazian DM, Schwartz TL, et al. Sequence of a probable potassium channel component encoded at *Shaker* locus of *Drosophila*. Science 1987;237:770—5.

70. Heginbotham L, Lu Z, Abramson T, et al. Mutations in the K channel signature sequence. Biophys J 1994;66:1061—7.

71. Curran ME, Splawski I, Timothy KW, et al. A molecular basis for cardiac arrhythmia: *HERG* mutations cause long QT syndrome. Cell 1995;80:795—804.

72. Kumar NM, Gilula NB. Cloning and characterization of human and rat liver cDNAs coding for a gap junction protein. J Cell Biol 1986;103:767—76.

73. Beyer EC, Paul DC, Goodenough DA. Connexin-43: a protein from rat heart homologous to a gap junction protein from liver. J Cell Biol 1989;105:2621—9.

74. Doyle DA, Cabral JM, Pfuetzner RA, et al. The structure of the potassium channel. Science 1998;280:69—77.

75. Gaskell WH. On the innervation of the heart. J Physiol 1884;4:43—78.

76. Coraboeuf E, deLozé C, Boistel J. Action de la digitale sur les potentials de membrane et d'action du tissu conducteur du coeur de chien etudee à l'aide de microelectrodes intracellulaires. CR Soc Biol 1953;147:1169—73.

77. Wittenberg SM, Streuli F, Klocke FJ. Acceleration of ventricular pacemakers by transient increases in heart rate in dogs during ouabain administration. Circ Res 1970;26:705—16.

78. Lederer WJ, Tsien RW. Transient inward current underlying arrhythmogenic effects of cardiac steroids in Purkinje fibers. J Physiol 1976;263:73—100.

79. Ferrier GR. Digitalis arrhythmias, arrhythmias, and oscillatory afterpotentials. Prog Cardiovasc Dis 1977;19:459—74.

80. January CT, Fozzard HA. Delayed afterpotentials in heart muscle: mechanisms and relevance. Pharmacol Rev 1989;40:219—27.

81. Sano T, Tsuchihashi H, Shimamoto T. Ventricular fibrillation studied by the microelectrode technique. Circ Res 1958;6:41—6.

82. Moe GK, Rheinholdt WC, Abildskov JA. A computer model of atrial fibrillation. Am Heart J 1964;67:200—21.

83. Allessie MA, Bonke FIM, Schopman FJG. Circus movement in rabbit atrial muscle as a mechanism of tachycardia. III. The "leading circle" concept. Circ Res 1977;41:9—18.

84. Litovsky S, Antzelevitch C. Transient outward current prominent in canine ventricular epicardium but not endocardium. Circ Res 1988;62:116—26.

85. Nagatomo T, January CT, Ye B, et al. Rate-dependent QT shortening mechanism for the LQT3 deltaKPQ mutant. Cardiovasc Res 2002;54:624—9.

86. Cachelin AB, dePeyer JE, Kokubun S, et al. Ca channel modulation by 8-bromocyclic AMP in cultured heart cells. Nature 1983;304:462—4.

87. Trimmer JS, Cooperman SS, Tomiko SA, et al. Primary structure and functional expression of a mammalian skeletal muscle sodium channel. Neuron 1989;3:33—49.

88. Witchel HJ, Hancox JC. Familial and acquired long qt syndrome and the cardiac rapid delayed rectifier potassium current. Clin Exp Pharmacol Physiol 2000;27:757—66.

Deciphering Arrhythmia Mechanisms: Tools of the Trade

Guy Salama, PhD[a],*, Fadi G. Akar, PhD[b]

KEYWORDS

- Arrhythmias • Repolarization • Calcium • Mapping
- Long QT syndrome • Heart failure • Alternans

Pathophysiological remodeling of cardiac function occurs at multiple levels, spanning the spectrum from molecular and subcellular changes to those occurring at the organ-system levels.[1–4] With the advent of gene expression profiling techniques, major advances have been made with regards to the characterization of the molecular and genetic fingerprints of the heart at various stages during disease development.[5–7] The combination of these high-throughput strategies with standard electrophysiological and molecular studies have led to a more comprehensive appreciation of the molecular basis of congenital and acquired cardiovascular disorders. Despite these advances, however, mechanisms by which molecular remodeling translates into altered electrophysiological properties at the tissue-organ level remain unclear. In fact, defining the exact nature of the electrophysiological substrate of the heart during disease progression and the mechanisms that promote arrhythmic triggers is currently an active subject of intense investigation in many laboratories across the world.[8–13] Understanding mechanisms by which molecular and cell signaling pathways promote ion channel dysfunction and alter key electrophysiological properties at the tissue-network level will ultimately facilitate the design of new pharmacologic as well as cell-based and gene-based approaches to combat arrhythmias in patients.

In this article, the authors illustrate how optical imaging techniques have been effectively exploited by various investigators to advance our basic understanding of arrhythmia mechanisms.

Specifically, the authors focus on a few studies in which optical mapping of ventricular repolarization gradients and intracellular calcium (Ca^{2+}) dynamics have allowed us to decipher arrhythmia mechanisms associated with a broad range of cardiovascular disorders, including the long QT syndrome (LQTS), heart failure (HF), and ischemia-reperfusion injury.

ALTERED REPOLARIZATION AND HEART FAILURE

Action potential (AP) prolongation is an electrophysiological hallmark of cells and tissues isolated from failing and hypertrophied hearts.[1,10,14–16] This fundamental change in myocyte biology is caused by the impaired repolarizing capacity of the cardiac cell.[15,17] Abnormal AP prolongation at the cellular level readily translates to the level of the intact organ resulting in a long and variable QT interval on the surface electrocardiogram (ECG).[18–20]

Key changes in the early and late phases of AP repolarization have been documented in numerous studies using the patch clamp technique in isolated cardiomyocytes from various small and large animal models of HF.[15,21,22] These cellular electrophysiological changes were mechanistically linked to overall downregulation of repolarizing potassium currents,[15,23,24] an increase in late Na current density, and major changes in intracellular Ca^{2+} handling proteins.[25–28] Notably, HF results in reduced Ca^{2+} load within the sarcoplasmic reticulum (SR). This is caused by defective

[a] University of Pittsburgh, School of Medicine, The Cardiovascular Institute, 3550 Terrace Street, Suite S628 Scaife Hall, Pittsburgh, PA 15261, USA
[b] Mount Sinai School of Medicine, New York, NY 10029, USA
* Corresponding author.
E-mail address: gsalama@pitt.edu

Card Electrophysiol Clin 3 (2011) 11–21
doi:10.1016/j.ccep.2010.10.013
1877-9182/11/$ — see front matter © 2011 Published by Elsevier Inc.

sequestration of Ca^{2+} by the SR Ca^{2+} ATPase (SERCA2a) coupled with increased diastolic SR Ca^{2+} leak via the ryanodine receptor (RYR2).[29-31] Abnormal intracellular Ca^{2+} cycling is exacerbated by an upregulation in the expression and function of the electrogenic Na^+-Ca^{2+} exchanger (NCX), which generates a net inward depolarizing current during the plateau phase of the AP, further delaying repolarization.[25,32] At the opposite end of the spectrum, studies in humans and animal models showed delayed global repolarization and enhanced temporal repolarization instability using clinical noninvasive metrics, such as the QT-interval variability index and T-wave alternans on the surface ECG. Rosenbaum, Berger, and others have successfully developed and used sophisticated algorithms that detect various ECG metrics of global cardiac repolarization to identify patients at high risk of developing sudden cardiac death (SCD).[33-42] Of note are recent findings of a multicenter clinical trial in which noninvasive T-wave alternans testing was shown to significantly enhance the predictability of impending SCD in subjects with HF when combined with standard electrophysiological testing in this high-risk population.[36]

These cellular and clinical studies highlight the importance of repolarization changes occurring at the tissue level for arrhythmia genesis in HF. Until recently, efforts to investigate the mechanistic link between repolarization changes and reentrant arrhythmias were hampered by technical difficulties in assessing spatiotemporal repolarization gradients across the heart. With the advent of optical imaging techniques using voltage-sensitive dyes, a high-resolution measurement of cardiac repolarization at a cellular level within the intact syncytium has become possible.[10,43-46] Importantly, a quantitative relationship between altered spatiotemporal repolarization gradients and the incidence of arrhythmias in various animal models of HF have recently emerged.[10,14] In what follows, the authors focus on the role of spatial heterogeneities of repolarization in the incidence of reentrant arrhythmias in animal models of HF and the long QT syndrome that are prone to arrhythmias. Specifically, the authors discuss changes in transmural and transepicardial repolarization gradients as mechanisms for sustained ventricular arrhythmias.

TRANSMURAL REPOLARIZATION GRADIENTS IN HF

Antzelevitch and colleagues[47,48] pioneered the notion that heterogeneities of cellular repolarization in different cell types (epicardial, midmyocardial, and endocardial) may represent a unifying mechanism underlying a host of arrhythmias in congenital or acquired cardiac diseases, such as the long QT, short QT,[49] Brugada,[50,51] Andersen-Tawil,[52] and Timothy syndromes.[53,54] Of particular importance was the role of midmyocardial (M) cells in the establishment of transmural repolarization heterogeneity under conditions of prolonged QT interval in various ex vivo models of the LQTS.[48,55,56] Indeed, the functional expression of transmural heterogeneity under conditions of prolonged QT interval has been confirmed in most mammalian species, with the possible exception of porcine myocardium.[57] In nonfailing human hearts, a marked transmural action potential duration (APD) heterogeneity was elegantly documented at slow pacing rates (0.5 Hz) as midmyocardial islands of cells with distinctly long APDs and steep local APD gradients were observed.[45] In contrast, human failing hearts exhibited surprisingly reduced transmural APD heterogeneity and lacked prominent local APD gradients.[45] Of note, nonfailing human wedges were extracted from donor hearts that were rejected for age, hypertrophy, atrial fibrillation, or coronary artery disease. As such, by necessity, both failing and nonfailing preparations were most likely remodeled, which is reflected by their long APD values.[45]

Although inherent differences in the electrophysiological and pharmacologic properties of cell types across the ventricular wall are well recognized, electrotonic flow of currents between cells is expected to reduce the functional expression of electrical heterogeneities across the heart.[58] This reduction in functional expression has called into question the functional significance of transmural heterogeneity in general and M cells in particular.[59] In fact, some elegant studies in which extracellular plunge electrode recordings were used have failed to detect these heterogeneities in vivo.[60,61] It is important to note, however, that these studies did not establish conditions favorable for the emergence of M cell behavior (marked QT interval prolongation by bradycardia or pharmacologic agents). To investigate the functional expression and significance of transmural heterogeneities in intact myocardium, the approach of transmural optical AP mapping was used.[10,43] This approach allowed a simultaneous high-resolution measurement of repolarization properties across all muscle layers of the ventricular wall in an intact preparation where the influence of cell-to-cell coupling was present. Furthermore, because QT interval prolongation represents an electrophysiological hallmark of the failing heart, it was hypothesized that LQTS and HF may share important phenotypic properties at the multicellular tissue level that predispose them to arrhythmias via similar mechanisms.[10] By assessing the functional expression of transmural repolarization heterogeneities in arterially perfused canine wedge preparations from normal and failing hearts, Akar and Rosenbaum confirmed the role of transmural repolarization gradients in the initiation and maintenance of arrhythmias.[10] As expected, HF was associated with a marked AP prolongation across all myocardial layers, consistent with findings in isolated myocytes and whole animals. Interestingly, however, AP prolongation was heterogeneous across the left ventricular wall, affecting midmyocardial and endocardial muscle layers more selectively, thereby increasing the effective transmural repolarization gradient by approximately 2-fold.[10] In support of transmural dispersion of repolarization as a mechanism for arrhythmias associated with various disease etiologies, Yan and colleagues[62] demonstrated that left ventricular hypertrophy in a rabbit model of renovascular hypertension was also associated with significant enhancement of transmural dispersion of repolarization because of selective prolongation of subendocardial APs in this model.

Mechanisms underlying increased transmural repolarization heterogeneity in HF remain unresolved. These changes, however, likely involve multiple factors, including heterogeneous remodeling of cell-to-cell coupling, ionic currents/exchangers, and Ca^{2+} handling proteins. In an elegant study, Li and colleagues[24] investigated the ionic basis of transmural AP remodeling in HF by measuring the density of key repolarizing potassium (K^+) currents, including the transient outward (I_{to}), the inward rectifier (I_{K1}), and both components of the delayed rectifier (I_K) currents. By enlarge, K current changes were uniform in epicardial, midmyocardial, and endocardial myocytes of failing hearts, indicating that transmural repolarization heterogeneity observed at the tissue level could not be readily explained by cell-type specific remodeling of repolarizing K^+ currents. In a subsequent study, Akar and colleagues measured the expression levels of key alpha and beta subunits encoding these K^+ currents in the 3 principal myocardial layers of normal and failing hearts.[63] In support of the findings of Li and colleagues,[24] they also did not find a K^+ channel molecular basis (neither at the mRNA or protein levels) for the enhanced transmural repolarization heterogeneity observed in the failing heart.[63]

Poelzing and colleagues[13] attributed the location of the maximum transmural repolarization gradient to increased electrical resistivity at that location. Furthermore, they were able to convert basal transmural APD gradients measured across normal preparations into ones that mimicked those in HF simply by perfusing normal preparations with the gap junction inhibitor Carbenoxolone.[13] These findings highlight the potential importance of gap junction uncoupling in the mechanism of increased transmural dispersion of repolarization in HF. The authors, and others, have investigated the molecular basis for gap junction uncoupling in HF and have found major changes in the expression, distribution, and phosphorylation state of the main ventricular gap junction protein, $C\times43$, that develops with varying time courses during disease progression.[9,11,14,64] Specifically, end-stage HF was associated with overall $C\times43$ downregulation, dephosphorylation, and lateralization. In addition, Jin and colleagues recently reported the loss of interaction between $C\times43$ and the cytoskeletal protein ZO-1as a potentially critical event underlying severe conduction slowing and therefore gap junction uncoupling at late stages of remodeling in a model of pressure overload hypertrophy.[14] Hyperphosphorylation of $C\times43$ also occurred at earlier stages of remodeling that were associated with a milder form of conduction slowing.[14] As such, disrupted phosphorylation (either increased or decreased) at critical residues within the carboxyl domain of $C\times43$ may lead to loss of gap junction function via distinct mechanisms. The individual contribution of these complex molecular changes to the establishment of transmural repolarization heterogeneity across the failing heart remains unclear and will require direct investigation.

ALTERED REPOLARIZATION AND THE ACQUIRED LONG QT SYNDROME

The long QT syndrome is characterized by QT-interval prolongation often resulting in sudden death caused by torsade de pointes (TdP) mediated arrhythmias.[43] To date, several distinct mutations in ion channel and cytoskeletal proteins that directly or indirectly modulate ventricular repolarization have been identified in patients with LQTS. Both triggered activity caused by early afterdepolarization-mediated beats and reentrant excitation have been implicated in the mechanism of TdP. Because of limitations of conventional electrophysiological recording techniques, an integrated understanding of the mechanistic relationship between genetically determined alterations of cellular repolarization, QT interval prolongation, and the underlying mechanism of TdP remained unclear for many years. Using transmural optical AP mapping in ex-vivo perfused canine wedge preparations, Akar and colleagues investigated the functional topography of M cells and their role in TdP.[43] These studies provided direct evidence that the topographic distribution of M cells promotes unidirectional block and reentrant excitation underlying TdP in this canine wedge model of LQTS.[43] Conduction slowing was not a requirement for reentry because the path length dictated by the M-cell refractory zone was sufficiently long to allow partial recovery of excitability at former sites of block. Because of the exquisite sensitivity of M cells to rate, the broad zones of block delineated by M cells collapsed into functional lines of block that shifted dynamically on successive beats.[43] It is noteworthy that similar topographic distributions of M cells have recently been uncovered in ventricular wedge preparations isolated from human myocardium.[45]

APEX-BASE GRADIENTS OF REPOLARIZATION

In addition to the transmural gradients of repolarization previously discussed, optical AP mapping revealed significant apex-base differences in repolarization properties across the heart. Despite species differences in the expression levels and subtypes of cardiac K^+ channels, a qualitatively consistent apico-basal APD gradient of repolarization (shorter APDs at the apex compared with the base) were observed in guinea pig,[65–67] rabbit,[68] mouse,[44,69] canine, and human[70] hearts. Although the myocardial activation sequence is a determinant of force generation, the apico-basal sequence of repolarization determines the direction of relaxation. This mechanical property appears to be common to all species tested so far and may be fundamental to cardiac mechanics. Moreover, in a novel rabbit heart preparation isolated with intact and functional autonomic innervation and combined with optical mapping, the repolarization sequence was shown to be reversed during bilateral sympathetic or parasympathetic nerve stimulation. The reversal of the repolarization sequence was in large part caused by a highly heterogeneous nerve distribution being considerably more dominant at the base than the apex of the heart.[71]

In acquired long QT type 2 elicited by drugs that inhibit the rapid component of the delayed rectifying K^+ current, I_{Kr}, AP prolongation across the heart was not uniform, as it was more pronounced at the apex compared with the base, resulting in large repolarization gradients and a reversal of the repolarization sequence. The heterogeneous effect of I_{Kr} blockers in terms of APD prolongation occurs because of the heterogeneous expression of ERG channels that exhibit a higher density at the apex than the base.[68]

REPOLARIZATION AND THE CONGENITAL LONG QT SYNDROME

As previously mentioned, congenital LQTS is caused by distinct mutations in ion channel related genes. To date, multiple gain-of-function and loss-of-function mutations affecting ion channel pore forming, accessory, or cytoskeletal proteins have been identified. To investigate the arrhythmia phenotype of congenital LQTS and gain a more comprehensive understanding of the role of individual ion channel genes in modulating the electrophysiological substrate, transgenic LQTS mouse models have been created.[72] The technique of optical AP imaging has provided a remarkable tool for deciphering arrhythmia mechanisms in these models.[44] Indeed, Salama and coworkers found that epicardial dispersion of repolarization and refractoriness are critical determinants of the arrhythmia phenotype of various congenital forms of LQTS. Importantly, they found that not all loss-of-function mutations affecting K^+ channel subunits are created equal. For example, genetic deletion of the K^+ channel accessory subunit minK, which participates in the formation of I_{Ks}, did not cause major changes in the electrophysiological substrate or the incidence of arrhythmias despite presence of marked neurologic abnormalities (deafness, loss of balance, spinning behavior) in these mice. The lack of cardiac phenotype in minK knockout mice is consistent with the minor role that I_{Ks} is thought to play in murine ventricular repolarization. Also, these data highlight the importance of investigating mutations that affect K^+ channel pore forming and not only auxiliary subunits.

In support of the notion that loss-of-function mutations affecting K^+ channel subunits can produce divergent outcomes, these investigators also found that genetic deletion of Kv4.2, which encodes a pore-forming subunit of I_{to}, a major murine repolarizing current resulted in a paradoxic suppression of the apico-basal repolarization gradient across the heart. This decrease in epicardial dispersion of repolarization, which occurred under a condition of prolonged QT (and APD) interval, was indeed protective against arrhythmias. In sharp contrast, deletion of Kv1.4, another I_{to} pore-forming subunit, led to a marked increase in epicardial dispersion of repolarization and a heightened susceptibility to programmed stimulation-induced arrhythmias. As such, these investigators elegantly provided compelling proof in favor of dispersion of repolarization and not

APD (or QT interval) prolongation as the mechanism of torsade de pointes in the intact heart. These findings further highlight the importance of investigating arrhythmia mechanisms in multicellular and intact preparations and not only in isolated myocytes because of the clear importance of regional gradients in repolarization properties that develop under conditions of LQTS, even within a single muscle layer (ie, epicardium).

Using optical AP imaging, Liu and colleagues[12] also uncovered the electrophysiological basis for sex differences in susceptibility to torsade de pointes. Specifically, they found that the greater predisposition of adult female rabbits to E4031-mediated arrhythmias was reversed in prepubertal animals, which exhibited a male predominance in terms of drug-induced APD prolongation, EAD formation, and arrhythmia induction. These findings highlight the dynamic nature of the electrophysiological substrate, revealing how a given agent (E4031) can produce highly divergent electrophysiological outcomes that are both age and sex dependent.[12]

THE CENTRAL ROLE OF Ca^{2+} IN THE GENESIS OF ARRHYTHMIAS

Excitation-contraction coupling (ECC) is the process by which Ca^{2+} cycling and force generation are tightly controlled by the AP. The reverse is also true, as the shape and duration of the AP depend on intracellular free Ca^{2+} (Ca_i). A host of ion channels give rise to this mechano-electrical coupling, including $I_{Ca,L}$, I_{NCX}, Ca^{2+}-sensitive Cl^- channels (I_{Cl}), and I_{Ks}. At steady state, Ca^{2+} influx must equal efflux across the plasma membrane and the SR; any imbalance can only be transiently tolerated. In fact, modifications that alter the balance of Ca^{2+} influx and efflux typically lead to rhythm or pump dysfunction.

There is now a growing appreciation that the balance of Ca^{2+} influx to efflux is compromised in a wide range of pathologic conditions that lead to lethal arrhythmias due to the interdependence of the AP and Ca_i cycling. Hence, aberrations in Ca_i cycling can be the result of (1) a metabolic deficit that compromises Ca^{2+} pump function that may occur in ischemia/reperfusion, (2) either a gain or a loss of function of a cardiac ion channel that may occur in congenital and acquired long QT syndrome, and (3) ion channel remodeling that directly or indirectly compromises the balance of Ca_i fluxes that may occur in heart failure.[73] The development of techniques to simultaneously map APs and Ca_i transients at high spatial (hundreds to thousands of site) and temporal (1–5 kHz) resolution has provided compelling evidence that aberrations of Ca_i transients can initiate arrhythmias and may influence the dynamics of ventricular fibrillation (VF).

SIMULTANEOUS OPTICAL MAPPING OF VOLTAGE AND INTRACELLULAR FREE Ca^{2+}

Although many excellent voltage-sensitive[74] and Ca^{2+} indicator[75] dyes were available for dual mapping, several problems had to be overcome: (1) The 2 probes needed to have the same excitation wavelength to avoid mechanical components for wavelength switching, which would reduce acquisition rates; (2) voltage The voltage (V_m) and Ca_i probes needed to have different Stokes's shifts to avoid cross-talk between V_m and Ca_i signals; (3) The probes had to yield large fluorescence changes during a cardiac beat with a high signal-to-noise ratio to eliminate the need to time average the signals. Fluorescent probes were chosen because they pick up less motion artifacts compared with absorption dyes.[76] The first apparatus was based on the combination of RH 237 and Rhod-2AM to measure V_m and Ca_i and a set of 2 photodiode arrays with 16×16 pixels (Hamamatsu America Inc, Model C4675-103, Bridgewater, NJ, USA).[65] A significant improvement in the signal-to-noise ratio was achieved by using a new voltage-sensitive dye with a longer emission wavelength Pittsburgh 1 (PGHI),[77,78] which can be excited at 540 nm (like Rhod-2) but fluoresces above 640 nm with a peak emission at 790 nm. As a result, a wider band pass interference filter (560–620 nm) can be used to pick up the Ca_i signals from Rhod-2 fluorescence and to pick up the V_m signals from PGHI with a cutoff filter at 630 nm with no cross talk between the two parameters. Another improvement in spatial resolution was achieved with the CMOS cameras (SciMedia, Costa Mesa, CA, USA, Model: Ultima One) with 100×100 pixels that can be scanned at up to 10,000 frames/s.[79] The CMOS cameras have a limited interval of uninterrupted recordings of tens of seconds such that in several applications the photodiode arrays with lower spatial resolution have the disadvantage of continuous recordings through a long-lasting experimental protocol. For example, with photodiode arrays it is possible to record V_m and Ca_i during an ischemia (12–15 minutes) followed by a reperfusion (30–45 minutes).[80] Another application more suitable for photodiode arrays are mapping studies during a period of sympathetic nerve stimulation followed by its recovery.[71,81] A recent review of methods used to simultaneously map V_m and Ca_i offers extensive technical details.[82] The need to better understand the role of Ca_i aberrations on cardiac arrhythmias was the driving force to develop a high-speed imaging system for V_m and Ca_i and the method is now routinely used by numerous investigators. Future developments to simultaneously map V_m and extracellular K^+ accumulation are not far behind and are expected to be equally promising.[83]

Ca^{2+} AND THE GENESIS OF EARLY AFTERDEPOLARIZATIONS

Early afterdepolarizations (EADs) are thought to trigger TdP under conditions of congenital and acquired LQTS. There is appreciable variability in the kinetics of EADs but those that exhibit rapid upstrokes are considered to trigger TdP because they can capture, propagate, and trigger propagating APs.[84] EADs in the setting of impaired repolarization have been classically attributed to the spontaneous reactivation of the L-type Ca^{2+} current, I_{CaL}, during the abnormally long plateau and repolarization phases of the AP.[85,86] Alternatively, EADs may be triggered by SR Ca^{2+} overload, leading to spontaneous SR Ca^{2+} release during phases 2 or 3 of the AP, and the activation of forward mode I_{NCX}.[87,88]

Simultaneous optical APs and Ca_i transient mapping in rabbit hearts demonstrated that perfusion with E4031 (0.5 μM) caused marked prolongation of APD, reversal of repolarization gradient, and a 3- to 5-fold increase in dispersion of refractoriness.[44,68] EADs developed rapidly (within minutes) and high-frequency Ca_i-mediated EAD firing evolved into TdP. Normally, AP upstrokes are followed (within approximately 10 milliseconds) by a rise of Ca_i. During an EAD, V_m followed the rise of Ca_i by only 4 to 6 milliseconds. To determine whether EADs were generated primarily by Purkinje fibers, liquid N_2 was used to cryoablate the conduction system and the endocardium to produce hearts with a thin layer of surviving epicardium (approximately 1 mm). After blocking I_{Kr}, EADs were elicited at the same frequency even after the ablation of Purkinje fibers. The dynamic relationship between Ca_i and V_m during an EAD supports the notion that SR Ca^{2+} overload and spontaneous SR Ca^{2+} release activates I_{NCX}, which triggers I_{CaL} to produce EADs. The role of spontaneous SR Ca^{2+} release as a trigger of EADs was further emphasized in adult female hearts paced at a bradycardic rate treated with the I_{Kr} blocker dofetilide as a model of acquired LQT2. In these conditions, Ca_i oscillations appeared during long APDs but before the onset of EADs and TdP. Such Ca_i oscillations and the subsequent TdP were abolished by perfusion with nifedipine, with low external Ca^{2+} or ryanodine plus thapsigargin.[89]

Ca^{2+} AND SEX DIFFERENCES IN ARRHYTHMIA RISK

Numerous studies have shown an increase of TdP in women versus men following an exposure to agents that block K^+ channel HERG and inhibit I_{Kr}.[90–93] The increase in vulnerability to sudden death in women has been reported for cardiac drugs[91,92] as well as numerous noncardiac drugs[94] and are the result of regulation of ionic channel by sex steroids.[95] In congenital LQT2, the underlying genetic defects of K^+ channels may be asymptomatic in some conditions but in the presence of a mild block of I_{Kr} may precipitate TdP in women more frequently than in men because of their reduced cardiac repolarization reserve.[96] Human registry data for congenital LQT2 showed that sex and age had differential effects on arrhythmia risk.[97,98] Adult females had significantly higher risk; whereas, in children (aged <14 years), boys had higher risk of cardiac events.[97]

Rabbit hearts exhibit the same sex and age differences of LQT2-related arrhythmias as humans. In LQT2 induced with E4031 (0.5 μM), adult female hearts fired EADs within 5 minutes that evolved to TdP (n = 24/24). In contrast, adult male hearts rarely had an EAD or TdP (n = 16/18).[99] In prepubertal rabbits, males were more prone to TdP than females, even though females had longer APDs.[12] In adult rabbit hearts, the arrhythmia risk was reversed and females were more prone to TdP than males.[12,99] Optical mapping of EADs showed that the first site to exhibit EADs were sites with greater Ca^{2+} overload and were located at the base of the ventricles in both adult female and prepubertal male hearts.[99] The reason for the greater Ca^{2+} overload at the base of the epicardium was investigated by measuring the current densities of $I_{Ca,L}$ and I_{NCX} in voltage-clamp experiments. Myocytes isolated from the base of adult female hearts were found to have a 25% to 30% greater peak $I_{Ca,L}$ compared with myocytes from the apex and from adult male myocytes (apex and base).[99] The higher $I_{Ca,L}$ density at the base of adult female myocytes was caused by higher expression levels of the main subunit of L-type Ca^{2+} channels, Cav1.2α.[99] Ongoing studies show that the higher expression levels of Cav1.2α are upregulated by estrogen by a regional genomic mechanism. This new link between arrhythmia risk and the higher expression of Cav1.2α provides compelling evidence for Ca_i overload as the mechanism for EADs and TdP.

In transgenic rabbits with congenital LQT2 through the overexpression of a nonfunctional human HERG channel females had more lethal arrhythmias than males.[100] Closer investigations of transgenic rabbit hearts revealed a greater dispersion of repolarization, slower AV conduction, and a propensity to discordant alternans rather than the typical EADs and LQT2-related TdP.[101,102]

SR Ca^{2+} RELEASE AND ARRHYTHMIAS

Besides LQTS, several other pathologies have been linked to anomalies in Ca_i handling. In myocytes, Ca^{2+} overload and abnormal SR Ca^{2+} release can be induced by rapid pacing, inhibition of the Na^+/K^+ pump or β-adrenergic agonists.[103] In human and animal models of heart failure, reduced amplitude and slower decay of Ca_i transients caused by reduced expression/function of SERCA2a are often accompanied by increased I_{NCX} and decreased I_{K1} amplitudes. Under these conditions, residual adrenergic activity may cause SR Ca^{2+} overload leading to spontaneous Ca^{2+} release events and triggered arrhythmias.[104–106] Ischemia, through an inhibition of oxidative metabolism, causes important changes in ionic concentrations: intracellular and extracellular acidosis, elevations of Ca_i, Na_i, Mg_i, and of external K^+.[107,108] During ischemia, excessive production of free radicals leads to oxidation of sulfhydryl groups on proteins and channels, including RyRs, resulting in increased channel activity.[108,109] Reperfusion also has dire consequences. The prompt recovery of pH_o creates an outward H^+ gradient, a rise of Na_i via Na/H exchange, and Ca^{2+} overload by Ca^{2+} entry via Na/Ca exchange. Substantial cellular evidence exists in support of this mechanistic scenario that causes Ca^{2+} overload and reperfusion arrhythmias.[110]

Indeed, optical mapping of V_m and Ca_i can provide evidence that spontaneous Ca_i elevation leads to triggered activity of sufficient magnitude to capture, propagate, and initiate arrhythmias. In a guinea pig model of ischemia/reperfusion, approximately 17% of electrical instabilities were preceded by spontaneous Ca_i oscillations implicating aberrant Ca_i cycling as a potentially important trigger of premature beats and bigeminal or trigeminal rhythms.[111] In a canine wedge model of drug-induced LQT1, Ca^{2+}-induced triggered activity was typically initiated on the endocardium.[112] In pig hearts, the interdependence of V_m and Ca_i during VF induced by burst pacing was analyzed using mutual information (MI), as a statistical measure of the extent to which one variable, V_m, predicts another, Ca_i.[113] MI was high during pacing and ventricular tachycardia but fell dramatically during VF, suggesting that spontaneous SR Ca_i release may sustain VF by promoting wave break formation.[113] Although the latter findings were not reproduced in nonischemic hearts in VF,[114,115] there is less controversy regarding the role of Ca_i overload in ischemia and hypoxia.[73]

SUMMARY

Pathophysiological remodeling of cardiac function occurs at multiple levels, spanning the spectrum from molecular and subcellular changes to those occurring at the organ-system levels. Of key importance to arrhythmias are changes in the electrophysiological substrate and the incidence of Ca^{2+}-mediated triggers. The role of Ca_i aberrations is central because any deviation between Ca^{2+} influx and efflux is poorly tolerated and can come about by several routes. In LQT2, APD prolongation lengthens the interval during which Ca^{2+} influx occurs despite a rapid phase of Ca^{2+}-dependent inactivation, because a small persistent level of Ca^{2+} influx is maintained throughout the plateau phase and is voltage-dependent. Thus, the higher the expression levels of $I_{Ca,L}$ (as in the female heart) the greater the propensity to Ca_i overload and Ca^{2+}-triggered EADs and arrhythmias. In ischemia and hypoxia, the metabolic deficit compromises ATP-dependent Ca^{2+} uptake by the SR pumps resulting in an accumulation of cytosolic Ca^{2+}. A compensatory response arising from lower ATP levels activates ATP-dependent K^+ channels, and shortens APDs thereby reducing Ca^{2+} influx. In reperfusion, oxidative stress causes SR Ca^{2+} leaks by activating ryanodine receptors or enhancing $I_{Ca,L}$. In HF, the weaker cardiac muscle arises partly due to slower and attenuated Ca_i transients, which has been attributed to SR Ca^{2+} leaks via RyR2. In VF induced by burst pacing, the high-firing frequencies reduce the diastolic intervals during which Ca^{2+} efflux would normally reset cellular Ca^{2+} levels. Hence, high-resolution optical imaging has been effectively used by various laboratories to decipher arrhythmia mechanisms across broad cardiovascular disorders.

REFERENCES

1. Hill JA. Electrical remodeling in cardiac hypertrophy. Trends Cardiovasc Med 2003;13:316.
2. Jin H, Lyon AR, Akar FG. Arrhythmia mechanisms in the failing heart. Pacing Clin Electrophysiol 2008;31:1048.
3. Tomaselli GF, Marban E. Electrophysiological remodeling in hypertrophy and heart failure. Cardiovasc Res 1999;42:270.
4. Tomaselli GF, Zipes DP. What causes sudden death in heart failure? Circ Res 2004;95:754.

5. Barth AS, Kuner R, Buness A, et al. Identification of a common gene expression signature in dilated cardiomyopathy across independent microarray studies. J Am Coll Cardiol 2006;48:1610.

6. Gao Z, Barth AS, DiSilvestre D, et al. Key pathways associated with heart failure development revealed by gene networks correlated with cardiac remodeling. Physiol Genomics 2008;35:222.

7. Kaab S, Barth AS, Margerie D, et al. Global gene expression in human myocardium-oligonucleotide microarray analysis of regional diversity and transcriptional regulation in heart failure. J Mol Med 2004;82:308.

8. Akar FG, Laurita KR, Rosenbaum DS. Cellular basis for dispersion of repolarization underlying reentrant arrhythmias. J Electrocardiol 2000;33:23.

9. Akar FG, Nass RD, Hahn S, et al. Dynamic changes in conduction velocity and gap junction properties during development of pacing-induced heart failure. Am J Physiol Heart Circ Physiol 2007;293:H1223.

10. Akar FG, Rosenbaum DS. Transmural electrophysiological heterogeneities underlying arrhythmogenesis in heart failure. Circ Res 2003;93:638.

11. Akar FG, Spragg DD, Tunin RS, et al. Mechanisms underlying conduction slowing and arrhythmogenesis in nonischemic dilated cardiomyopathy. Circ Res 2004;95:717.

12. Liu T, Choi BR, Drici MD, et al. Sex modulates the arrhythmogenic substrate in prepubertal rabbit hearts with Long QT 2. J Cardiovasc Electrophysiol 2005;16:516.

13. Poelzing S, Rosenbaum DS. Altered connexin43 expression produces arrhythmia substrate in heart failure. Am J Physiol Heart Circ Physiol 2004;287:H1762.

14. Jin H, Chemaly ER, Lee A, et al. Mechanoelectrical remodeling and arrhythmias during progression of hypertrophy. FASEB J 2010;24:451.

15. Kaab S, Nuss HB, Chiamvimonvat N, et al. Ionic mechanism of action potential prolongation in ventricular myocytes from dogs with pacing-induced heart failure. Circ Res 1996;78:262.

16. Nattel S, Maguy A, Le Bouter S, et al. Arrhythmogenic ion-channel remodeling in the heart: heart failure, myocardial infarction, and atrial fibrillation. Physiol Rev 2007;87:425.

17. Kleiman RB, Houser SR. Outward currents in normal and hypertrophied feline ventricular myocytes. Am J Physiol 1989;256:H1450.

18. Atiga WL, Calkins H, Lawrence JH, et al. Beat-to-beat repolarization lability identifies patients at risk for sudden cardiac death. J Cardiovasc Electrophysiol 1998;9:899.

19. Pak PH, Nuss HB, Tunin RS, et al. Repolarization abnormalities, arrhythmia and sudden death in canine tachycardia induced cardiomyopathy. J Am Coll Cardiol 1997;30:576.

20. Tomaselli GF, Beuckelmann DJ, Calkins HG, et al. Sudden cardiac death in heart failure. The role of abnormal repolarization. Circulation 1994;90:2534.

21. Akar FG, Tomaselli GF. Ion channels as novel therapeutic targets in heart failure. Ann Med 2005;37:44.

22. Nass RD, Aiba T, Tomaselli GF, et al. Mechanisms of disease: ion channel remodeling in the failing ventricle. Nat Clin Pract Cardiovasc Med 2008;5:196.

23. Beuckelmann DJ, Nabauer M, Erdmann E. Alterations of K+ currents in isolated human ventricular myocytes from patients with terminal heart failure. Circ Res 1993;73:379.

24. Li GR, Lau CP, Ducharme A, et al. Transmural action potential and ionic current remodeling in ventricles of failing canine hearts. Am J Physiol Heart Circ Physiol 2002;283:H1031.

25. Bers DM, Pogwizd SM, Schlotthauer K. Upregulated Na/Ca exchange is involved in both contractile dysfunction and arrhythmogenesis in heart failure. Basic Res Cardiol 2002;97(Suppl 1):I36.

26. Beuckelmann DJ, Nabauer M, Erdmann E. Intracellular calcium handling in isolated ventricular myocytes from patients with terminal heart failure. Circulation 1992;85:1046.

27. Hasenfuss G, Meyer M, Schillinger W, et al. Calcium handling proteins in the failing human heart. Basic Res Cardiol 1997;92:87.

28. O'Rourke B, Kass DA, Tomaselli GF, et al. Mechanisms of altered excitation-contraction coupling in canine tachycardia-induced heart failure, I: experimental studies. Circ Res 1999;84:562.

29. Lehnart SE, Wehrens XH, Marks AR. Defective ryanodine receptor interdomain interactions may contribute to intracellular Ca2+ leak: a novel therapeutic target in heart failure. Circulation 2005;111:3342.

30. Marks AR, Priori S, Memmi M, et al. Involvement of the cardiac ryanodine receptor/calcium release channel in catecholaminergic polymorphic ventricular tachycardia. J Cell Physiol 2002;190:1.

31. Wehrens XH, Lehnart SE, Reiken S, et al. Ryanodine receptor/calcium release channel PKA phosphorylation: a critical mediator of heart failure progression. Proc Natl Acad Sci U S A 2006;103:511.

32. Bers DM, Despa S, Bossuyt J. Regulation of Ca2+ and Na+ in normal and failing cardiac myocytes. Ann N Y Acad Sci 2006;1080:165.

33. Amit G, Costantini O, Rosenbaum DS. Can we alternate between T-wave alternans testing methods? Heart Rhythm 2009;6:338.

34. Amit G, Rosenbaum DS, Super DM, et al. Microvolt T-wave alternans and electrophysiological testing predict distinct arrhythmia substratoo: implications for identifying patients at risk for sudden cardiac death. Heart Rhythm 2010;7(6):763—8.

35. Costantini O, Drabek C, Rosenbaum DS. Can sudden cardiac death be predicted from the T wave of the ECG? A critical examination of T wave alternans and QT interval dispersion. Pacing Clin Electrophysiol 2000;23:1407.

36. Costantini O, Hohnloser SH, Kirk MM, et al. The ABCD (Alternans Before Cardioverter Defibrillator) Trial: strategies using T-wave alternans to improve efficiency of sudden cardiac death prevention. J Am Coll Cardiol 2009;53:471.

37. Cutler MJ, Rosenbaum DS. Explaining the clinical manifestations of T wave alternans in patients at risk for sudden cardiac death. Heart Rhythm 2009;6:S22.

38. Cutler MJ, Rosenbaum DS. Risk stratification for sudden cardiac death: is there a clinical role for T wave alternans? Heart Rhythm 2009;6:S56.

39. Laurita KR, Rosenbaum DS. Cellular mechanisms of arrhythmogenic cardiac alternans. Prog Biophys Mol Biol 2008;97:332.

40. Rosenbaum DS. T-wave alternans in the sudden cardiac death in heart failure trial population: signal or noise? Circulation 2008;118:2015.

41. Rosenbaum DS, Jackson LE, Smith JM, et al. Electrical alternans and vulnerability to ventricular arrhythmias. N Engl J Med 1994;330:235.

42. Wilson LD, Jeyaraj D, Wan X, et al. Heart failure enhances susceptibility to arrhythmogenic cardiac alternans. Heart Rhythm 2009;6:251.

43. Akar FG, Yan GX, Antzelevitch C, et al. Unique topographical distribution of M cells underlies reentrant mechanism of torsade de pointes in the long-QT syndrome. Circulation 2002;105:1247.

44. Baker LC, London B, Choi BR, et al. Enhanced dispersion of repolarization and refractoriness in transgenic mouse hearts promotes reentrant ventricular tachycardia. Circ Res 2000;86:396.

45. Glukhov AV, Fedorov VV, Lou Q, et al. Transmural dispersion of repolarization in failing and nonfailing human ventricle. Circ Res 2010;106:981.

46. Salama G, Baker L, Wolk R, et al. Arrhythmia phenotype in mouse models of human long QT. J Interv Card Electrophysiol 2009;24:77.

47. Antzelevitch C. Role of spatial dispersion of repolarization in inherited and acquired sudden cardiac death syndromes. Am J Physiol Heart Circ Physiol 2007;293:H2024.

48. Antzelevitch C, Shimizu W, Yan GX, et al. The M cell: its contribution to the ECG and to normal and abnormal electrical function of the heart. J Cardiovasc Electrophysiol 1999;10:1124.

49. Antzelevitch C. Cardiac repolarization. The long and short of it. Europace 2005;7(Suppl 2):3.

50. Antzelevitch C, Brugada P, Brugada J, et al. Brugada syndrome: from cell to bedside. Curr Probl Cardiol 2005;30:9.

51. Brugada P, Brugada R, Antzelevitch C, et al. The Brugada Syndrome. Arch Mal Coeur Vaiss 2005;98:115.

52. Tsuboi M, Antzelevitch C. Cellular basis for electrocardiographic and arrhythmic manifestations of Andersen-Tawil syndrome (LQT7). Heart Rhythm 2006;3:328.

53. Sicouri S, Glass A, Ferreiro M, et al. Transseptal dispersion of repolarization and its role in the development of torsade de pointes arrhythmias. J Cardiovasc Electrophysiol 2010;21(4):441–7.

54. Sicouri S, Timothy KW, Zygmunt AC, et al. Cellular basis for the electrocardiographic and arrhythmic manifestations of Timothy syndrome: effects of ranolazine. Heart Rhythm 2007;4:638.

55. Antzelevitch C, Yan GX, Shimizu W. Transmural dispersion of repolarization and arrhythmogenicity: the Brugada syndrome versus the long QT syndrome. J Electrocardiol 1999;32(Suppl):158.

56. Yan GX, Shimizu W, Antzelevitch C. Characteristics and distribution of M cells in arterially perfused canine left ventricular wedge preparations. Circulation 1998;98:1921.

57. Coronel R, Wilms-Schopman FJ, Opthof T, et al. Dispersion of repolarization and arrhythmogenesis. Heart Rhythm 2009;6:537.

58. Viswanathan PC, Shaw RM, Rudy Y. Effects of IKr and IKs heterogeneity on action potential duration and its rate dependence: a simulation study. Circulation 1999;99:2466.

59. Anyukhovsky EP, Sosunov EA, Gainullin RZ, et al. The controversial M cell. J Cardiovasc Electrophysiol 1999;10:244.

60. Opthof T, Coronel R, Janse MJ. Is there a significant transmural gradient in repolarization time in the intact heart? Repolarization gradients in the intact heart. Circ Arrhythm Electrophysiol 2009;2:89.

61. Voss F, Opthof T, Marker J, et al. There is no transmural heterogeneity in an index of action potential duration in the canine left ventricle. Heart Rhythm 2009;6:1028.

62. Yan GX, Rials SJ, Wu Y, et al. Ventricular hypertrophy amplifies transmural repolarization dispersion and induces early afterdepolarization. Am J Physiol Heart Circ Physiol 2001;281:H1968.

63. Akar FG, Wu RC, Juang GJ, et al. Molecular mechanisms underlying K+ current downregulation in canine tachycardia-induced heart failure. Am J Physiol Heart Circ Physiol 2005;288:H2887.

64. Qu J, Volpicelli FM, Garcia LI, et al. Gap junction remodeling and spironolactone-dependent reverse remodeling in the hypertrophied heart. Circ Res 2009;104:365.

65. Choi BR, Salama G. Simultaneous maps of optical action potentials and calcium transients in guinea-pig hearts: mechanisms underlying concordant alternans. J Physiol 2000;529(Pt 1):171.

66. Efimov IR, Ermentrout B, Huang DT, et al. Activation and repolarization patterns are governed by different structural characteristics of ventricular

myocardium: experimental study with voltage-sensitive dyes and numerical simulations. J Cardiovasc Electrophysiol 1996;7:512.

67. Salama G, Lombardi R, Elson J. Maps of optical action potentials and NADH fluorescence in intact working hearts. Am J Physiol 1987;252:H384.

68. Choi BR, Burton F, Salama G. Cytosolic Ca2+ triggers early afterdepolarizations and Torsade de Pointes in rabbit hearts with type 2 long QT syndrome. J Physiol 2002;543:615.

69. London B, Baker LC, Petkova-Kirova P, et al. Dispersion of repolarization and refractoriness are determinants of arrhythmia phenotype in transgenic mice with long QT. J Physiol 2007;578:115.

70. Szentadrassy N, Banyasz T, Biro T, et al. Apico-basal inhomogeneity in distribution of ion channels in canine and human ventricular myocardium. Cardiovasc Res 2005;65:851.

71. Mantravadi R, Gabris B, Liu T, et al. Autonomic nerve stimulation reverses ventricular repolarization sequence in rabbit hearts. Circ Res 2007; 100:e72.

72. Salama G, London B. Mouse models of long QT syndrome. J Physiol 2007;578:43.

73. Salama G. Arrhythmia genesis: aberrations of voltage or Ca2+ cycling? Heart Rhythm 2006;3:67.

74. Loew LM, Cohen LB, Dix J, et al. A naphthyl analog of the aminostyryl pyridinium class of potentiometric membrane dyes shows consistent sensitivity in a variety of tissue, cell, and model membrane preparations. J Membr Biol 1992;130:1.

75. Del Nido PJ, Glynn P, Buenaventura P, et al. Fluorescence measurement of calcium transients in perfused rabbit heart using rhod 2. Am J Physiol 1998;274:H728.

76. Morad M, Salama G. Optical probes of membrane potential in heart muscle. J Physiol 1979;292:267.

77. Patrick MJ, Ernst LA, Waggoner AS, et al. Enhanced aqueous solubility of long wavelength voltage-sensitive dyes by covalent attachment of polyethylene glycol. Org Biomol Chem 2007;5: 3347.

78. Salama G, Choi BR, Azour G, et al. Properties of new, long-wavelength, voltage-sensitive dyes in the heart. J Membr Biol 2005;208:125.

79. Choi BR, Jang W, Salama G. Spatially discordant voltage alternans cause wavebreaks in ventricular fibrillation. Heart Rhythm 2007;4:1057.

80. Choi BR, Liu T, Salama G. Calcium transients modulate action potential repolarizations in ventricular fibrillation. Conf Proc IEEE Eng Med Biol Soc 2006;1:2264.

81. Ng GA, Mantravadi R, Walker WH, et al. Sympathetic nerve stimulation produces spatial heterogeneities of action potential restitution. Heart Rhythm 2009;6:696.

82. Salama G, Hwang SM. Simultaneous optical mapping of intracellular free calcium and action potentials from Langendorff perfused hearts. Curr Protoc Cytom 2009;Chapter 12:Unit 12.17.

83. Kim JJ, Chakraborty SK, Gabris B, et al. Optical measurements of extracellular potassium accumulation (EKA) during ischemia with new potassium sensitive dyes. Heart Rhythm 2010;7(5):P04.

84. Cranefield PF. Action potentials, afterpotentials, and arrhythmias. Circ Res 1977;41:415.

85. January CT, Riddle JM. Early afterdepolarizations: mechanism of induction and block. A role for L-type Ca2+ current. Circ Res 1989;64:977.

86. Viswanathan PC, Rudy Y. Pause induced early afterdepolarizations in the long QT syndrome: a simulation study. Cardiovasc Res 1999;42:530.

87. Szabo B, Jackman WM, Lazzara R. New theories on the genesis of early and delayed afterdepolarizations. Armonk (NY): Futura Publishing Company; 1999.

88. Volders PG, Vos MA, Szabo B, et al. Progress in the understanding of cardiac early afterdepolarizations and torsades de pointes: time to revise current concepts. Cardiovasc Res 2000;46:376.

89. Nemec J, Kim JJ, Gabris B, et al. Calcium oscillations and T-wave lability precede ventricular arrhythmias in acquired long QT type 2. Heart Rhythm 2010;7(11):1686.

90. Kuhlkamp V, Mermi J, Mewis C, et al. Efficacy and proarrhythmia with the use of d, l-sotalol for sustained ventricular tachyarrhythmias. J Cardiovasc Pharmacol 1997;29:373.

91. Lehmann MH, Hardy S, Archibald D, et al. JTc prolongation with d, l-sotalol in women versus men. Am J Cardiol 1999;83:354.

92. Makkar RR, Fromm BS, Steinman RT, et al. Female gender as a risk factor for torsades de pointes associated with cardiovascular drugs. JAMA 1993;270:2590.

93. Pratt CM, Camm AJ, Cooper W, et al. Mortality in the Survival With ORal D-sotalol (SWORD) trial: why did patients die? Am J Cardiol 1998;81:869.

94. Drici MD, Burklow TR, Haridasse V, et al. Sex hormones prolong the QT interval and downregulate potassium channel expression in the rabbit heart. Circulation 1996;94:1471.

95. Drici MD, Clement N. Is gender a risk factor for adverse drug reactions? The example of drug-induced long QT syndrome. Drug Saf 2001;24:575.

96. Roden DM. Long QT syndrome: reduced repolarization reserve and the genetic link. J Intern Med 2006;259:59.

97. Goldenberg I, Moss AJ, Peterson DR, et al. Risk factors for aborted cardiac arrest and sudden cardiac death in children with the congenital long-QT syndrome. Circulation 2008;117:2184.

98. Zareba W, Moss AJ, Locati EH, et al. Modulating effects of age and gender on the clinical course of long QT syndrome by genotype. J Am Coll Cardiol 2003;42:103.

99. Sims C, Reisenweber S, Viswanathan PC, et al. Sex, age, and regional differences in L-type calcium current are important determinants of arrhythmia phenotype in rabbit hearts with drug-induced long QT type 2. Circ Res 2008;102:e86.

100. Brunner M, Peng X, Liu GX, et al. Mechanisms of cardiac arrhythmias and sudden death in transgenic rabbits with long QT syndrome. J Clin Invest 2008;118:2246.

101. Odening KE, Kirk M, Brunner M, et al. Electrophysiological studies of transgenic long QT type 1 and 2 rabbits reveal genotype-specific differences in ventricular refractoriness and his conduction. Am J Physiol Heart Circ Physiol 2010;299(3):H643–55.

102. Ziv O, Morales E, Song YK, et al. Origin of complex behaviour of spatially discordant alternans in a transgenic rabbit model of type 2 long QT syndrome. J Physiol 2009;587:4661.

103. Pogwizd SM, Bers DM. Cellular basis of triggered arrhythmias in heart failure. Trends Cardiovasc Med 2004;14:61.

104. Gwathmey JK, Copelas L, MacKinnon R, et al. Abnormal intracellular calcium handling in myocardium from patients with end-stage heart failure. Circ Res 1987;61:70.

105. London B, Baker LC, Lee JS, et al. Calcium-dependent arrhythmias in transgenic mice with heart failure. Am J Physiol Heart Circ Physiol 2003;284:H431.

106. Pogwizd SM, Schlotthauer K, Li L, et al. Arrhythmogenesis and contractile dysfunction in heart failure: Roles of sodium-calcium exchange, inward rectifier potassium current, and residual beta-adrenergic responsiveness. Circ Res 2001;88:1159.

107. Bers DM. Excitation-contraction coupling and cardiac contractile force. Dordrecht/Boston/. 2nd edition. London: Kluwer Academic Publishers; 2001.

108. Carmeliet E. Cardiac ionic currents and acute ischemia: from channels to arrhythmias. Physiol Rev 1999;79:917.

109. Menshikova EV, Salama G. Cardiac ischemia oxidizes regulatory thiols on ryanodine receptors: captopril acts as a reducing agent to improve Ca^{2+} uptake by ischemic sarcoplasmic reticulum. J Cardiovasc Pharmacol 2000;36:656.

110. Karmazyn M. The role of the myocardial sodium-hydrogen exchanger in mediating ischemic and re-perfusion injury. From amiloride to cariporide. Ann N Y Acad Sci 1999;874:326.

111. Lakireddy V, Bub G, Baweja P, et al. The kinetics of spontaneous calcium oscillations and arrhythmogenesis in the in vivo heart during ischemia/reperfusion. Heart Rhythm 2006;3:58.

112. Katra RP, Laurita KR. Cellular mechanism of calcium-mediated triggered activity in the heart. Circ Res 2005;96:535.

113. Omichi C, Lamp ST, Lin SF, et al. Intracellular Ca dynamics in ventricular fibrillation. Am J Physiol Heart Circ Physiol 2004;286:H1836.

114. Warren M, Huizar JF, Shvedko AG, et al. Spatiotemporal relationship between intracellular Ca^{2+} dynamics and wave fragmentation during ventricular fibrillation in isolated blood-perfused pig hearts. Circ Res 2007;101:e90.

115. Warren M, Zaitsev AV. Evidence against the role of intracellular calcium dynamics in ventricular fibrillation. Circ Res 2008;102:e103.

Overview of Basic Mechanisms of Cardiac Arrhythmia

Charles Antzelevitch, PhD, FHRS*,
Alexander Burashnikov, PhD, FHRS

KEYWORDS

- Electrophysiology • Pharmacology • Ventricular tachycardia
- Ventricular fibrillation

A cardiac arrhythmia simply defined is a variation from the normal heart rate and/or rhythm that is not physiologically justified. Recent years have witnessed important advances in our understanding of the electrophysiologic mechanisms underlying the development of a variety of cardiac arrhythmias. The mechanisms responsible for cardiac arrhythmias are generally divided into 2 major categories: (1) enhanced or abnormal impulse formation (ie, focal activity) and (2) conduction disturbances (ie, reentry) (**Fig. 1**).

ABNORMAL IMPULSE FORMATION
Normal Automaticity

Automaticity is the property of cardiac cells to generate spontaneous action potentials. Spontaneous activity is the result of diastolic depolarization caused by a net inward current during phase 4 of the action potential, which progressively brings the membrane potential to threshold. The sinoatrial (SA) node normally displays the highest intrinsic rate. All other pacemakers are referred to as subsidiary or latent pacemakers because they take over the function of initiating excitation of the heart only when the SA node is unable to generate impulses or when these impulses fail to propagate.

The Voltage and Calcium Clocks

The terms sarcolemma voltage or Ca clocks have been used by Maltsev and colleagues[1] to describe the mechanisms of SA node automaticity. The voltage clock refers to voltage-sensitive membrane currents, such as the hyperpolarization-activated pacemaker current (I_f).[3] This current is also referred to as a "funny" current because, unlike most voltage-sensitive currents, it is activated by hyperpolarization rather than depolarization. At the end of the action potential, the I_f is activated and depolarizes the sarcolemmal membrane.[3] I_f is a mixed Na-K inward current modulated by the autonomic nervous system through cAMP. The depolarization activates $I_{Ca,L}$, which provides Ca to activate the cardiac ryanodine receptor (RyR2). The activation of RyR2 initiates sarcoplasmic reticulum (SR) Ca release (Ca-induced Ca release), leading to contraction of the heart, a process known as EC coupling. Intracellular Ca (Ca_i) is then pumped back into SR by the SR Ca-ATPase (SERCA2a) and completes this Ca cycle. In addition to I_f, multiple time- and voltage-dependent ionic currents have been identified in cardiac pacemaker cells, which contribute to diastolic depolarization. These currents include (but are not limited to) I_{Ca-L}, I_{Ca-T}, I_{ST}, and various types of delayed rectifier K currents.[2] Many of these membrane currents are known to respond to β-adrenergic stimulation. All these membrane ionic currents contribute to the regulation of SA node automaticity by altering membrane potential.

Conflict of interest: None.
Financial support: Supported by grant HL47678 from the National Heart, Lung, and Blood Institute (CA) and NYS and Florida Masons.
Masonic Medical Research Laboratory, 2150 Bleecker Street, Utica, NY 13501, USA
* Corresponding author.
E-mail address: ca@mmrl.edu

Card Electrophysiol Clin 3 (2011) 23–45
doi:10.1016/j.ccep.2010.10.012

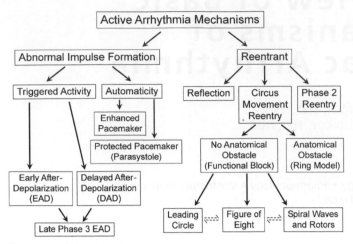

Fig. 1. Classification of active cardiac arrhythmias.

Another important ionic current capable of depolarizing the cell is the sodium-calcium exchanger current (I_{NCx}). In its forward mode, I_{NCx} exchanges 3 extracellular Na^+ with 1 intracellular Ca^{2+}, resulting in a net intracellular charge gain. This electrogenic current is active during late phase 3 and phase 4 because the Ca_i decline outlasts the SA node action potential duration. Recent studies showed that I_{NCx} may participate in normal pacemaker activity.[4] The sequence of events includes spontaneous rhythmic SR Ca release, Ca_i elevation, the activation of I_{NCx}, and membrane depolarization. This process is highly regulated by cAMP and the autonomic nervous system.[2] These studies suggest that sympathetic stimulation accelerates heart rate by phosphorylation of proteins that regulate Ca_i balance and spontaneous SR Ca cycling. These proteins include phospholamban (PLB, an SR membrane protein regulator of SERCA2a), L-type Ca channels, and RyR2. Phosphorylation of these proteins controls the phase and extent of subsarcolemmal SR Ca releases.

Subsidiary Pacemakers

In addition to the SA node, the atrioventicular (AV) node and Purkinje system are also capable of generating automatic activity. The contribution of I_f and I_K differs in SA node/AV nodes and Purkinje fiber because of the different potential ranges of these two pacemaker types (ie, −70 to −35 mV and −90 to −65 mV, respectively). The contribution of other voltage-dependent currents can also differ among the different cardiac cell types. Whether or not the Ca clock plays a role in pacemaking of AV node and Purkinje cells remains unclear.

SA nodal cells possess the fastest intrinsic rates, making them the primary pacemakers in the normal heart. When impulse generation or conduction in the SA node is impaired, latent or subsidiary pacemakers within the atria or ventricles take control of pacing the heart. The intrinsically slower rates of these latent pacemakers generally result in bradycardia. Both atrial and AV junctional subsidiary pacemakers are under autonomic control, with the sympathetic system increasing and parasympathetic system slowing the pacing rate. Although acetylcholine produces little in the way of a direct effect, it can significantly reduce Purkinje automaticity by means of the inhibition of the sympathetic influence, a phenomenon termed *accentuated antagonism*.[5] Simultaneous recording of cardiac sympathetic and parasympathetic activity in ambulatory dogs confirmed that sympathetic activation followed by vagal activation may be associated with significant bradycardia.[6,7]

AUTOMATICITY AS A MECHANISM OF CARDIAC ARRHYTHMIAS

Abnormal automaticity includes both reduced automaticity, which causes bradycardia, and increased automaticity, which causes tachycardia. Arrhythmias caused by abnormal automaticity can result from diverse mechanisms (see **Fig. 1**). Alterations in sinus rate can be accompanied by shifts of the origin of the dominant pacemaker within the sinus node or to subsidiary pacemaker sites elsewhere in the atria. Impulse conduction out of the SA mode can be impaired or blocked as a result of disease or increased vagal activity leading to development of bradycardia. AV junctional rhythms occur when AV junctional pacemakers located either in the AV node or in the His bundle accelerate to exceed the rate of

SA node, or when the SA nodal activation rate was too slow to suppress the AV junctional pacemaker.

Bradycardia can occur in structurally normal hearts because of genetic mutations that result in abnormalities of either membrane clock or Ca clock mechanisms of automaticity. One example is the mutation of hyperpolarization-activated nucleotide-gated channel (HCN4), which is part of the channels that carry I_f. Mutations of the HCN4 may cause familial bradycardia as well.[8,9]

Secondary SA Node Dysfunction

Common diseases, such as heart failure and atrial fibrillation, may be associated with significant SA node dysfunction. Malfunction of both membrane voltage and Ca clocks might be associated with both of these common diseases. Zicha and colleagues[10] reported that down-regulation of HCN4 expression contributes to heart failure-induced sinus node dysfunction. An A450 V missense loss of function mutation in *HCN4* has recently been shown to underlie familial sinus bradycardia in several unrelated probands of Moroccan Jewish descent.[9,11–13]

Enhanced Automaticity

Atrial and ventricular myocardial cells do not display spontaneous diastolic depolarization or automaticity under normal conditions, but can develop these characteristics when depolarized, resulting in the development of repetitive impulse initiation, a phenomenon termed *depolarization-induced automaticity*.[14] The membrane potential at which abnormal automaticity develops ranges between −70 and −30 mV. The rate of abnormal automaticity is substantially higher than that of normal automaticity and is a sensitive function of resting membrane potential (ie, the more depolarized resting potential the faster the rate). Similar to normal automaticity, abnormal automaticity is enhanced by β-adrenergic agonists and by reduction of external potassium.

Depolarization of membrane potential associated with disease states is most commonly a result of (1) an increase in extracellular potassium, which reduces the reversal potential for I_{K1}, the outward current that largely determines the resting membrane or maximum diastolic potential; (2) a reduced number of I_{K1} channels; (3) a reduced ability of the I_{K1} channel to conduct potassium ions; or (4) electrotonic influence of neighboring cells in the depolarized zone. Because the conductance of I_{K1} channels is sensitive to extracellular potassium concentration, hypokalemia can lead to major reduction in I_{K1}, leading to depolarization and the development of enhanced or abnormal automaticity, particularly in Purkinje pacemakers. A reduction in I_{K1} can also occur secondary to a mutation in *KCNJ2*, the gene that encodes for this channel, leading to increased automaticity and extrasystolic activity presumably arising from the Purkinje system.[15,16] Loss of function KCNJ2 mutation gives rise to Andersen-Tawil syndrome, which is characterized among other things by a marked increase in extrasystolic activity.[17–20]

Overdrive Suppression of Automaticity

Automatic activity of most pacemakers within the heart is inhibited when they are overdrive paced,[21] owing to a mechanism termed *overdrive suppression*. Under normal conditions, all subsidiary pacemakers are overdrive-suppressed by SA nodal activity. A possible mechanism of overdrive suppression is intracellular accumulation of Na leading to enhanced activity of the sodium pump (sodium-potassium adenosine triphosphatase [Na^+-K^+ ATPase]), which generates a hyperpolarizing electrogenic current that opposes phase 4 depolarization.[22] The faster the overdrive rate or the longer the duration of overdrive, the greater the enhancement of sodium pump activity, so that the period of quiescence after cessation of overdrive is directly related to the rate and duration of overdrive.

Parasystole and Modulated Parasystole

Latent pacemakers throughout the heart are generally reset by the propagating wavefront initiated by the dominant pacemaker. An exception to this rule occurs when the pacemaking tissue is protected from the impulse of sinus nodal origin. A region of entrance block arises when cells exhibiting automaticity are surrounded by ischemic, infarcted, or otherwise compromised cardiac tissues that prevent the propagating wave from invading the focus, but which permit the spontaneous beat generated within the automatic focus to exit and activate the rest of the myocardium. A pacemaker region exhibiting entrance block, and exit conduction is referred to as a parasystolic focus. The ectopic activity generated by a parasystolic focus is characterized by premature ventricular complexes with variable coupling intervals, fusion beats, and inter-ectopic intervals that are multiples of a common denominator. This rhythm is relatively rare and is usually considered benign, although a premature ventricular activation of parasystolic origin can induce malignant ventricular rhythms in the ischemic myocardium or in the presence of a suitable myocardial substrate.

Modulated parasystole, a variant of classical parasystole, was described by Jalife and colleagues.[23,24] This variant of the arrhythmia results from incomplete entrance block of the parasystolic focus. Electrotonic influences arriving early in the pacemaker cycle delayed and those arriving late in the cycle accelerated the firing of the parasystolic pacemaker, so that ventricular activity could entrain the partially protected pacemaker. As a consequence, at select heart rate, extrasystolic activity generated by the entrained parasystolic pacemaker can mimic reentry, generating extrasystolic activity with fixed coupling.[23–27]

AFTERDEPOLARIZATION AND TRIGGERED ACTIVITY

Depolarizations that attend or follow the cardiac action potential and depend on preceding transmembrane activity for their manifestation are referred to as afterdepolarizations (**Fig. 2**). Two subclasses are traditionally recognized: (1) early, and (2) delayed. Early afterdepolarization (EAD) interrupts or retards repolarization during phase 2 and/or phase 3 of the cardiac action potential, whereas delayed afterdepolarization (DAD) occurs after full repolarization. When EAD or DAD amplitude suffices to bring the membrane to its threshold potential, a spontaneous action potential referred to as a triggered response is the result (see **Fig. 2**). These triggered events give rise to extrasystoles, which can precipitate tachyarrhythmias.

Early Afterdepolarizations and Triggered Activity

EADs are typically observed in cardiac tissues exposed to injury, altered electrolytes, hypoxia, acidosis, catecholamines, and pharmacologic agents, including antiarrhythmic drugs. Ventricular hypertrophy and heart failure also predispose

to the development of EADs.[28] EAD characteristics vary as a function of animal species, tissue or cell type, and the method by which the EAD is elicited. Although specific mechanisms of EAD induction can differ, a critical prolongation of repolarization accompanies most, but not all, EADs. Drugs that inhibit potassium currents or which augment inward currents predispose to the development of EADs.[29] Phase 2 and phase 3 EADs sometimes appear in the same preparation.

EAD-induced triggered activity is sensitive to stimulation rate. Antiarrhythmic drugs with class III action generally induce EAD activity at slow stimulation rates.[14] In contrast, β-adrenergic agonist–induced EADs are fast rate-dependent.[30] In the presence of rapidly activating delayed rectifier current (rapid outward potassium current [I_{Kr}]) blockers, β-adrenergic agonists, and/or acceleration from an initially slow rate transiently facilitate the induction of EAD activity in ventricular M cells, but not in epicardium or endocardium and rarely in Purkinje fibers.[31]

Cellular Origin of Early Afterdepolarizations

EADs develop more commonly in midmyocardial M cells and Purkinje fibers than in epicardial or endocardial cells when exposed to action potential duration (APD)-prolonging agents. This is because of the presence of a weaker I_{Ks} and stronger late I_{Na} in M cells.[32,33] Block of I_{Ks} with chromanol 293B permits the induction of EADs in canine epicardial and endocardial tissues in response to I_{Kr} blockers such as E-4031 or sotalol.[34] The predisposition of cardiac cells to the development of EADs depends principally on the reduced availability of I_{Kr} and I_{Ks} as occurs in many forms of cardiomyopathy. Under these conditions, EADs can appear in any part of the ventricular myocardium.[35]

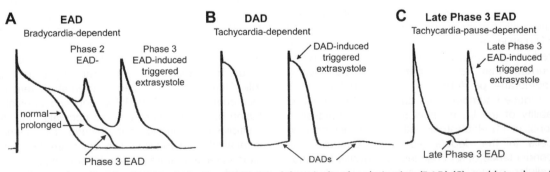

Fig. 2. Examples of early afterdepolarization (EAD) (*A*), delayed afterdepolarization (DAD) (*B*), and late phase 3 EAD (*C*). (*Modified from* Burashnikov A, Antzelevitch C. Late-phase 3 EAD. A unique mechanism contributing to initiation of atrial fibrillation. Pacing Clin Electrophysiol 2006;29:290–5; with permission.)

Ionic Mechanisms Responsible for the EAD

EADs develop when the balance of current active during phase 2 and/or 3 of the action potential shifts in the inward direction. If the change in current-voltage relation results in a region of net inward current during the plateau range of membrane potentials, it leads to a depolarization or EAD. Most pharmacologic interventions or pathophysiological conditions associated with EADs can be categorized as acting predominantly through 1 of 4 different mechanisms: (1) A reduction of repolarizing potassium currents (I_{Kr}, class IA and III antiarrhythmic agents; I_{Ks}, chromanol 293B or I_{K1}); (2) an increase in the availability of calcium current (Bay K 8644, catecholamines); (3) an increase in the sodium-calcium exchange current (I_{NCx}) caused by augmentation of Ca_i activity or upregulation of the I_{NCx}; and (4) an increase in late sodium current (late I_{Na}) (aconitine, anthopleurin-A, and ATX-II). Combinations of these interventions (ie, calcium loading and I_{Kr} reduction) or pathophysiological states can act synergistically to facilitate the development of EADs.

Delayed Afterdepolarization-Induced Triggered Activity

DADs and DAD-induced triggered activity are observed under conditions that augment intracellular calcium, $[Ca^{2+}]_i$, such as after exposure to toxic levels of cardiac glycosides (digitalis)[36–38] or catecholamines.[30,39,40] This activity is also manifest in hypertrophied and failing hearts[41,42] as well as in Purkinje fibers surviving myocardial infarction.[43] In contrast to EADs, DADs are always induced at relatively rapid rates.

Role of Delayed Afterdepolarization-Induced Triggered Activity in the Development of Cardiac Arrhythmias

An example of DAD-induced arrhythmia is the catecholaminergic polymorphic ventricular tachycardia (CPVT), which may be caused by the mutation of either the type 2 ryanodine receptor (RyR2) or the calsequestrin (CSQ2).[44] The principal mechanism underlying these arrhythmias is the "leaky" ryanodine receptor, which is aggravated during catecholamine stimulation. A typical clinical phenotype of CPVT is bidirectional ventricular tachycardia, which is also seen in digitalis toxicity. Wehrens and colleagues[45] demonstrated that heterozygous mutation of FKBP12.6 leads to leaky RyR2 and exercise-induced VT and VF, simulating the human CPVT phenotype. RyR2 stabilization with a derivative of 1,4-benzothiazepine (JTV519) increased the affinity of calstabin2 for RyR2, which stabilized the closed state of RyR2 and prevented the Ca leak that triggers arrhythmias. Other studies indicate that delayed afterdepolarization-induced extrasystoles serve to trigger catecholamine-induced VT/VF, but that the epicardial origin of these ectopic beats increases transmural dispersion of repolarization, thus providing the substrate for the development of reentrant tachyarrhythmias, which underlie the rapid polymorphic VT/VF.[46] Heart failure is associated with structural and electrophysiological remodeling, leading to tissue heterogeneity that enhances arrhythmogenesis and the propensity of sudden cardiac death.[47]

Late Phase 3 Early Afterdepolarizations and Their Role in the Initiation of Fibrillation

In 2003, Burashnikov and Antzelevitch[48,49] described a novel mechanism giving rise to triggered activity, termed "late phase 3 EAD," which combines properties of both EAD and DAD, but has its own unique character (see **Fig. 2**). Late phase 3 EAD-induced triggered extrasystoles represent a new concept of arrhythmogenesis in which abbreviated repolarization permits "normal SR calcium release" to induce an EAD-mediated closely coupled triggered response, particularly under conditions permitting intracellular calcium loading.[48,49] These EADs are distinguished by the fact that they interrupt the final phase of repolarization of the action potential (late phase 3). In contrast to previously described DAD or Ca_i-dependent EAD, it is *normal,* not spontaneous SR calcium release that is responsible for the generation of the EAD. Two principal conditions are required for the appearance of late phase 3 EAD: an APD abbreviation and a strong SR calcium release.[48] Such conditions may occur when both parasympathetic and sympathetic influences are combined. Simultaneous sympathovagal activation is also known to be the primary trigger of paroxysmal atrial tachycardia and AF episodes in dogs with intermittent rapid pacing.[6]

Late phase 3 EAD-induced extrasystoles have been shown to initiate AF in canine atria, particularly following spontaneous termination of the arrhythmia (IRAF, immediate reinduction of AF).[48] The appearance of late phase 3 EAD immediately following termination of AF or rapid pacing has been reported by in the canine atria in vivo[50] and pulmonary veins in vitro.[51] In addition to the atrial arrhythmias, late phase 3 EAD may also be responsible for the development recurrent VF in failing hearts.[52]

REENTRANT ARRHYTHMIAS

Reentry is fundamentally different from automaticity or triggered activity in the mechanism by which it initiates and sustains cardiac arrhythmias. Circus movement reentry occurs when an activation wavefront propagates around an anatomic or functional obstacle or core, and reexcites the site of origin (**Fig. 3**). In this type of reentry, all cells take turns in recovering from excitation so that they are ready to be excited again when the next wavefront arrives. In contrast, reflection and phase 2 reentry occur in a setting in which large differences of recovery from refractoriness exist between one site and another. The site with delayed recovery serves as a virtual electrode that excites its already recovered neighbor, resulting in a reentrant reexcitation. In addition, reentry can also be classified as anatomic and functional, although there is a gray zone in which both functional and anatomic factors are important in determining the characteristics of reentrant excitation.

Circus Movement Reentry Around an Anatomic Obstacle

The ring model is the prototypical example of reentry around an anatomic obstacle (see **Fig. 3**). It first emerged as a concept shortly after the turn of the last century when Mayer[53] reported the results of experiments involving the subumbrella tissue of a jellyfish (*Sychomedusa cassiopeia*). The muscular disk did not contract until ringlike cuts were made and pressure and a stimulus applied. This caused the disc to "spring into rapid rhythmic pulsation so regular and sustained as to recall the movement of clockwork."[p25] Mayer demonstrated similar circus movement excitation in rings cut from the ventricles of turtle hearts, but he did not consider this to be a plausible mechanism for the development of cardiac

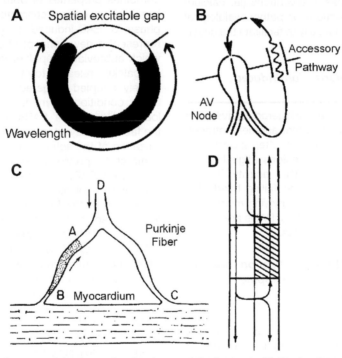

Fig. 3. Ring models of reentry. (*A*) Schematic of a ring model of reentry. (*B*) Mechanism of reentry in the Wolf-Parkinson-White syndrome involving the AV node and an atrioventricular accessory pathway (AP). (*C*) A mechanism for reentry in a Purkinje-muscle loop proposed by Schmitt and Erlanger. The diagram shows a Purkinje bundle (D) that divides into 2 branches, both connected distally to ventricular muscle. Circus movement was considered possible if the stippled segment, A → B, showed unidirectional block. An impulse advancing from D would be blocked at A, but would reach and stimulate the ventricular muscle at C by way of the other terminal branch. The wavefront would then reenter the Purkinje system at B traversing the depressed region slowly so as to arrive at A following expiration of refractoriness. (*D*) Schematic representation of circus movement reentry in a linear bundle of tissue as proposed by Schmitt and Erlanger. The upper pathway contains a depressed zone (shaded) that serves as a site of unidirectional block and slow conduction. Anterograde conduction of the impulse is blocked in the upper pathway but succeeds along the lower pathway. Once beyond the zone of depression, the impulse crosses over through lateral connections and reenters through the upper pathway. (*C* and *D from* Schmitt FO, Erlanger J. Directional differences in the conduction of the impulse through heart muscle and their possible relation to extrasystolic and fibrillary contractions. Am J Physiol 1928;87:326–47.)

arrhythmias. His experiments proved valuable in identifying 2 fundamental conditions necessary for the initiation and maintenance of circus movement excitation: (1) unidirectional block—the impulse initiating the circulating wave must travel in one direction only; and (2) for the circus movement to continue, the circuit must be long enough to allow each site in the circuit to recover before the return of the circulating wave. G. R. Mines[54] was the first to develop the concept of circus movement reentry as a mechanism responsible for cardiac arrhythmias. He confirmed Mayer's observations and suggested that the recirculating wave could be responsible for clinical cases of tachycardia.[55] The following 3 criteria developed by Mines for identification of circus movement reentry remains in use today:

1. An area of unidirectional block must exist.
2. The excitatory wave progresses along a distinct pathway, returning to its point of origin and then following the same path again.
3. Interruption of the reentrant circuit at any point along its path should terminate the circus movement.

It was recognized that successful reentry could occur only when the impulse was sufficiently delayed in an alternate pathway to allow for expiration of the refractory period in the tissue proximal to the site of unidirectional block. Both conduction velocity and refractoriness determine the success or failure of reentry, and the general rule is that the length of the circuit (path length) must exceed or equal that of the wavelength, the wavelength being defined as the product of the conduction velocity and the refractory period or that part of the path length occupied by the impulse and refractory to reexcitation. The theoretical minimum path length required for development of reentry was therefore dependent on both the conduction velocity and the refractory period. Reduction of conduction velocity or APD can both significantly reduce the theoretical limit of the path length required for the development or maintenance of reentry.

Circus Movement Reentry without an Anatomic Obstacle

In 1914, Garrey[56] suggested that reentry could be initiated without the involvement of anatomic obstacles and that "natural rings are not essential for the maintenance of circus contractions."(p409) Nearly 50 years later, Allessie and coworkers[57] provided direct evidence in support of this hypothesis in experiments in which they induced a tachycardia in isolated preparations of rabbit left atria by applying properly timed premature extra-stimuli.

Using multiple intracellular electrodes, they showed that although the basic beats elicited by stimuli applied near the center of the tissue spread normally throughout the preparation, premature impulses propagate only in the direction of shorter refractory periods. An arc of block thus develops around which the impulse is able to circulate and reexcite its site of origin. Recordings near the center of the circus movement showed only subthreshold responses. The investigators proposed the term "leading circle" to explain their observation.[58] They argued that the functionally refractory region that develops at the vortex of the circulating wavefront prevents the centripetal waves from short circuiting the circus movement and thus serves to maintain the reentry. The investigators also proposed that the refractory core was maintained by centripetal wavelets that collide with each other. Because the head of the circulating wavefront usually travels on relatively refractory tissue, a fully excitable gap of tissue may not be present; unlike other forms of reentry, the leading circle model may not be readily influenced by extraneous impulses initiated in areas outside the reentrant circuit and thus may not be easily entrained. Although the leading circle reentry for a while was widely accepted as a mechanism of functional reentry, there is significant conceptual limitation to this model of reentry. For example, the centripetal wavelet was difficult to demonstrate either by experimental studies with high-resolution mapping or with computer simulation studies.

Weiner and Rosenblueth[59] in 1946 introduced the concept of spiral waves (rotors) to describe reentry around an anatomic obstacle; the term *spiral wave reentry* was later adopted to describe circulating waves in the absence of an anatomic obstacle.[60] Spiral wave theory has advanced our understanding of the mechanisms responsible for the functional form of reentry. Although leading circle and spiral wave reentry are considered by some to be similar, a number of distinctions have been suggested. The curvature of the spiral wave is the key to the formation of the core.[61] The term *spiral wave* is usually used to describe reentrant activity in 2 dimensions. The center of the spiral wave is called the *core* and the distribution of the core in 3 dimensions is referred to as the *filament*. The 3-dimensional form of the spiral wave forms a scroll wave. In its simplest form, the scroll wave has a straight filament spanning the ventricular wall (ie, from epicardium to endocardium). Theoretical studies have described 3 major scroll wave configurations with curved filaments (L-, U-, and O-shaped), although numerous variations of these 3-dimensional filaments in space and time are assumed to exist during cardiac arrhythmias.

Spiral wave activity has been used to explain the electrocardiographic patterns observed during monomorphic and polymorphic cardiac arrhythmias as well as during fibrillation. Monomorphic VT results when the spiral wave is anchored and not able to drift within the ventricular myocardium. In contrast, a meandering or drifting spiral wave causes polymorphic VT- and VF-like activity.[62] VF seems to be the most complex representation of rotating spiral waves in the heart. VF is often preceded by VT. One of the theories suggests that VF develops when a single spiral wave responsible for VT breaks up, leading to the development of multiple spirals that are continuously extinguished and re-created.[63]

Figure 8 Reentry

In the late 1980s, El-Sherif and coworkers[64] delineated a figure 8 reentry in the surviving epicardial layer overlying an area of infarction produced by occlusion of the left anterior descending artery in canine hearts. The same patterns of activation can also be induced by creating artificial anatomic obstacles in the ventricles,[65] or during functional reentry induced by a single premature ventricular stimulation.[66] In the figure 8 model, the reentrant beat produces a wavefront that circulates in both directions around a line of conduction block rejoining on the distal side of the block. The wavefront then breaks through the arc of block to reexcite the tissue proximal to the block. The reentrant activation continues as 2 circulating wavefronts that travel in clockwise and counterclockwise directions around the 2 arcs in a pretzellike configuration.

Reflection

Reentry can occur without circus movement. Reflection and phase 2 reentry are 2 examples of non—circus movement reentry. The concept of reflection was first suggested by studies of the propagation characteristics of slow action potential responses in K^+-depolarized Purkinje fibers.[67] In strands of Purkinje fiber, Wit and coworkers[67] demonstrated a phenomenon similar to that observed by Schmitt and Erlanger[68] in which slow anterograde conduction of the impulse was at times followed by a retrograde wavefront that produced a "return extrasystole." They proposed that the nonstimulated impulse was caused by circuitous reentry at the level of the syncytial interconnections, made possible by longitudinal dissociation of the bundle, as the most likely explanation for the phenomenon but also suggested the possibility of reflection. Direct evidence in support of reflection as a mechanism of arrhythmogenesis was provided by Antzelevitch and colleagues[69,70] in the early 1980s. A number of models of reflection have been developed. The first of these involves use of *ion-free* isotonic sucrose solution to create a narrow (1.5 to 2 mm) central inexcitable zone (gap) in unbranched Purkinje fibers mounted in a 3-chamber tissue bath (**Fig. 4**).[71] In the sucrose-gap model, stimulation of the proximal (P) segment elicits an action potential that propagates to the proximal border of the sucrose gap. Active propagation across the sucrose gap is not possible because of the ion-depleted extracellular milieu, but local circuit current continues to flow through the intercellular

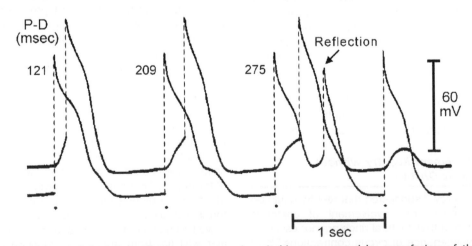

Fig. 4. Delayed transmission and reflection across an inexcitable gap created by superfusion of the central segment of a Purkinje fiber with an *ion-free* isotonic sucrose solution. The 2 traces were recorded from proximal (P) and distal (D) active segments. P—D conduction time (indicated in the upper portion of the figure, in ms) increased progressively with a 4:3 Wenckebach periodicity. The third stimulated proximal response was followed by a reflection. (*From* Antzelevitch C. Clinical applications of new concepts of parasystole, reflection, and tachycardia. Cardiol Clin 1983;1:39—50; with permission.)

low-resistance pathways (an Ag/AgCl extracellular shunt pathway is provided). This local circuit or electrotonic current, very much reduced on emerging from the gap, gradually discharges the capacity of the distal (D) tissue, thus giving rise to a depolarization that manifests as a either a subthreshold response (last distal response) or a foot-potential that brings the distal excitable tissue to its threshold potential. Active impulse propagation stops and then resumes after a delay that can be as long as several hundred milliseconds. When anterograde (P to D) transmission time is sufficiently delayed to permit recovery of refractoriness at the proximal end, electrotonic transmission of the impulse in the retrograde direction is able to reexcite the proximal tissue, thus generating a closely coupled reflected reentry. Reflection therefore results from the to-and-fro electrotonically mediated transmission of the impulse across the same inexcitable segment; neither longitudinal dissociation nor circus movement need be invoked to explain the phenomenon.

A second model of reflection involved the creation of an inexcitable zone permitting delayed conduction by superfusion of a central segment of a Purkinje bundle with a solution designed to mimic the extracellular milieu at a site of ischemia.[70] The gap was shown to be largely composed of an inexcitable cable across which conduction of impulses was electrotonically mediated. Reflected reentry has been demonstrated in isolated atrial and ventricular myocardial tissues as well.[72–74] Reflection has also been demonstrated in Purkinje fibers in which a functionally inexcitable zone is created by focal depolarization of the preparation with long duration constant current pulses.[75] Reflection is also observed in isolated canine Purkinje fibers homogeneously depressed with high K^+ solution as well as in branched preparations of *normal* Purkinje fibers.[76]

Phase 2 Reentry

Another reentrant mechanism that does not depend on circus movement and can appear to be of focal origin is Phase 2 reentry.[77–79] Phase 2 reentry occurs when the dome of the action potential, most commonly epicardial, propagates from sites at which it is maintained to sites at which it is abolished, causing local reexcitation of the epicardium and the generation of a closely coupled extrasystole. Severe spatial dispersion of repolarization is needed for phase 2 reentry to occur.

Phase 2 reentry has been proposed as the mechanism responsible for the closely coupled extrasystole that precipitates ventricular tachycardia/ventricular fibrillation (VT/VF) associated with Brugada and early repolarization syndromes.[80,81]

Spatial Dispersion of Repolarization

Studies conducted over the past 20 years have established that ventricular myocardium is electrically heterogeneous and composed of at least 3 electrophysiologically and functionally distinct cell types: epicardial, M, and endocardial cells.[82,83] These 3 principal ventricular myocardial cell types differ with respect to phase 1 and phase 3 repolarization characteristics (**Fig. 5**). Ventricular epicardial and M, but not endocardial, cells generally display a prominent phase 1, because of a large 4-aminopyridine (4-AP)-sensitive transient outward current (I_{to}), giving the action potential a spike and dome or notched configuration. These regional differences in I_{to}, first suggested on the basis of action potential data,[84] have now been directly demonstrated in ventricular myocytes from a wide variety of species including canine,[85] feline,[86] guinea pig,[87] swine,[88] rabbit,[89] and humans.[90,91] Differences in the magnitude of the action potential notch and corresponding differences in I_{to} have also been described between right and left ventricular (LV) epicardium.[92] Similar interventricular differences in I_{to} have also been described for canine ventricular M cells.[93] This distinction is thought to form the basis for why the Brugada syndrome is a right ventricular disease.

Myocytes isolated from the epicardial region of the LV wall of the rabbit show a higher density of cAMP-activated chloride current when compared with endocardial myocytes.[94] I_{to2}, initially ascribed to a K^+ current, is now thought to be largely composed of a calcium-activated chloride current ($I_{Cl(Ca)}$) that contributes to the action potential notch, but it is not known whether this current differs among the 3 ventricular myocardial cell types.[95]

Between the surface epicardial and endocardial layers are transitional cells and M cells. M cells are distinguished by the ability of their action potential to prolong disproportionately relative to the action potential of other ventricular myocardial cells in response to a slowing of rate and/or in response to APD-prolonging agents.[82,96,97] In the dog, the ionic basis for these features of the M cell includes the presence of a smaller slowly activating delayed rectifier current (I_{Ks}),[32] a larger late sodium current (late I_{Na}),[33] and a larger Na-Ca exchange current (I_{NCx}).[98] In the canine heart, the rapidly activating delayed rectifier (I_{Kr}) and inward rectifier (I_{K1}) currents are similar in the 3 transmural cell types. Transmural and apical-basal differences in the density of I_{Kr} channels have been described in the ferret heart.[99] Amplification of transmural heterogeneities normally present in the early and late phases of the action potential can lead to the development of a variety of arrhythmias, including Brugada, long QT, and short QT syndromes, as well as catecholaminergic VT. The genetic mutations associated with these inherited channelopathies are listed in **Table 1**. The resulting gain or loss of function underlies the development of the arrhythmogenic substrate and triggers.

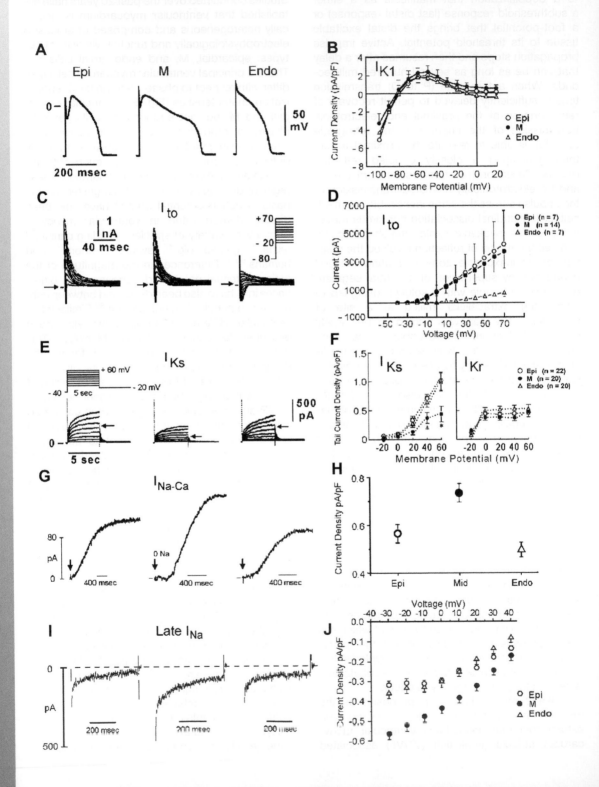

MECHANISMS UNDERLYING CHANNELOPATHIES

In the following sections we briefly discuss how the reentrant and triggered mechanisms described previously contribute to development of VT/VF associated with the long QT, short QT, and J wave syndromes.

J Wave Syndromes

Because they share a common arrhythmic platform related to amplification of I_{to}-mediated J waves, and because of similarities in ECG characteristics, clinical outcomes and risk factors, congenital and acquired forms of Brugada syndrome (BrS) and early repolarization syndrome (ERS) have been grouped together under the heading of J wave syndromes.[80]

Brugada syndrome

In 1992, Pedro and Josep Brugada[100] reported a new syndrome associated with ST elevation in ECG leads V1-V3, right bundle branch appearance during sinus rhythm, and a high incidence of VF and sudden cardiac death. BrS has been associated with mutations in 7 different genes. Mutations in SCN5A (Na$_v$1.5, BrS1) have been reported in 11% to 28% of BrS probands, CACNA1C (Ca$_v$1.2, BrS3) in 6.7%, CACNB2b (Ca$_v$β2b, BrS4) in 4.8%, and mutations in Glycerol-3-phophate dehydrogenase 1—like enzyme gene (GPD1L, BrS2), SCN1B (β$_1$-subunit of sodium channel, BrS5), KCNE3 (MiRP2; BrS6), and SCN3B (β3-subunit of sodium channel, BrS7) are much more rare.[101–105] The newest gene associated with BrS is CACNA2D1 (Ca$_v$α2δ, BrS8).[106]

The mechanisms of arrhythmogenesis in BrS can be explained by the heterogeneous shortening of the APD on the right ventricular epicardium (Fig. 6).[81]

In regions of the myocardium exhibiting a prominent I_{to}, such as the right ventricular outflow tract epicardium, accentuation of the action potential notch secondary to a reduction of calcium or sodium channel current or an increase in outward current, results in a transmural voltage gradient that leads to coved ST segment elevation, which is the only form of ST segment elevation diagnostic of BrS (see Fig. 6B). Under these conditions, there is little in the way of an arrhythmogenic substrate. However, a further outward shift of the currents active during the early phase of the action potential can lead to loss of the action potential dome, thus creating a dispersion of repolarization between epicardium and endocardium as well as within epicardium, between regions at which the dome is maintained and regions where it is lost (see Fig. 6C). The extent to which the action potential notch is accentuated leading to loss of the dome depends on the initial level of I_{to}.[107–109] When I_{to} is prominent, as it is in the right ventricular epicardium,[92,107,109] an outward shift of current causes phase 1 of the action potential to progress to more negative potentials at which the L-type calcium current ($I_{Ca,L}$) fails to activate, leading to an all-or-none repolarization and loss of the dome (see Fig. 6C). Because loss of the action potential dome is usually heterogeneous, the result is a marked abbreviation of action potential at some sites but not others. The epicardial action potential dome can then propagate from regions where it is maintained to regions where it is lost, giving rise to a very closely coupled extrasystole via phase 2 reentry (see Fig. 6D).[77] The extrasystole produced via phase 2 reentry often occurs on the preceding T wave resulting in an R-on-T

Fig. 5. (A) Ionic distinctions among epicardial, M, and endocardial cells. Action potentials recorded from myocytes isolated from the epicardial, endocardial, and M regions of the canine left ventricle. (B) I-V relations for I_{K1} in epicardial, endocardial, and M region myocytes. Values are mean ± SD. (C) Transient outward current (I_{to}) recorded from the 3 cell types (current traces recorded during depolarizing steps from a holding potential of −80 mV to test potentials ranging between −20 and +70 mV). (D) The average peak current-voltage relationship for I_{to} for each of the 3 cell types. Values are mean ± SD. (E) Voltage-dependent activation of the slowly activating component of the delayed rectifier K$^+$ current (I_{Ks}) (currents were elicited by the voltage pulse protocol shown in the inset; Na$^+$-, K$^+$-, and Ca^{2+}- free solution). (F) Voltage dependence of I_{Ks} (current remaining after exposure to E-4031) and I_{Kr} (E-4031-sensitive current). Values are mean ± SE. *P < .05 compared with Epi or Endo. (G) Reverse-mode sodium-calcium exchange currents recorded in potassium- and chloride-free solutions at a voltage of −80 mV. I_{Na-Ca} was maximally activated by switching to sodium-free external solution at the time indicated by the arrow. (H) Midmyocardial sodium-calcium exchanger density is 30% greater than endocardial density, calculated as the peak outward I_{Na-Ca} normalized by cell capacitance. Endocardial and epicardial densities were not significantly different. (I) TTX-sensitive late sodium current. Cells were held at −80 mV and briefly pulsed to −45 mV to inactivate fast sodium current before stepping to −10 mV. (J) Normalized late sodium current measured 300 msec into the test pulse was plotted as a function of test pulse potential. (Data from Zygmunt AC, Goodrow RJ, Antzelevitch C. INaCa contributes to electrical heterogeneity within the canine ventricle. Am J Physiol Heart Circ Physiol 2000;278:H1671;8; and Refs.[32,84,97])

Table 1
Genetic disorders causing cardiac arrhythmias in the absence of structural heart disease (Primary Electrical Disease)

		Rhythm	Inheritance	Locus	Ion Channel	Gene
LQTS	(RW)	TdP	AD			
	LQT1	(Andersen-Tawil Syndrome) (Timothy Syndrome)		11p15	I_{Ks}	KCNQ1, KvLQT1
	LQT2			7q35	I_{Kr}	KCNH2, HERG
	LQT3			3p21	I_{Na}	SCN5A, $Na_v1.5$
	LQT4			4q25		ANKB, ANK2
	LQT5			21q22	I_{Ks}	KCNE1, minK
	LQT6			21q22	I_{Kr}	KCNE2, MiRP1
	LQT7			17q23	I_{K1}	KCNJ2, Kir 2.1
	LQT8			6q8A	I_{Ca}	CACNA1C, $Ca_v1.2$
	LQT9			3p25	I_{Na}	CAV3, Caveolin-3
	LQT10			11q23.3	I_{Na}	SCN4B. Na_vb4
	LQT11			7q21-q22	I_{Ks}	AKAP9, Yotiao
	LQT12			20q11.2	I_{Na}	SNTA1, $\alpha-1$ Syntrophin
	LQT13			11q24	IK-ACh	KCNJ5, Kir3.4
LQTS	(JLN)	TdP	AR	11p15	I_{Ks}	KCNQ1, KvLQT1
				21q22	I_{Ks}	KCNE1, minK
BrS	BrS1	PVT	AD	3p21	I_{Na}	SCN5A, $Na_v1.5$
	BrS2	PVT	AD	3p24	I_{Na}	GPD1L
	BrS3	PVT	AD	12p13.3	I_{Ca}	CACNA1C, $Ca_v1.2$
	BrS4	PVT	AD	10p12.33	I_{Ca}	CACNB2b, $Ca_v\beta_{2b}$
	BrS5	PVT	AD	19q13.1	I_{Na}	SCN1B, $Na_v\beta1$
	BrS6	PVT	AD	11q13-14	I_{Ca}	KCNE3. MiRP2
	BrS7	PVT	AD	11q23.3	I_{Na}	SCN3B, Navb3
	BrS8	PVT	AD	7q21.11	I_{Ca}	CACNA2D1, $Ca_v\alpha2\delta$
ERS	ERS1	PVT	AD	12p11.23	IK-ATP	KCNJ8, Kir6.1
	ERS2	PVT	AD	12p13.3	I_{Ca}	CACNA1C, $Ca_v1.2$
	ERS3	PVT	AD	10p12.33	I_{Ca}	CACNB2b, $Ca_v\beta_{2b}$
	ERS4	PVT	AD	7q21.11	I_{Ca}	CACNA2D1, $Ca_v\alpha2\delta$
SQTS	SQT1	VT/VF	AD	7q35	I_{Kr}	KCNH2, HERG
	SQT2			11p15	I_{Ks}	KCNQ1, KvLQT1
	SQT3		AD	17q23.1-24.2	I_{K1}	KCNJ2, Kir2.1
	SQT4			12p13.3	I_{Ca}	CACNA1C, $Ca_v1.2$
	SQT5		AD	10p12.33	I_{Ca}	CACNB2b, $Ca_v\beta_{2b}$
Catecholaminergic Polymorphic VT						
	CPVT1	VT	AD	1q42-43		RyR2
	CPVT2	VT	AR	1p13-21		CASQ2

Abbreviations: AD, autosomal dominant; AR, autosomal recessive; BrS, Brugada syndrome; ERS, early repolarization syndrome; JLN, Jervell and Lange −Nielsen; LQTS, long QT syndrome; RW, Romano-Ward; SQTS, short QT syndrome; TdP, Torsade de Pointes; VF, ventricular fibrillation; VT, ventricular tachycardia.

phenomenon. This in turn can initiate polymorphic VT or VF (see **Fig. 6**E, F).

Potent sodium channel blockers like procainamide, pilsicainide, propafenone, and flecainide can be used to induce or unmask ST segment elevation in patients with concealed J-wave syndromes because they facilitate an outward shift of currents active in the early phases of the action potential.[110–112] Sodium channel blockers like quinidine, which also inhibits I_{to}, reduce the magnitude of the J wave and normalize ST segment elevation.[107,113]

Recent studies point to a prominent role of depolarization impairment resulting in local conduction delay in the RV[114]; however, the role of conduction delay in the RV in the electrocardiographic and arrhythmic manifestations of BrS remains a matter of debate.[115]

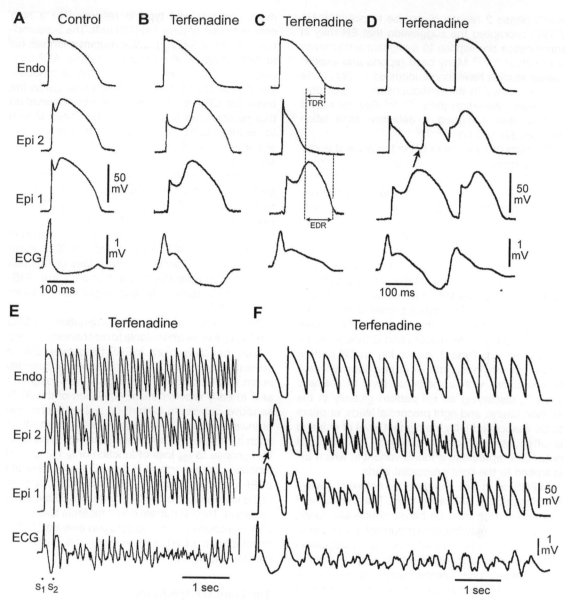

Fig. 6. Cellular basis for electrocardiographic and arrhythmic manifestation of BrS. Each panel shows transmembrane action potentials from 1 endocardial (*top*) and 2 epicardial sites together with a transmural ECG recorded from a canine coronary-perfused right ventricular wedge preparation. (*A*) Control (basic cycle length (BCL) 400 msec). (*B*) Combined sodium and calcium channel block with terfenadine (5 μM) accentuates the epicardial action potential notch creating a transmural voltage gradient that manifests as an ST segment elevation or exaggerated J wave in the ECG. (*C*) Continued exposure to terfenadine results in all-or-none repolarization at the end of phase 1 at some epicardial sites but not others, creating a local epicardial dispersion of repolarization (EDR) as well as a transmural dispersion of repolarization (TDR). (*D*) Phase 2 reentry occurs when the epicardial action potential dome propagates from a site where it is maintained to regions where it has been lost giving rise to a closely coupled extrasystole. (*E*) Extrastimulus (S1–S2 = 250 msec) applied to epicardium triggers a polymorphic VT. (*F*) Phase 2 reentrant extrasystole triggers a brief episode of polymorphic VT. (*Modified from* Fish JM, Antzelevitch C. Role of sodium and calcium channel block in unmasking the Brugada syndrome. Heart Rhythm 2004;1:210–17; with permission.)

Early repolarization syndrome

An early repolarization (ER) pattern, consisting of a J point elevation, a notch or slur on the QRS (J wave), and tall/symmetric T waves, is commonly found in healthy young males and has traditionally been regarded as totally benign.[116,117] A report in 2000 that an ER pattern in the coronary-perfused wedge preparation can easily convert to one in which phase 2 reentry gives rise to polymorphic VT/VF, prompted the suggestion that ER may in some cases predispose to malignant arrhythmias in the clinic.[80,118] Many case reports and experimental studies have long suggested a critical role for the J wave in the pathogenesis of idiopathic ventricular fibrillation (IVF).[119-127] Several recent studies have provided a definitive association between ER and IVF.[128-132]

The high prevalence of ER in the general population suggests that it is not a sensitive marker for sudden cardiac death (SCD), but that it is a marker of a genetic predisposition for the development of VT/VF via an ERS. Thus, when observed in patients with syncope or malignant family history of sudden cardiac death, ER may be prognostic of risk. We recently proposed a classification scheme for ERS based on the available data pointing to an association of risk with spatial localization of the ER pattern.[80] In this scheme, Type 1 is associated with ER pattern predominantly in the lateral precordial leads; this form is very prevalent among healthy male athletes and is thought to be largely benign. Type 2, displaying an ER pattern predominantly in the inferior or inferolateral leads, is associated with a moderate level of risk and Type 3, displaying an ER pattern globally in the inferior, lateral, and right precordial leads, appears to be associated with the highest level of risk and is often associated with electrical storms.[80] Of note, BrS represents a fourth variant in which ER is limited to the right precordial leads.

In ERS, as in BrS, the dynamic nature of J wave manifestation is well recognized. The amplitude of J waves, which may be barely noticeable during sinus rhythm, may become progressively accentuated with increased vagal tone and bradycardia and still further accentuated following successive extrasystoles and compensatory pauses giving rise to short long short sequences that precipitate VT/VF.[80,129,133]

Studies examining the genetic and molecular basis for ERS are few and data are very limited (see **Table 1**). Haissaguerre and colleagues[134] were the first to associate KCNJ8 with ERS. Functional expression of the S422L missense mutation in KCNJ8 was not available at the time but was recently reported by Medeiros-Domingo and colleagues.[135] The investigators genetically screened 101 probands with BrS and ERS and found one BrS and one ERS proband with an S422L-KCNJ8 (Kir6.1) mutation; the variation was absent in 600 controls. The investigators co-expressed the KCNJ8 mutation with ATP regulatory subunit SUR2A in COS-1 cells and measured I_{K-ATP} using whole cell patch clamp techniques. A significantly larger I_{K-ATP} was recorded for the

mutant versus wild type in response to a high concentration of pinacidil (100 µM). The presumption is that the S422L-KCNJ8 mutant channels fail to close properly at normal intracellular ATP concentrations, thus resulting in a gain of function. The prospect of a gain of function in I_{K-ATP} as the basis for ERS is supported by the observation that pinacidil, an I_{K-ATP} opener, has been shown to induce both the electrocardiographic and arrhythmic manifestation of ERS in LV wedge preparations.[80]

Recent studies from our group have identified 4 probands in whom mutations in highly conserved residues of CACNA1C, CACNB2, and CACNA2D1 were found to be associated with ERS.[106] Preliminary studies involving heterologous expression of these genes in HEK293 cells indicate that these mutations are associated with a loss of function of I_{Ca}, supporting the thesis that all 3 are ERS-susceptibility genes (Barajas, unpublished observation, 2010).

The ECG and arrhythmic manifestations of ERS are thought to be attributable to mechanisms similar to those operative in BrS. In ERS, the outward shift of current may extend beyond the action potential notch, thus leading to an elevation of the ST segment akin to early repolarization. Activation of the ATP-sensitive potassium current (I_{K-ATP}) or depression of inward calcium channel current (I_{Ca}) can effect such a change.[106] Transmural gradients generated in response to I_{Ca} loss of function or I_{K-ATP} gain of function could manifest in the ECG as a diversity of ER patterns including J point elevation, slurring of the terminal part of the QRS, and mild ST segment elevation. The ER pattern could facilitate loss of the dome because of other factors and thus lead to the development of ST segment elevation, phase 2 reentry, and VT/VF.

The Long QT Syndrome

The long QT syndromes (LQTS) are phenotypically and genotypically diverse, but have in common the appearance of long QT interval in the ECG, an atypical polymorphic ventricular tachycardia known as Torsade de Pointes (TdP), and, in many but not all cases, a relatively high risk for sudden cardiac death.[136-138] Congenital LQTS has been associated with 13 genes in at least 7 different ion genes and a structural anchoring protein located on chromosomes 3, 4, 6, 7, 11, 17, 20, and 21 (see **Table 1**).[139-146] Timothy syndrome, also referred to as LQT8, is a rare congenital disorder characterized by multiorgan dysfunction including prolongation of the QT interval, lethal arrhythmias, webbing of fingers and toes, congenital heart disease, immune deficiency, intermittent hypoglycemia, cognitive abnormalities, and autism. Timothy syndrome has been linked to loss of voltage-dependent inactivation owing to mutations in $Ca_v1.2$, the gene that encodes for an α subunit of the calcium channel.[147] The most recent gene associated with LQTS is *KCNJ5,* which encodes Kir3.4 protein, the protein that encodes the α subunit of the I_{K-ACh} channel. Mutations in this gene produce a loss of function that produces an LQT phenotype via a mechanism that is not clearly understood.[148]

Two patterns of inheritance have been identified in LQTS: (1) a rare autosomal recessive disease associated with deafness (Jervell and Lange-Nielsen), caused by 2 genes that encode for the slowly activating delayed rectifier potassium channel (KCNQ1 and KCNE1); and (2) a much more common autosomal dominant form known a the Romano Ward syndrome, caused by mutations in 13 different genes (see **Table 1**).

Acquired LQTS refers to a syndrome similar to the congenital form but caused by exposure to drugs that prolong the duration of the ventricular action potential[149] or QT prolongation secondary to cardiomyopathies, such as dilated or hypertrophic cardiomyopathy, as well as to abnormal QT prolongation associated with bradycardia or electrolyte imbalance.[150–154] The acquired form of the disease is far more prevalent than the congenital form, and in some cases may have a genetic predisposition.

Amplification of spatial dispersion of repolarization within the ventricular myocardium has been identified as the principal arrhythmogenic substrate in both acquired and congenital LQTS. The accentuation of spatial dispersion, typically secondary to an increase of transmural, trans-septal, or apico-basal dispersion of repolarization, and the development of early afterdepolarization (EAD)-induced triggered activity underlie the substrate and trigger for the development of TdP arrhythmias observed under LQTS conditions.[155,156] Models of the LQT1, LQT2, and LQT3, and LQT7 forms of the long QT syndrome have been developed using the canine arterially perfused left ventricular wedge preparation (**Fig. 7**).[16,157,158] Data from these studies suggest that in LQTS, preferential prolongation of the M cell APD leads to an increase in the QT interval as well as an increase in transmural dispersion of repolarization (TDR), which contributes to the development of spontaneous as well as stimulation-induced TdP.[159–161] The unique characteristics of the M cells, ie, the ability of their action potential to prolong more than that of epicardium or endocardium in response to a slowing of rate,[96,162,163] is at the heart of this mechanism.- **Fig. 7** presents our working hypothesis for our understanding of the mechanisms underlying LQTS-related TdP based on available data. The hypothesis presumes the presence of electrical heterogeneity in the form of transmural dispersion of repolarization under baseline conditions and the amplification of TDR by agents that reduce net repolarizing current via a reduction in I_{Kr} or I_{Ks} or augmentation of I_{Ca} or late I_{Na}. Conditions leading to a reduction in I_{Kr} or augmentation of late I_{Na} lead to a preferential prolongation of the M cell action potential. As a consequence, the QT interval prolongs and is accompanied by a dramatic increase in transmural dispersion of repolarization, thus creating a vulnerable window for the development of reentry. The reduction in net repolarizing current also predisposes to the development of

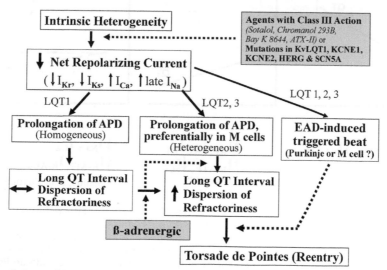

Fig. 7. Proposed cellular and ionic mechanisms for the long QT syndrome.

EAD-induced triggered activity in M and Purkinje cells, which provide the extrasystole that triggers TdP when it falls within the vulnerable period. β adrenergic agonists further amplify transmural heterogeneity (transiently) in the case of I_{Kr} block, but reduce it in the case of I_{Na} agonists.[161,164]

Short QT Syndrome

The short QT syndrome (SQTS), first proposed as a clinical entity by Gussak and colleagues[165] in 2000, is an inherited syndrome characterized by a QTc of 360 msec or less and high incidence of VT/VF in infants, children, and young adults.[166,167] The familial nature of this sudden death syndrome was highlighted by Gaita and colleagues[168] in 2003. Mutations in 5 genes have been associated with SQTS: *KCNH2, KCNJ2, KCNQ1, CACNA1c,* and *CACNB2b.*[102,169–171] Mutations in these genes cause either a gain of function in outward potassium channel currents (I_{Kr}, I_{Ks} and I_{K1}) or a loss of function in inward calcium channel current (I_{Ca}).

Experimental studies suggest that the abbreviation of the action potential in SQTS is heterogeneous with preferential abbreviation of either ventricular epicardium or endocardium, giving rise to an increase in TDR.[172,173] In the atria, the I_{Kr} agonist PD118057 causes a much greater abbreviation of the action potential in epicardium when compared with cristae terminalis, thus creating a marked dispersion of repolarization in the right atrium.[174] Dispersion of repolarization and refractoriness serve as substrates for reentry by promoting unidirectional block. The marked abbreviation of wavelength (product of refractory period and conduction velocity) is an additional factor promoting the maintenance of reentry. T_{peak}-T_{end} interval and T_{peak}-T_{end} /QT ratio, an electrocardiographic index of spatial dispersion of ventricular repolarization, and perhaps TDR, have been reported to be significantly augmented in cases of SQTS.[175,176] Interestingly, this ratio is more amplified in patients who are symptomatic.[177]

Evidence supporting the role of augmented TDR in atrial and ventricular arrhythmogenesis in SQTS derives from experimental studies involving the canine left ventricular wedge and atrial preparations.[172–174,178]

The Role of Spatial Dispersion of Repolarization in Channelopathy-Mediated Sudden Death

The inherited and acquired sudden death syndromes discussed previously differ with respect to the behavior of the QT interval (**Fig. 8**).

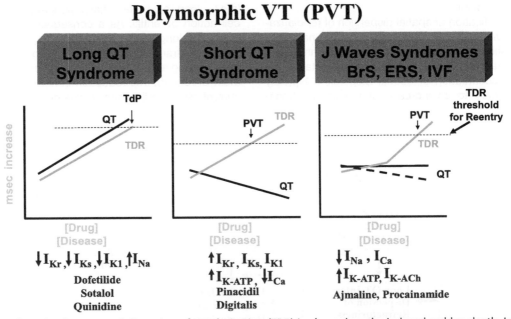

Polymorphic VT (PVT)

Fig. 8. The role of transmural dispersion of repolarization (TDR) in channelopathy-induced sudden death. In the long QT syndrome, QT increases as a function of disease or drug concentration. In the J wave syndromes (Brugada and early repolarization syndromes), it remains largely unchanged or is moderately abbreviated, and in the short QT syndrome, QT interval decreases as a function of disease or drug. The 3 syndromes have in common the ability to amplify TDR, which results in the development of polymorphic VT (PVT) or Torsade de Pontes (TdP) when dispersion reaches the threshold for reentry.

In the long QT syndrome, QT increases as a function of disease or drug concentration. In the Brugada and early repolarization syndromes, it remains largely unchanged or is abbreviated, and in the short QT syndrome, QT interval decreases as a function of disease or drug. What these syndromes have in common is an amplification of TDR, which results in the development of polymorphic VT when TDR reaches the threshold for reentry. In the setting of a prolonged QT, we refer to it as TdP. It is noteworthy that the threshold for reentry decreases as APD and refractoriness are reduced, thus requiring a shorter path length for reentry, making it easier to induce.

REFERENCES

1. Maltsev VA, Vinogradova TM, Lakatta EG. The emergence of a general theory of the initiation and strength of the heartbeat. J Pharmacol Sci 2006;100:338–69.
2. Lakatta EG. A paradigm shift for the heart's pacemaker. Heart Rhythm 2010;7:559–64.
3. DiFrancesco D. The pacemaker current I_f plays an important role in regulating SA node pacemaker activity. Cardiovasc Res 1995;30:307–8.
4. Huser J, Blatter LA, Lipsius SL. Intracellular Ca^{2+} release contributes to automaticity in cat atrial pacemaker cells. J Physiol 2000;524(Pt 2):415–22.
5. Levy MN. Sympathetic-parasympathetic interactions in the heart. Circ Res 1971;29:437–45.
6. Tan AY, Zhou S, Ogawa M, et al. Neural mechanisms of paroxysmal atrial fibrillation and paroxysmal atrial tachycardia in ambulatory canines. Circulation 2008;118:916–25.
7. Ogawa M, Zhou S, Tan AY, et al. Left stellate ganglion and vagal nerve activity and cardiac arrhythmias in ambulatory dogs with pacing-induced congestive heart failure. J Am Coll Cardiol 2007;50:335–43.
8. Schulze-Bahr E, Neu A, Friederich P, et al. Pacemaker channel dysfunction in a patient with sinus node disease. J Clin Invest 2003; 111:1537–45.
9. Nof E, Luria D, Brass D, et al. Point mutation in the *HCN4* cardiac ion channel pore affecting synthesis, trafficking, and functional expression is associated with familial asymptomatic sinus bradycardia. Circulation 2007;116:463–70.
10. Zicha S, Fernandez-Velasco M, Lonardo G, et al. Sinus node dysfunction and hyperpolarization-activated (HCN) channel subunit remodeling in a canine heart failure model. Cardiovasc Res 2005;66:472–81.
11. Laish-Farkash A, Marek D, Brass D, et al. A novel mutation in the HCN4 gene causes familial sinus bradycardia in two unrelated Moroccan families [abstract]. Heart Rhythm 2008;5S:S275.
12. Laish-Farkash A, Glikson M, Brass D, et al. A novel mutation in the HCN4 gene causes symptomatic sinus bradycardia in Moroccan Jews. J Cardiovasc Electrophysiol, in press.
13. Nof E, Antzelevitch C, Glickson M. The contribution of HCN4 to normal sinus nose function in humans and animal models. Pacing Clin Electrophysiol 2010;33:100–6.
14. Wit AL, Rosen MR. Afterdepolarizations and triggered activity: distinction from automaticity as an arrhythmogenic mechanism. In: Fozzard HA, Haber E, Jenning RB, et al, editors. The heart and cardiovascular system. New York: Raven Press; 1992. p. 2113–64.
15. Zhang L, Benson DW, Tristani-Firouzi M, et al. Electrocardiographic features in Andersen-Tawil syndrome patients with KCNJ2 mutations: characteristic T-U-wave patterns predict the KCNJ2 genotype. Circulation 2005;111:2720–6.
16. Tsuboi M, Antzelevitch C. Cellular basis for electrocardiographic and arrhythmic manifestations of Andersen-Tawil syndrome (LQT7). Heart Rhythm 2006;3:328–35.
17. Barajas-Martínez H, Hu D, Ontiverod G, et al. Biophysical characterization of a novel KCNJ2 mutation associated with Andersen-Tawil syndrome and CPVT mimicry [abstract]. Biophys J 2009;96: 260a.
18. Tristani-Firouzi M. Andersen-Tawil syndrome: an ever-expanding phenotype? Heart Rhythm 2006; 3:1351–2.
19. Tristani-Firouzi M, Etheridge SP. Kir 2.1 channelopathies: the Andersen-Tawil syndrome. Pflugers Arch, in press.
20. Tristani-Firouzi M, Jensen JL, Donaldson MR, et al. Functional and clinical characterization of KCNJ2 mutations associated with LQT7 (Andersen syndrome). J Clin Invest 2002;110:381–8.
21. Vassalle M. The relationship among cardiac pacemakers. Overdrive suppression. Circ Res 1977;41: 269–77.
22. Gadsby DC, Cranefield PF. Electrogenic sodium extrusion in cardiac Purkinje fibers. J Gen Physiol 1979;73:819–37.
23. Jalife J, Moe GK. A biological model of parasystole. Am J Cardiol 1979;43:761–72.
24. Jalife J, Antzelevitch C, Moe GK. The case for modulated parasystole. Pacing Clin Electrophysiol 1982;5:911–26.
25. Nau GJ, Aldariz AE, Acunzo RS, et al. Modulation of parasystolic activity by nonparasystolic beats. Circulation 1982;66:462–9.
26. Antzelevitch C, Bernstein MJ, Feldman HN, et al. Parasystole, reentry, and tachycardia: a canine preparation of cardiac arrhythmias occurring

across inexcitable segments of tissue. Circulation 1983;68:1101–15.

27. Jalife J, Moe GK. Effect of electrotonic potentials on pacemaker activity of canine Purkinje fibers in relation to parasystole. Circ Res 1976;39:801–8.

28. Roden DM. Drug-induced prolongation of the QT interval. N Engl J Med 2004;350:1013–22.

29. Roden DM. Long QT syndrome: reduced repolarization reserve and the genetic link. J Intern Med 2006;259:59–69.

30. Priori SG, Corr PB. Mechanisms underlying early and delayed afterdepolarizations induced by catecholamines. Am J Physiol 1990;258: H1796–805.

31. Burashnikov A, Antzelevitch C. Acceleration-induced action potential prolongation and early afterdepolarizations. J Cardiovasc Electrophysiol 1998;9:934–48.

32. Liu DW, Antzelevitch C. Characteristics of the delayed rectifier current (I_{Kr} and I_{Ks}) in canine ventricular epicardial, midmyocardial, and endocardial myocytes. A weaker I_{Ks} contributes to the longer action potential of the M cell. Circ Res 1995;76: 351–65.

33. Zygmunt AC, Eddlestone GT, Thomas GP, et al. Larger late sodium conductance in M cells contributes to electrical heterogeneity in canine ventricle. Am J Physiol 2001;281:H689–97.

34. Burashnikov A, Antzelevitch C. Prominent IKs in epicardium and endocardium contributes to development of transmural dispersion of repolarization but protects against development of early afterdepolarizations. J Cardiovasc Electrophysiol 2002;13: 172–7.

35. Aiba T, Tomaselli GF. Electrical remodeling in the failing heart. Curr Opin Cardiol 2010;25:29–36.

36. Ferrier GR, Saunders JH, Mendez C. A cellular mechanism for the generation of ventricular arrhythmias by acetylstrophanthidin. Circ Res 1973;32:600–9.

37. Rosen MR, Gelband H, Merker C, et al. Mechanisms of digitalis toxicity—effects of ouabain on phase four of canine Purkinje fiber transmembrane potentials. Circulation 1973;47:681–9.

38. Saunders JH, Ferrier GR, Moe GK. Conduction block associated with transient depolarizations induced by acetylstrophanthidin in isolated canine Purkinje fibers. Circ Res 1973;32:610–7.

39. Rozanski GJ, Lipsius SL. Electrophysiology of functional subsidiary pacemakers in canine right atrium. Am J Physiol 1985;249:H594–603.

40. Wit AL, Cranefield PF. Triggered and automatic activity in the canine coronary sinus. Circ Res 1977;41:435–45.

41. Aronson RS. Afterpotentials and triggered activity in hypertrophiod myocardium from rats with renal-hypertension. Circ Res 1981;48:720–7.

42. Vermeulen JT, McGuire MA, Opthof T, et al. Triggered activity and automaticity in ventricular trabeculae of failing human and rabbit hearts. Cardiovasc Res 1994;28:1547–54.

43. Lazzara R, El-Sherif N, Scherlag BJ. Electrophysiological properties of canine Purkinje cells in one-day-old myocardial infarction. Circ Res 1973;33: 722–34.

44. Priori SG, Napolitano C, Tiso N, et al. Mutations in the cardiac ryanodine receptor gene (hRyR2) underlie catecholaminergic polymorphic ventricular tachycardia. Circulation 2001;103:196–200.

45. Wehrens XH, Lehnart SE, Reiken SR, et al. Protection from cardiac arrhythmia through ryanodine receptor-stabilizing protein calstabin2. Science 2004;304:292–6.

46. Nam GB, Burashnikov A, Antzelevitch C. Cellular mechanisms underlying the development of catecholaminergic ventricular tachycardia. Circulation 2005;111:2727–33.

47. Tomaselli GF, Zipes DP. What causes sudden death in heart failure? Circ Res 2004;95:754–63.

48. Burashnikov A, Antzelevitch C. Reinduction of atrial fibrillation immediately after termination of the arrhythmia is mediated by late phase 3 early afterdepolarization-induced triggered activity. Circulation 2003;107:2355–60.

49. Burashnikov A, Antzelevitch C. Late-phase 3 EAD. A unique mechanism contributing to initiation of atrial fibrillation. Pacing Clin Electrophysiol 2006; 29:290–5.

50. Watanabe I, Okumura Y, Ohkubo K, et al. Steady-state and nonsteady-state action potentials in fibrillating canine atrium: alternans of action potential and late phase 3 early afterdepolarization as a precursor of atrial fibrillation [abstract]. Heart Rhythm 2005;2:S259.

51. Patterson E, Po SS, Scherlag BJ, et al. Triggered firing in pulmonary veins initiated by in vitro autonomic nerve stimulation. Heart Rhythm 2005;2: 624–31.

52. Ogawa M, Morita N, Tang L, et al. Mechanisms of recurrent ventricular fibrillation in a rabbit model of pacing-induced heart failure. Heart Rhythm 2009;6:784–92.

53. Mayer AG. Rhythmical pulsations is scyphomedusae. Washington, DC: Publication 47 of the Carnegie Institute; 1906. p. 1–62.

54. Mines GR. On circulating excitations in heart muscles and their possible relation to tachycardia and fibrillation. Trans R Soc Can 1914;8: 43–52.

55. Mines GR. On dynamic equilibrium in the heart. J Physiol 1913;46:350–83.

50. Garrey WE. The nature of fibrillatory contraction of the heart—its relation to tissue mass and form. Am J Physiol 1914;33:397–414.

57. Allessie MA, Bonke FIM, Schopman JG. Circus movement in rabbit atrial muscle as a mechanism of tachycardia. Circ Res 1973;33:54–62.

58. Allessie MA, Bonke FIM, Schopman JG. Circus movement in rabbit atrial muscle as a mechanism of tachycardia. III. The "leading circle" concept: a new model of circus movement in cardiac tissue without the involvement of an anatomical obstacle. Circ Res 1977;41:9–18.

59. Weiner N, Rosenblueth A. The mathematical formulation of the problem of conduction of impulses in a network of connected excitable elements, specifically in cardiac muscle. Arch Inst Cardiol Mex 1946;16:205–65.

60. Davidenko JM, Cohen L, Goodrow RJ, et al. Quinidine-induced action potential prolongation, early afterdepolarizations, and triggered activity in canine Purkinje fibers. Effects of stimulation rate, potassium, and magnesium. Circulation 1989;79: 674–86.

61. Jalife J, Delmar M, Davidenko JM, et al. Basic cardiac electrophysiology for the clinician. Armonk (NY): Futura Publishing; 1999.

62. Gray RA, Jalife J, Panfilov AV, et al. Mechanisms of cardiac fibrillation. Science 1995;270:1222–3.

63. Garfinkel A, Kim YH, Voroshilovsky O, et al. Preventing ventricular fibrillation by flattening cardiac restitution. Proc Natl Acad Sci U S A 2000;97: 6061–6.

64. El-Sherif N, Smith RA, Evans K. Canine ventricular arrhythmias in the late myocardial infarction period. 8. Epicardial mapping of reentrant circuits. Circ Res 1981;49:255–65.

65. Valderrabano M, Kim YH, Yashima M, et al. Obstacle-induced transition from ventricular fibrillation to tachycardia in isolated swine right ventricles: insights into the transition dynamics and implications for the critical mass. J Am Coll Cardiol 2000;36:2000–8.

66. Chen PS, Wolf PD, Dixon EG, et al. Mechanism of ventricular vulnerability to single premature stimuli in open-chest dogs. Circ Res 1988;62:1191–209.

67. Wit AL, Cranefield PF, Hoffman BF. Slow conduction and reentry in the ventricular conducting system. II. Single and sustained circus movement in networks of canine and bovine Purkinje fibers. Circ Res 1972;30:11–22.

68. Schmitt FO, Erlanger J. Directional differences in the conduction of the impulse through heart muscle and their possible relation to extrasystolic and fibrillary contractions. Am J Physiol 1928;87:326–47.

69. Antzelevitch C, Jalife J, Moe GK. Characteristics of reflection as a mechanism of reentrant arrhythmias and its relationship to parasystole. Circulation 1980;61:182–91.

70. Antzelevitch C, Moe GK. Electrotonically-mediated delayed conduction and reentry in relation to "slow responses" in mammalian ventricular conducting tissue. Circ Res 1981;49:1129–39.

71. Antzelevitch C. Clinical applications of new concepts of parasystole, reflection, and tachycardia. Cardiol Clin 1983;1:39–50.

72. Rozanski GJ, Jalife J, Moe GK. Reflected reentry in nonhomogeneous ventricular muscle as a mechanism of cardiac arrhythmias. Circulation 1984;69: 163–73.

73. Lukas A, Antzelevitch C. Reflected reentry, delayed conduction, and electrotonic inhibition in segmentally depressed atrial tissues. Can J Physiol Pharmacol 1989;67:757–64.

74. Davidenko JM, Antzelevitch C. The effects of milrinone on action potential characteristics, conduction, automaticity, and reflected reentry in isolated myocardial fibers. J Cardiovasc Pharmacol 1985; 7:341–9.

75. Rosenthal JE, Ferrier GR. Contribution of variable entrance and exit block in protected foci to arrhythmogenesis in isolated ventricular tissues. Circulation 1983;67:1–8.

76. Antzelevitch C, Lukas A. Reflection and circus movement reentry in isolated atrial and ventricular tissues. In: Dangman KH, Miura DS, editors. Electrophysiology and pharmacology of the heart. A clinical guide. New York: Marcel Dekker; 1991. p. 251–75.

77. Krishnan SC, Antzelevitch C. Flecainide-induced arrhythmia in canine ventricular epicardium. Phase 2 reentry? Circulation 1993;87:562–72.

78. Lukas A, Antzelevitch C. Phase 2 reentry as a mechanism of initiation of circus movement reentry in canine epicardium exposed to simulated ischemia. Cardiovasc Res 1996;32:593–603.

79. Di Diego JM, Antzelevitch C. Pinacidil-induced electrical heterogeneity and extrasystolic activity in canine ventricular tissues. Does activation of ATP-regulated potassium current promote phase 2 reentry? Circulation 1993;88:1177–89.

80. Antzelevitch C, Yan GX. J wave syndromes. Heart Rhythm 2010;7:549–58.

81. Antzelevitch C. Brugada syndrome. Pacing Clin Electrophysiol 2006;29:1130–59.

82. Antzelevitch C, Sicouri S, Litovsky SH, et al. Heterogeneity within the ventricular wall. Electrophysiology and pharmacology of epicardial, endocardial, and M cells. Circ Res 1991;69:1427–49.

83. Antzelevitch C, Sicouri S, Lukas A, et al. Clinical implications of electrical heterogeneity in the heart: the electrophysiology and pharmacology of epicardial, M, and endocardial cells. In: Podrid PJ, Kowey PR, editors. Cardiac arrhythmia: mechanism, diagnosis and management. Baltimore (MD): William & Wilkins; 1995. p. 88–107.

84. Litovsky SH, Antzelevitch C. Transient outward current prominent in canine ventricular epicardium but not endocardium. Circ Res 1988;62:116–26.

85. Liu DW, Gintant GA, Antzelevitch C. Ionic bases for electrophysiological distinctions among epicardial, midmyocardial, and endocardial myocytes from the free wall of the canine left ventricle. Circ Res 1993;72:671–87.

86. Furukawa T, Myerburg RJ, Furukawa N, et al. Differences in transient outward currents of feline endocardial and epicardial myocytes. Circ Res 1990;67:1287–91.

87. Sicouri S, Quist M, Antzelevitch C. Evidence for the presence of M cells in the guinea pig ventricle. J Cardiovasc Electrophysiol 1996;7:503–11.

88. Stankovicova T, Szilard M, De Scheerder I, et al. M cells and transmural heterogeneity of action potential configuration in myocytes from the left ventricular wall of the pig heart. Cardiovasc Res 2000;45:952–60.

89. McIntosh MA, Cobbe SM, Smith GL. Heterogeneous changes in action potential and intracellular Ca2+ in left ventricular myocyte sub-types from rabbits with heart failure. Cardiovasc Res 2000;45:397–409.

90. Wettwer E, Amos GJ, Posival H, et al. Transient outward current in human ventricular myocytes of subepicardial and subendocardial origin. Circ Res 1994;75:473–82.

91. Nabauer M, Beuckelmann DJ, Uberfuhr P, et al. Regional differences in current density and rate-dependent properties of the transient outward current in subepicardial and subendocardial myocytes of human left ventricle. Circulation 1996;93:168–77.

92. Di Diego JM, Sun ZQ, Antzelevitch C. I_{to} and action potential notch are smaller in left vs. right canine ventricular epicardium. Am J Physiol 1996;271:H548–61.

93. Volders PG, Sipido KR, Carmeliet E, et al. Repolarizing K+ currents ITO1 and IKs are larger in right than left canine ventricular midmyocardium. Circulation 1999;99:206–10.

94. Takano M, Noma A. Distribution of the isoprenaline-induced chloride current in rabbit heart. Pflugers Arch 1992;420:223–6.

95. Zygmunt AC. Intracellular calcium activates chloride current in canine ventricular myocytes. Am J Physiol 1994;267:H1984–95.

96. Sicouri S, Antzelevitch C. A subpopulation of cells with unique electrophysiological properties in the deep subepicardium of the canine ventricle. The M cell. Circ Res 1991;68:1729–41.

97. Anyukhovsky EP, Sosunov EA, Rosen MR. Regional differences in electrophysiologic properties of epicardium, midmyocardium and endocardium: in vitro and in vivo correlations. Circulation 1996;94:1981–8.

98. Zygmunt AC, Goodrow RJ, Antzelevitch C. I_{NaCa} contributes to electrical heterogeneity within the canine ventricle. Am J Physiol Heart Circ Physiol 2000;278:H1671–8.

99. Brahmajothi MV, Morales MJ, Rasmusson RL, et al. Heterogeneity in K+ channel transcript expression detected in isolated ferret cardiac myocytes. Pacing Clin Electrophysiol 1997;20:388–96.

100. Brugada P, Brugada J. Right bundle branch block, persistent ST segment elevation and sudden cardiac death: a distinct clinical and electrocardiographic syndrome: a multicenter report. J Am Coll Cardiol 1992;20:1391–6.

101. Schulze-Bahr E, Eckardt L, Breithardt G, et al. Sodium channel gene (SCN5A) mutations in 44 index patients with Brugada syndrome: different incidences in familial and sporadic disease. Hum Mutat 2003;21:651–2.

102. Antzelevitch C, Pollevick GD, Cordeiro JM, et al. Loss-of-function mutations in the cardiac calcium channel underlie a new clinical entity characterized by ST-segment elevation, short QT intervals, and sudden cardiac death. Circulation 2007;115:442–9.

103. London B, Michalec M, Mehdi H, et al. Mutation in glycerol-3-phosphate dehydrogenase 1 like gene (GPD1-L) decreases cardiac Na+ current and causes inherited arrhythmias. Circulation 2007;116:2260–8.

104. Watanabe H, Koopmann TT, Le Scouarnec S, et al. Sodium channel β1 subunit mutations associated with Brugada syndrome and cardiac conduction disease in humans. J Clin Invest 2008;118:2260–8.

105. Hu D, Barajas-Martinez H, Burashnikov E, et al. A mutation in the β3 subunit of the cardiac sodium channel associated with Brugada ECG phenotype. Circ Cardiovasc Genet 2009;2:270–8.

106. Burashnikov E, Pfeifer R, Barajas-Martinez H, et al. Mutations in the cardiac L-type calcium channel associated J wave syndrome and sudden cardiac death. Heart Rhythm, in press.

107. Yan GX, Antzelevitch C. Cellular basis for the Brugada syndrome and other mechanisms of arrhythmogenesis associated with ST segment elevation. Circulation 1999;100:1660–6.

108. Antzelevitch C, Shimizu W, Yan GX. Electrical heterogeneity and the development of arrhythmias. In: Olsson SB, Yuan S, Amlie JP, editors. Dispersion of ventricular repolarization: state of the art. Armonk (NY): Futura Publishing Company, Inc; 2000. p. 3–21.

109. Yan GX, Lankipalli RS, Burke JF, et al. Ventricular repolarization components on the electrocardiogram: cellular basis and clinical significance. J Am Coll Cardiol 2003;42:401–9.

110. Shimizu W, Antzelevitch C, Suyama K, et al. Effect of sodium channel blockers on ST segment, QRS duration, and corrected QT interval in patients with Brugada syndrome. J Cardiovasc Electrophysiol 2000;11:1320–9.

111. Brugada R, Brugada J, Antzelevitch C, et al. Sodium channel blockers identify risk for sudden death in patients with ST-segment elevation and right bundle branch block but structurally normal hearts. Circulation 2000;101:510–5.

112. Morita H, Morita ST, Nagase S, et al. Ventricular arrhythmia induced by sodium channel blocker in patients with Brugada syndrome. J Am Coll Cardiol 2003;42:1624–31.

113. Gussak I, Antzelevitch C, Bjerregaard P, et al. The Brugada syndrome: clinical, electrophysiologic and genetic aspects. J Am Coll Cardiol 1999;33: 5–15.

114. Postema PG, van Dessel PF, Kors JA, et al. Local depolarization abnormalities are the dominant pathophysiologic mechanism for type 1 electrocardiogram in Brugada syndrome: a study of electrocardiograms, vectorcardiograms, and body surface potential maps during ajmaline provocation. J Am Coll Cardiol 2010;55:789–97.

115. Wilde AA, Postema PG, Di Diego JM, et al. The pathophysiological mechanism underlying Brugada syndrome: depolarization versus repolarization. J Mol Cell Cardiol 2010;49:543–53.

116. Wasserburger RH, Alt WJ. The normal RS-T segment elevation variant. Am J Cardiol 1961;8: 184–92.

117. Mehta MC, Jain AC. Early repolarization on scalar electrocardiogram. Am J Med Sci 1995;309:305–11.

118. Gussak I, Antzelevitch C. Early repolarization syndrome: clinical characteristics and possible cellular and ionic mechanisms. J Electrocardiol 2000;33:299–309.

119. Bjerregaard P, Gussak I, Kotar SL, Gessler JE. Recurrent syncope in a patient with prominent J-wave. Am Heart J 1994;127:1426–30.

120. Yan GX, Antzelevitch C. Cellular basis for the electrocardiographic J wave. Circulation 1996;93: 372–9.

121. Geller JC, Reek S, Goette A, et al. Spontaneous episode of polymorphic ventricular tachycardia in a patient with intermittent Brugada syndrome. J Cardiovasc Electrophysiol 2001;12:1094.

122. Daimon M, Inagaki M, Morooka S, et al. Brugada syndrome characterized by the appearance of J waves. Pacing Clin Electrophysiol 2000;23: 405–6.

123. Kalla H, Yan GX, Marinchak R. Ventricular fibrillation in a patient with prominent J (Osborn) waves and ST segment elevation in the inferior electrocardiographic leads: a Brugada syndrome variant? J Cardiovasc Electrophysiol 2000;11:95–8.

124. Komiya N, Imanishi R, Kawano H, et al. Ventricular fibrillation in a patient with prominent J wave in the inferior and lateral electrocardiographic leads after gastrostomy. Pacing Clin Electrophysiol 2006;29: 1022–4.

125. Shinohara T, Takahashi N, Saikawa T, et al. Characterization of J wave in a patient with idiopathic ventricular fibrillation. Heart Rhythm 2006;3:1082–4.

126. Riera AR, Ferreira C, Schapachnik E, et al. Brugada syndrome with atypical ECG: downsloping ST-segment elevation in inferior leads. J Electrocardiol 2004;37:101–4.

127. Shu J, Zhu T, Yang L, et al. ST-segment elevation in the early repolarization syndrome, idiopathic ventricular fibrillation, and the Brugada syndrome: cellular and clinical linkage. J Electrocardiol 2005; 38:26–32.

128. Haissaguerre M, Derval N, Sacher F, et al. Sudden cardiac arrest associated with early repolarization. N Engl J Med 2008;358:2016–23.

129. Nam GB, Kim YH, Antzelevitch C. Augmentation of J waves and electrical storms in patients with early repolarization. N Engl J Med 2008;358:2078–9.

130. Rosso R, Kogan E, Belhassen B, et al. J-point elevation in survivors of primary ventricular fibrillation and matched control subjects: incidence and clinical significance. J Am Coll Cardiol 2008;52:1231–8.

131. Tikkanen JT, Anttonen O, Junttila MJ, et al. Long-term outcome associated with early repolarization on electrocardiography. N Engl J Med 2009;361: 2529–37.

132. Sinner MF, Reinhard W, Muller M, et al. Association of early repolarization pattern on ECG with risk of cardiac and all-cause mortality: a population-based prospective cohort study (MONICA/KORA). PLoS Med 2010;7:e1000314.

133. Nam GB, Ko KH, Kim J, et al. Mode of onset of ventricular fibrillation in patients with early repolarization pattern vs. Brugada syndrome. Eur Heart J 2010;31:330–9.

134. Haissaguerre M, Chatel S, Sacher F, et al. Ventricular fibrillation with prominent early repolarization associated with a rare variant of KCNJ8/K_{ATP} channel. J Cardiovasc Electrophysiol 2009;20:93–8.

135. Medeiros-Domingo A, Tan BH, Crotti L, et al. Gain-of-function mutation, S422L, in the KCNJ8-encoded cardiac K ATP channel kir6.1 as a pathogenic substrate for J wave syndromes. Heart Rhythm 2010;7(10):1466–71.

136. Schwartz PJ. The idiopathic long QT syndrome: progress and questions. Am Heart J 1985;109: 399–411.

137. Moss AJ, Schwartz PJ, Crampton RS, et al. The long QT syndrome: prospective longitudinal study of 328 families. Circulation 1991;84:1136–44.

138. Zipes DP. The long QT interval syndrome. A rosetta stone for sympathetic related ventricular tachyarrhythmias. Circulation 1991;84:1414–9.

139. Plaster NM, Tawil R, Tristani-Firouzi M, et al. Mutations in Kir2.1 cause the developmental and episodic electrical phenotypes of Andersen's syndrome. Cell 2001;105:511–9.

140. Wang Q, Shen J, Splawski I, et al. *SCN5A* mutations associated with an inherited cardiac arrhythmia, long QT syndrome. Cell 1995;80:805–11.

141. Mohler PJ, Schott JJ, Gramolini AO, et al. Ankyrin-B mutation causes type 4 long-QT cardiac arrhythmia and sudden cardiac death. Nature 2003;421:634–9.

142. Curran ME, Splawski I, Timothy KW, et al. A molecular basis for cardiac arrhythmia: HERG mutations cause long QT syndrome. Cell 1995;80:795–803.

143. Wang Q, Curran ME, Splawski I, et al. Positional cloning of a novel potassium channel gene: *KVLQT1* mutations cause cardiac arrhythmias. Nat Genet 1996;12:17–23.

144. Splawski I, Tristani-Firouzi M, Lehmann MH, et al. Mutations in the hminK gene cause long QT syndrome and suppress I_{Ks} function. Nat Genet 1997;17:338–40.

145. Ye B, Tester DJ, Vatta M, et al. Molecular and functional characterization of novel cav3-encoded caveolin-3 mutations in congenital long QT syndrome [abstract]. Heart Rhythm 2006;3:S1.

146. Domingo AM, Kaku T, Tester DJ, et al. Sodium channel ß4 subunit mutation causes congenital long QT syndrome. Heart Rhythm 2006;3:S34.

147. Splawski I, Timothy KW, Sharpe LM, et al. Ca$_v$1.2 calcium channel dysfunction causes a multisystem disorder including arrhythmia and autism. Cell 2004;119:19–31.

148. Yang Y, Yang Y, Liang B, et al. Identification of a Kir3.4 mutation in congenital long QT syndrome. Am J Hum Genet 2010;86:872–80.

149. Bednar MM, Harrigan EP, Anziano RJ, et al. The QT interval. Prog Cardiovasc Dis 2001;43:1–45.

150. Tomaselli GF, Marban E. Electrophysiological remodeling in hypertrophy and heart failure. Cardiovasc Res 1999;42:270–83.

151. Sipido KR, Volders PG, De Groot SH, et al. Enhanced Ca^{2+} release and Na/Ca exchange activity in hypertrophied canine ventricular myocytes: potential link between contractile adaptation and arrhythmogenesis. Circulation 2000;102:2137–44.

152. Volders PG, Sipido KR, Vos MA, et al. Downregulation of delayed rectifier K(+) currents in dogs with chronic complete atrioventricular block and acquired torsades de pointes. Circulation 1999;100:2455–61.

153. Undrovinas AI, Maltsev VA, Sabbah HN. Repolarization abnormalities in cardiomyocytes of dogs with chronic heart failure: role of sustained inward current. Cell Mol Life Sci 1999;55:494–505.

154. Maltsev VA, Sabbah HN, Higgins RS, et al. Novel, ultraslow inactivating sodium current in human ventricular cardiomyocytes. Circulation 1998;98:2545–52.

155. Belardinelli L, Antzelevitch C, Vos MA. Assessing predictors of drug-induced torsade de pointes. Trends Pharmacol Sci 2003;24:619–25.

156. Antzelevitch C, Shimizu W. Cellular mechanisms underlying the long QT syndrome. Curr Opin Cardiol 2002;17:43–51.

157. Shimizu W, Antzelevitch C. Effects of a K$^+$ channel opener to reduce transmural dispersion of repolarization and prevent torsade de pointes in LQT1, LQT2, and LQT3 models of the long-QT syndrome. Circulation 2000;102:706–12.

158. Antzelevitch C. Heterogeneity of cellular repolarization in LQTS: the role of M cells. Eur Heart J Suppl 2001;3:K2–16.

159. Shimizu W, Antzelevitch C. Cellular basis for the ECG features of the LQT1 form of the long QT syndrome: effects of β-adrenergic agonists and antagonists and sodium channel blockers on transmural dispersion of repolarization and torsade de pointes. Circulation 1998;98:2314–22.

160. Shimizu W, Antzelevitch C. Sodium channel block with mexiletine is effective in reducing dispersion of repolarization and preventing torsade de pointes in LQT2 and LQT3 models of the long-QT syndrome. Circulation 1997;96:2038–47.

161. Shimizu W, Antzelevitch C. Differential effects of beta-adrenergic agonists and antagonists in LQT1, LQT2 and LQT3 models of the long QT syndrome. J Am Coll Cardiol 2000;35:778–86.

162. Antzelevitch C, Shimizu W, Yan GX, et al. The M cell: its contribution to the ECG and to normal and abnormal electrical function of the heart. J Cardiovasc Electrophysiol 1999;10:1124–52.

163. Anyukhovsky EP, Sosunov EA, Gainullin RZ, et al. The controversial M cell. J Cardiovasc Electrophysiol 1999;10:244–60.

164. Li GR, Feng J, Yue L, et al. Transmural heterogeneity of action potentials and Ito1 in myocytes isolated from the human right ventricle. Am J Physiol 1998;275:H369–77.

165. Gussak I, Brugada P, Brugada J, et al. Idiopathic short QT interval: a new clinical syndrome? Cardiology 2000;94:99–102.

166. Gussak I, Brugada P, Brugada J, et al. ECG phenomenon of idiopathic and paradoxical short QT intervals. Card Electrophysiol Rev 2002;6:49–53.

167. Patel C, Yan GX, Antzelevitch C. Short QT syndrome: from bench to bedside. Circ Arrhythm Electrophysiol 2010;3:401–8.

168. Gaita F, Giustetto C, Bianchi F, et al. Short QT syndrome: a familial cause of sudden death. Circulation 2003;108:965–70.

169. Bellocq C, Van Ginneken AC, Bezzina CR, et al. Mutation in the KCNQ1 gene leading to the short QT-interval syndrome. Circulation 2004;109:2394–7.

170. Brugada R, Hong K, Dumaine R, et al. Sudden death associated with short-QT syndrome linked to mutations in HERG. Circulation 2004;109: 30–5.

171. Priori SG, Pandit SV, Rivolta I, et al. A novel form of short QT syndrome (SQT3) is caused by a mutation in the KCNJ2 gene. Circ Res 2005;96:800–7.

172. Extramiana F, Antzelevitch C. Amplified transmural dispersion of repolarization as the basis for arrhythmogenesis in a canine ventricular-wedge model of short QT syndrome. Circulation 2004; 110:3661–6.

173. Patel C, Antzelevitch C. Cellular basis for arrhythmogenesis in an experimental model of the SQT1 form of the short QT syndrome. Heart Rhythm 2008;5:585–90.

174. Nof E, Burashnikov A, Antzelevitch C. Cellular basis for atrial fibrillation in an experimental model of short QT1: implications for a pharmacological approach to therapy. Heart Rhythm 2010;7:251–7.

175. Anttonen O, Vaananen H, Junttila J, et al. Electrocardiographic transmural dispersion of repolarization in patients with inherited short QT syndrome. Ann Noninvasive Electrocardiol 2008;13:295–300.

176. Gupta P, Patel C, Patel H, et al. T_{p-e}/QT ratio as an index of arrhythmogenesis. J Electrocardiol 2008; 41:567–74.

177. Anttonen O, Junttila MJ, Maury P, et al. Differences in twelve-lead electrocardiogram between symptomatic and asymptomatic subjects with short QT interval. Heart Rhythm 2009;6:267–71.

178. Milberg P, Tegelkamp R, Osada N, et al. Reduction of dispersion of repolarization and prolongation of postrepolarization refractoriness explain the antiarrhythmic effects of quinidine in a model of short QT syndrome. J Cardiovasc Electrophysiol 2007;18: 658–64.

The J Wave Syndromes and Their Role in Sudden Cardiac Death

Dongqi Wang, MD, PhD[a], Gan-Xin Yan, MD, PhD[a,b],
Charles Antzelevitch, PhD, FHRS[c],*

KEYWORDS

- Sudden cardiac death • Transient outward current
- Early repolarization syndrome • ST segment elevation
- Brugada syndrome

The electrocardiographic J wave, also referred to as the "Osborn wave," is a deflection with a dome or hump morphology at the junction between the QRS complex and the ST segment on the body surface electrocardiogram (ECG). Earlier studies attributed the J wave to a variety of factors including hypoxia, injury current, acidosis, delayed ventricular depolarization, and early ventricular repolarization.[1] Clinical and arrhythmogenic significance of the J wave abnormalities had largely been ignored until 1996 when Yan and Antzelevitch[2] published a study elucidating the ionic and cellular basis of the J wave, indicating that a prominent I_{to}-mediated action potential notch in ventricular epicardium but not endocardium may produce a transmural voltage gradient during early ventricular repolarization that could register as a J wave or J point elevation in the ECG. Growing evidence has since been advanced indicating that J wave abnormalities, which are often accompanied by early repolarization and ST segment elevation on the ECG, are in some cases associated with a risk of sudden cardiac death. The J wave syndromes, which represent a variable spectrum of phenotypic expression with accentuation of the J wave, can be inherited or acquired.[3–6] This article summarizes current knowledge about J wave syndromes, linking bench work with the bedside.

HISTORICAL PERSPECTIVE OF J WAVE AND J WAVE SYNDROMES

Tomaszewski[7] first described J wave as a slowly inscribed deflection between QRS complex and earliest part of ST segment on the ECG in an accidentally frozen man in 1938. Similar descriptions of hypothermic J waves followed in which the J wave was described as a widening secondary deflection of QRS complex. Osborn[8] in 1953 described what he called "current of injury" in hypothermic dogs that later fibrillated. This so-called "current of injury" was in fact a J wave that was later named the Osborn J wave.[9]

Appearance of the J wave or J point elevation is often associated with an early repolarization pattern and ST segment elevation. The early repolarization pattern and ST segment elevation was first reported by evaluating the four-lead ECG of 200 healthy young men and women in 1936 by Shipley and Hallaran. This electrocardiographic phenomenon was ascribed to accelerated ventricular repolarization.[10,11] In subsequent years, several investigators attempted to characterize the clinical importance of early repolarization pattern and failed to find any immediate and long-term consequences.[12,13]

A shift away from a benign view of the J wave began in 1984 when Otto and coworkers[14]

a The First Affiliated Hospital, Medical School of Xi'an Jiaotong University, Xi'an, China
b Lankenau Institute for Medical Research and Main Line Health Heart Center, Wynnewood, PA, USA
c Masonic Medical Research Laboratory, 2150 Bleecker Street, Utica, NY 13501, USA
* Corresponding author.
E-mail address: ca@mmrl.edu

Card Electrophysiol Clin 3 (2011) 47–56
doi:10.1016/j.ccep.2010.10.014

presented three cases of ventricular fibrillation (VF) that occurred during sleep in young male Southeast Asian refugees who had structurally normal hearts. In one of three patients, a prominent J wave with ST segment elevation appeared after termination of VF. More interestingly, inducible VF in this patient was inhibited by quinidine, a drug that inhibits I_{to}, but not procainamide. This indicates that I_{to}-mediated J wave may play a role in the sudden unexpected nocturnal death. Sudden unexpected nocturnal death was reported in the literatures as early as the 1950s to 1960s.[15] In the Philippine capital city Manila, a total of 722 apparently healthy young men died during sleep between 1948 and 1982, a disease called "Bangungut" (to rise and moan during sleep) in their native language.[16] Sudden unexpected nocturnal death is fairly common in Southeast Asian and Pacific Rim countries and its etiology remained a mystery for many decades.[17,18]

In 1992, Pedro and Josep Brugada published a landmark study describing eight similar patients with sudden cardiac death in whom the ECG revealed "right bundle branch block" and ST segment elevation limited to the precordial leads V1 to V3 in the absence of ischemic or other structural disease.[19] In 1994, Bjerregaard and colleagues[20] reported that a 47-year-old African American woman presented with recurrent syncope and a similar ECG pattern to that reported by the Brugada brothers. In this report, Bjerregaard and colleagues[20] suggested that the so-called "right bundle branch block" described by the Brugada brothers in 1992 was in fact a prominent J wave. This was the first report in which the contribution of J wave to VF was discussed. This entity was later named "Brugada syndrome."[2,21]

In 2000 Gussak and Antzelevitch[22] suggested that in some cases ER may be malignant, based on observations that an ER pattern in arterially perfused wedge preparations can easily convert to one in which phase 2 reentry gives rise to polymorphic ventricular tachycardia (VT) and VF. Evidence in support of this hypothesis was provided by Kalla and colleagues[23] and Takagi and colleagues[24] in 2000. Kalla and colleagues[23] reported a case of idiopathic VF in a 29-year-old Vietnamese man whose ECG showed prominent J wave with ST segment elevation in the inferior ECG leads and first postulated that it may represent a variant of the Brugada syndrome. Shortly thereafter, Takagi and colleagues[24] provided additional evidence in support of this hypothesis. In 2004, Qi and colleagues[25] reported that a young Chinese man with structurally normal heart survived from recurrent VF and his ECG exhibited prominent J waves, early repolarization, and ST segment elevation in all of 12 ECG leads. This interesting case triggered a debate in China whether "J wave syndromes" should be used to cover all clinical entities derived from accentuated J waves.[3] Additional supporting evidence was provided by two reports in the New England Journal of Medicine in 2008. Both Haissaguerre and coworkers[26] and Nam and coworkers[27] demonstrated a clear association between J waves with early repolarization pattern and VF.

In 2010, Antzelevitch and Yan[6] further defined J wave syndromes and divided them into four subtypes based on their ECG features and relative risk potentials of sudden cardiac death (**Table 1**).

IONIC AND CELLULAR BASIS OF J WAVE AND ITS ARRHYTHMOGENESIS

The fact that the J wave immediately follows the completion of ventricular activation (QRS complex) indicates the presence of a transient transmural voltage gradient during early ventricular repolarization. In the late 1980s, Antzelevitch and colleagues first proposed that a difference in repolarization phases 1 and 2 of the action potential between canine ventricular epicardium and endocardium form the basis for the ECG J wave.[28,29] Ventricular epicardium commonly displays action potentials with a prominent notch (spike and dome) largely mediated by a 4-aminopyridine–sensitive transient outward current (I_{to}). The absence of a prominent notch in the endocardium is the consequence of a much smaller I_{to}. A prominent I_{to}-mediated action potential notch in ventricular epicardium but not endocardium produces a transmural voltage gradient during early ventricular repolarization that registers as a J wave or J point elevation in the ECG. Direct evidence in support of this hypothesis was obtained in the arterially perfused canine ventricular wedge preparation.[2] The data obtained from the wedge preparation have demonstrated a linear correlation between the J wave size and I_{to}-mediated action potential notch in epicardium (**Fig. 1**). Factors that influence I_{to} kinetics and ventricular activation sequence can modify the J wave on the ECG. With a normal ventricular activation sequence from endocardium to epicardium, an acceleration of heart rate reduces I_{to} because of its slow recovery from inactivation, resulting in a decrease in the J wave size.[23,30] This property of the J wave is particularly useful in distinguishing the J wave from the terminal part of a notched QRS complex. Because a notched QRS is the consequence of altered ventricular activation, an increase in heart rate generally exaggerates its manifestation. Similarly, sodium channel blockers like quinidine, which inhibit I_{to}, act to reduce the size of the

Table 1
J wave syndromes: similarities and differences

	Inherited				Acquired	
	Early Repolarization in Lateral Leads (ERS Type 1)	Early Repolarization in Inferior or Inferolateral Leads (ERS Type 2)	Global Early Repolarization (ERS Type 3)	Brugada Syndrome	Ischemia-mediated	Hypothermia-mediated
Anatomic location responsible for chief EP manifestation	Anterolateral left ventricle	Inferior left ventricle	Left and right ventricles	Right ventricle	Left and right ventricles	Left and right ventricles
Leads displaying J point/J wave abnormalities	I, V4–V6	II, III, aVF	Global	V1–V3	Any of 12 leads	Any of the 12 leads
Response of J wave amplitude/ST elevation to: bradycardia Na+ channel blockers	Increase Limited data	Increase Limited data	Increase Limited data	Increase Increase	N/A N/A	N/A N/A
Gender dominance	Male	Male	Male	Male	Male	Either gender
VF	Rare	Yes	Yes, VF storms	Yes	Yes	Yes
Response to quinidine	Normalization of J point elevation and inhibition of VT/VF	Normalization of J point elevation and inhibition of VT/VF	Limited data; normalization of J point elevation and inhibition of VT/VF	Normalization of J point elevation and inhibition of VT/VF	Limited data	Inhibition of VT/VF
Response to isoproterenol	Normalization of J point elevation and inhibition of VT/VF	Normalization of J point elevation and inhibition of VT/VF	Limited data	Normalization of J point elevation and inhibition of VT/VF	N/A	N/A
Gene mutations	CACNA1C, CACNB2B	KCNJ8, CACNA1C, CACNB2B	CACNA1C	SCN5A, CACNA1C, CACNB2B, GPD1-L, SCN1B, KCNE3, SCN3B, KCNJ8	SCN5A	N/A

Abbreviations: EP, electrophysiology; ERS, early repolarization syndrome; N/A, not available; VF, ventricular fibrillation; VT, ventricular tachycardia.
Reprinted from Antzelevitch C, Yan GX. J wave syndromes. Heart Rhythm 2010;7:549–58; with permission.

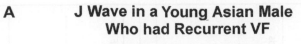

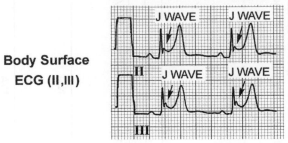

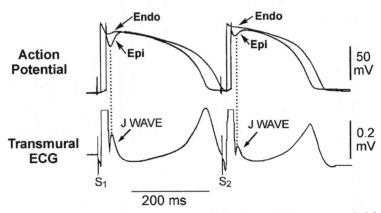

Fig. 1. Cellular basis for the J wave. (*A*) Prominent J waves in leads II and III were recorded from a young Asian man who had recurrent VF. (*B*) Simultaneous recording of transmembrane action potentials from epicardial (Epi) and endocardial (Endo) regions and a transmural ECG in a coronary-perfused canine ventricular wedge preparation. An I_{to}-mediated action potential notch in the epicardium but not endocardium is associated with a J wave. A premature stimulus (S_1-S_2 = 300 ms) caused a parallel decrease in the amplitude of the epicardial action potential notch and of the J wave. (*Modified from* Yan GX, Antzelevitch C. Cellular basis for the electrocardiographic J wave. Circulation 1996;93:372–9; with permission.)

J wave[31,32] but do not reduce the magnitude of QRS notching. The prominent J wave induced by hypothermia is the result of a marked accentuation of the spike and dome morphology of epicardial action potentials probably caused by the effect of cold temperatures to slow the activation kinetic of I_{to} less than that of the L-type Ca^{2+} current.[2]

The I_{to}-mediated epicardial action potential notch including spike and dome is sensitive to changes in net repolarizing current. An increase in net repolarizing current, caused by either a decrease of inward current or augmentation of outward current, accentuates the notch leading to augmentation of the J wave. A further increase in net repolarizing current can further enhance the epicardial action potential notch, so that $I_{Ca,L}$ activation is influenced, resulting in partial or complete loss of the action potential dome at phase 2 that can manifest as early repolarization and ST segment elevation on the ECG.[30,31,33]

Depending on the extent of epicardial action potential phase 2 depression (partial vs complete loss of the dome), the ST segment may behave differently. Partial loss of the epicardial action potential dome manifests as early repolarization with or without ST segment elevation. ST segment elevation caused by partial loss of the epicardial action potential is concave upward or saddle-back-like.[30,34] Complete loss of the epicardial action potential dome in response to an increase in outward current (eg, I_{to} or I_{K-ATP}) or a decrease in inward current (eg, I_{Na} or I_{Ca}), particularly in the right ventricle where the I_{to}-mediated phase 1 is prominent, results in coved ST segment elevation as often seen in the Brugada syndrome (**Fig. 2**).[31,33]

Loss of the dome is usually heterogeneous, occurring at some sites but not others, leading to a marked dispersion of repolarization on the epicardial surface (**Fig. 3**). The epicardial action potential

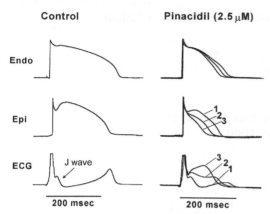

Control   **Pinacidil (2.5 μM)**

Endo

Epi   1
                                       2
                                       3

ECG   J wave   3 2
                                     1

200 msec   200 msec

Fig. 2. Pinacidil, a K_{ATP} channel opener, causes loss of action potential plateau in the canine right ventricular epicardium. Dynamic change in the epicardial action potential plateau is associated with different types of ST segment elevation. Epi, epicardial; Endo, endocardial. (*Modified from* Yan GX, Antzelevitch C. Cellular basis for the Brugada syndrome and other mechanisms of arrhythmogenesis associated with ST segment elevation. Circulation 1999;100:1660–6; with permission.)

dome[35] may then propagate from epicardial sites where it is maintained to sites at which it was lost, thus producing local re-excitation, termed "phase 2 reentry." The closely coupled extrasystole produced by phase 2 reentry always occurs on the descending limb of T wave producing an R-on-T phenomenon, which can initiate polymorphic VT or VF (see **Fig. 3**).

SUBTYPES OF J WAVE SYNDROMES AND THEIR CLINICAL FEATURES

Inherited J wave syndromes can be divided into four subtypes based on their ECG features and relative risk for contributing to sudden cardiac death. Gene mutations have been identified in all four subtypes (see **Table 1**).[6]

Type 1 is a distinct J wave or J point elevation accompanied by early repolarization pattern with or without concave upward ST segment elevation that is limited to the left precordial leads V4 to V6. This pattern has previously been referred to as "early repolarization syndrome," and generally considered to be a benign ECG phenomenon seen in healthy individuals, particularly athletes. Its prevalence is estimated at 5.8% in adults.[36] Type 1 ER pattern is rarely associated with VT-VF and sudden cardiac death.

Type 2 is a prominent J wave or J point elevation with an ER pattern occurring predominantly in inferior leads II, III, and aVF. The prevalence of type 2 is estimated to be 3.5% in adults,[36] but it is probably more prevalent in Asian men. There is mounting evidence that type 2 is associated with moderate risk for sudden cardiac death.[14,23,24,26,27]

Type 3 is rare and its true prevalence is unknown. This type of ECG is characterized by global J waves or J point elevation with marked ST segment elevation, particularly in the period immediately preceding the development of VT-VF (**Fig. 4**). Patients with type 3 often present with recurrent VF, often characterized as electrical storms.[25,27]

Type 4 is the Brugada syndrome in which prominent J waves and ST segment elevation are limited to the right precordial leads V1 to V3. The initial publication in 1992 by Pedro and Josep Brugada described eight similar patients with sudden cardiac death.[19] Because the ECG pattern of the Brugada syndrome can be dynamic and is often concealed, it is difficult to estimate the true prevalence of the disease in the general population. In two Asian studies, Brugada type ECG (coved ST segment elevation) was observed in 12 of 10,000 inhabitants; types 2 and 3 ST segment elevation, which are not diagnostic of Brugada syndrome, were much more prevalent, appearing in 58 of 10,000 inhabitants.[37,38]

The common clinical features of the J wave syndromes include (1) modulation of J wave and associated ST segment elevation by heart rate and autonomic tone, tachycardia or increased sympathetic tone lead to reduction in the magnitude of the J wave and normalization of the ST segment, whereas bradycardia or increases vagal tone augment the magnitude of the J wave and cause ST segment elevation[21,23]; (2) J wave syndromes predominate in men; and (3) arrhythmic events are more likely to occur between the ages of 20 and 40 with a median age in the mid-30s.[16–18,39]

Among the J wave syndromes, Brugada syndrome has been the most widely studied. Consensus reports published in 2002 and 2005 delineated diagnostic criteria, risk stratification schemes, and approaches to therapy.[40,41] The Brugada syndrome is definitively diagnosed when a spontaneous or drug-induced type 1 or coved ST segment elevation is observed in more than one right precordial lead (V1–V3) in conjunction with one of the following: documented VF, polymorphic VT, a family history of sudden cardiac death at less than 45 years old, coved-type ECGs in family members, inducibility of VT with programmed electrical stimulation, syncope, or nocturnal agonal respiration.[41] Diagnosis of the Brugada syndrome is also established when a type 2 or 3 ST-segment elevation in more than one right precordial leads under baseline conditions is converted to the diagnostic type 1 pattern on exposure to a sodium channel blocker (ST-segment elevation should be ≥2 mm). One or more of the clinical criteria described previously should also be present.

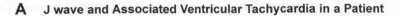

A J wave and Associated Ventricular Tachycardia in a Patient

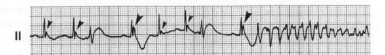

B Phase 2 Reentry and Ventricualr Tachycardia in a Canine
Ventricular Preparation

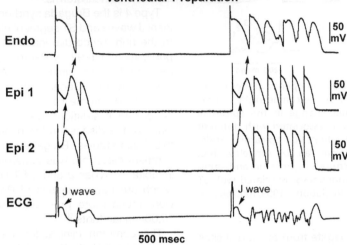

Fig. 3. The mechanism responsible for J wave–related arrhythmogenesis. (*A*) Development of VF in a patient with the prominent J waves in lead II. (*From* Aizawa Y, Tamura M, Chinushi M, et al. Idiopathic ventricular fibrillation and bradycardia-dependent intraventricular block. Am Heart J 1993;126:1473–4; with permission.) (*B*) VF initiated by phase 2 reentry in a canine right ventricular wedge in the presence of 2.5 μmol/L of pinacidil. Action potentials were simultaneously recorded from two epicardial sites (Epi$_1$ and Epi$_2$) and one Endo site. Loss of the AP dome in Epi$_1$ but not in Epi$_2$ led to phase 2 reentry capable of initiating VF. Epi, epicardial; Endo, endocardial. (*Modified from* Yan GX, Lankipalli RS, Burke JF, et al. Ventricular repolarization components on the electrocardiogram: cellular basis and clinical significance. J Am Coll Cardiol 2003;42:401–9; with permission.)

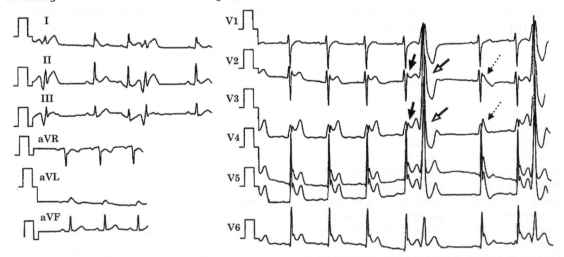

Fig. 4. ECG obtained from a 34-year-old Chinese man with a structurally normal heart who survived cardiac arrest displaying characteristics of the type 3 early repolarization syndrome. Prominent J waves and ST segment elevation were observed in almost all ECG leads, including an early repolarization pattern in leads of I, II, aVL, aVF, and V4 to V6 and a saddleback ST segment elevation suggestive of Brugada in V$_2$ to V$_3$ (*thick arrows*). R-on-T extrasystoles, likely caused by phase 2 reentry (*open arrows*), were seen and the postextrasystolic beat displayed a coved ST segment elevation characteristic of Brugada type 1 wave (*thin arrows*). (*Reprinted from* Qi X, Sun F, An X, et al. A case of Brugada syndrome with ST segment elevation through entire precordial leads. Chin J Cardiol 2004;32:272–3; with permission.)

Implantable cardioverter defibrillator (ICD) implantation is the only proved effective treatment for the Brugada syndrome. Survivors of cardiac arrest with Brugada syndrome and other types of J wave syndromes are at a high risk for recurrence and should be protected by an ICD.

Other treatment options involve the use of pharmacologic agents, including I_{to} blockers, such as quinidine.[42–44] Antiarrhythmic agents, such as amiodarone and β-blockers, have been shown to be ineffective. The presence of a prominent I_{to} is critical to the mechanism underlying the Brugada syndrome. Consequently, the most prudent approach to therapy, regardless of the ionic or genetic basis for the disease,

is to inhibit I_{to}. Cardioselective and I_{to}-specific blockers are currently not available. An agent currently on the market in the United States and other regions of the world with significant I_{to} blocking properties is quinidine, and this agent was proposed for the treatment of BrS in 1999.[42] Belhassen and Viskin[43] reported on the efficacy of quinidine in a prospective study of 25 patients. After a follow-up period of 6 months to 22.2 years, of 19 patients treated with oral quinidine for 6 to 219 months (56 ± 67 months) none developed arrhythmic events. The effectiveness of quinidine has been demonstrated in a number of studies[45] (for references), the most recent of which involves its use in children with Brugada syndrome.[46]

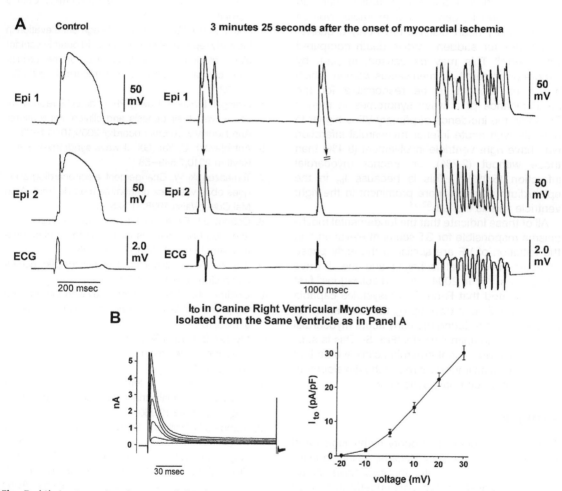

Fig. 5. (A) Acute regional myocardial ischemia resulting in complete loss of the action potential dome at Epi_2 within the ischemic zone but not at Epi_1 by perfused side of the ischemic border, leading to propagation of the dome at Epi_1 to Epi_2 (phase 2 reentry). Phase 2 reentry and probably its transmural propagation manifested as a closely coupled R-on-T extrasystole on the ECG that was able to initiate VF. BCL = 2000 ms. (B) I_{to} traces recorded at step voltages from −20 to +30 mV in canine right ventricular epicardial myocytes isolated from the same ventricle from which the ventricular wedge in A was isolated. I-V relationships (*right*): averaged I_{to} density (30.3 pA/pF) was normalized by cell membrane capacitance in four myocytes. (*Reprinted from* Yan GX, Yao QH, Wang DQ, et al. Electrocardiographic J wave and J wave syndromes. Chin J Cardiac Arrhyth 2004;8:360–5; with permission.)

Oral quinidine therapy is also a reasonable "bridge therapy" or adjunct to ICD therapy.[47] A prospective registry for asymptomatic patients with Brugada has been created with the aim of tracking the effectiveness of empiric therapy with quinidine.[48] There is a clear need for development of a more cardioselective and I_{to}-specific blocker.

ST SEGMENT ELEVATION AND PHASE 2 REENTRY IN ACUTE MYOCARDIAL ISCHEMIA

Whether I_{to}-mediated phase 2 reentry plays an important role in initiating VF during early acute myocardial ischemia is not clear, but clinical observations suggest some association of risk of primary VF during acute myocardial infarction with increased I_{to} density. For example, women with coronary heart disease have only a quarter of the risk for sudden cardiac death compared with men.[49] This may be caused, in part, by a more prominent I_{to} in men versus women, which has been thought to be responsible for the predominance of J wave syndromes in men.[50] Similarly, the incidence of primary VF is higher in patients with acute inferior myocardial infarction who have right ventricle involvement (8.4%) than those without (2.7%), or anterior myocardial infarction (5.0%).[51] This is because I_{to} in the epicardium is much more prominent in the right ventricle versus the left.[52,53]

All of these indicate that the fundamental mechanisms responsible for ST segment elevation and the initiation of VF are similar in the early phase of acute myocardial ischemia and the J wave syndromes.[31,34] In 2004, Yan and colleagues[3] first demonstrated that R-on-T extrasystoles capable of initiating VF can develop by the mechanism of phase 2 reentry during the early acute myocardial ischemia in an animal model (**Fig. 5**). This is supported by more recent emerging clinical data that J wave plays an important role in the development of VF in acute coronary syndrome.[54–56]

SUMMARY

Advances in modern laboratory technologies and techniques over the past decade, including electrophysiologic and genetic analyses, have uncovered many novel mechanisms underlying sudden cardiac death, the J wave being one example. J wave syndromes include a spectrum of disorders that involve accentuation of the I_{to}-mediated epicardial action potential notch in different regions of the heart, leading to the development of prominent J waves, early repolarization, and ST segment elevation on the ECG. Phase 2 reentry has been identified as the trigger in the J wave syndromes,

and enhanced dispersion of repolarization as the substrate, giving rise to polymorphic VT and VF and sudden death.

REFERENCES

1. Gussak I, Bjerregaard P, Egan TM, et al. ECG phenomenon called the J wave. History, pathophysiology, and clinical significance. J Electrocardiol 1995;28:49–58.
2. Yan GX, Antzelevitch C. Cellular basis for the electrocardiographic J wave. Circulation 1996;93:372–9.
3. Yan GX, Yao QH, Wang DQ, et al. Electrocardiographic J wave and J wave syndromes. Chin J Cardiac Arrhyth 2004;8:360–5.
4. Shu J, Zhu T, Yang L, et al. ST-segment elevation in the early repolarization syndrome, idiopathic ventricular fibrillation, and the Brugada syndrome: cellular and clinical linkage. J Electrocardiol 2005;38:26–32.
5. Hlaing T, Dimino T, Kowey PR, et al. ECG repolarization waves: their genesis and clinical implications. Ann Noninvasive Electrocardiol 2005;10:211–23.
6. Antzelevitch C, Yan GX. J wave syndromes. Heart Rhythm 2010;7:549–58.
7. Tomaszewski W. Changement electrocardiographiques observes chez un homme mort de froid. Arch Mal Coeur Vaiss 1938;31:525–8.
8. Osborn JJ. Experimental hypothermia: respiratory and blood pH changes in relation to cardiac function. Am J Physiol 1953;175:389–98.
9. Abbott JA, Cheitlin MD. The nonspecific camelhump sign. JAMA 1976;235:413–4.
10. Goldman MJ. RS-T segment elevation in mid- and left precordial leads as a normal variant. Am Heart J 1953;46:817–20.
11. Myers GB, Koein HA, Stofer BE, et al. Normal variations in multiple precordial leads. Am Heart J 1947;34:785–808.
12. Fenichel NN. A long term study of concave RS-T elevation: a normal variant of the electrocardiogram. Angiology 1962;13:360–6.
13. Kambara H, Phillips J. Long-term evaluation of early repolarization syndrome (normal variant RS-T segment elevation). Am J Cardiol 1976;38:157–61.
14. Otto CM, Tauxe RV, Cobb LA, et al. Ventricular fibrillation causes sudden death in Southeast Asian immigrants. Ann Intern Med 1984;101:45–7.
15. Aponte GE. The enigma of "bangungut." Ann Intern Med 1960;52:1258–63.
16. Munger RG, Booton EA. Bangungut in Manila: sudden and unexplained death in sleep of adult Filipinos. Int J Epidemiol 1998;27:677–84.
17. Centers for Disease Control (CDC). Sudden, unexpected, nocturnal deaths among Southeast Asian

refugees. MMWR Morb Mortal Wkly Rep 1981;30: 581–4.

18. Parrish RG, Tucker M, Ing R, et al. Sudden unexplained death syndrome in Southeast Asian refugees: a review of CDC surveillance. MMWR CDC Surveill Summ 1987;36:43SS–53SS.

19. Brugada P, Brugada J. Right bundle branch block, persistent ST segment elevation and sudden cardiac death: a distinct clinical and electrocardiographic syndrome: a multicenter report. J Am Coll Cardiol 1992;20:1391–6.

20. Bjerregaard P, Gussak I, Kotar SL, et al. Recurrent synocope in a patient with prominent J-wave. Am Heart J 1994;127:1426–30.

21. Miyazaki T, Mitamura H, Miyoshi S, et al. Autonomic and antiarrhythmic drug modulation of ST segment elevation in patients with Brugada syndrome. J Am Coll Cardiol 1996;27:1061–70.

22. Gussak I, Antzelevitch C. Early repolarization syndrome: clinical characteristics and possible cellular and ionic mechanisms. J Electrocardiol 2000;33:299–309.

23. Kalla H, Yan GX, Marinchak R. Ventricular fibrillation in a patient with prominent J (Osborn) waves and ST segment elevation in the inferior electrocardiographic leads: a Brugada syndrome variant? J Cardiovasc Electrophysiol 2000;11:95–8.

24. Takagi M, Aihara N, Takaki H, et al. Clinical characteristics of patients with spontaneous or inducible ventricular fibrillation without apparent heart disease presenting with J wave and ST segment elevation in inferior leads. J Cardiovasc Electrophysiol 2000;11: 844–8.

25. Qi X, Sun F, An X, et al. A case of Brugada syndrome with ST segment elevation through entire precordial leads. Chin J Cardiol 2004;32:272–3.

26. Haissaguerre M, Derval N, Sacher F, et al. Sudden cardiac arrest associated with early repolarization. N Engl J Med 2008;358:2016–23.

27. Nam GB, Kim YH, Antzelevitch C. Augmentation of J waves and electrical storms in patients with early repolarization. N Engl J Med 2008;358:2078–9.

28. Litovsky SH, Antzelevitch C. Transient outward current prominent in canine ventricular epicardium but not endocardium. Circ Res 1988;62:116–26.

29. Antzelevitch C, Sicouri S, Litovsky SH, et al. Heterogeneity within the ventricular wall. Electrophysiology and pharmacology of epicardial, endocardial, and M cells. Circ Res 1991;69:1427–49.

30. Yan GX, Lankipalli RS, Burke JF, et al. Ventricular repolarization components on the electrocardiogram: cellular basis and clinical significance. J Am Coll Cardiol 2003;42:401–9.

31. Yan GX, Antzelevitch C. Cellular basis for the Brugada syndrome and other mechanisms of arrhythmogenesis associated with ST segment elevation. Circulation 1999;100:1660–6.

32. Gussak I, Antzelevitch C, Bjerregaard P, et al. The Brugada syndrome: clinical, electrophysiologic and genetic aspects. J Am Coll Cardiol 1999;33:5–15.

33. Antzelevitch C, Yan GX. Cellular and ionic mechanisms responsible for the Brugada syndrome. J Electrocardiol 2000;33(Suppl):33–9.

34. Yan GX, Kowey PR. ST segment elevation and sudden cardiac death: from the Brugada syndrome to acute myocardial ischemia. J Cardiovasc Electrophysiol 2000;11:1330–2.

35. Yan GX, Wu Y, Liu T, et al. Phase 2 early after depolarization as a trigger of polymorphic ventricular tachycardia in acquired long-qt syndrome: direct evidence from intracellular recordings in the intact left ventricular wall. Circulation 2001;103:2851–6.

36. Tikkanen JT, Anttonen O, Junttila MJ, et al. Longterm outcome associated with early repolarization on electrocardiography. N Engl J Med 2009;361: 2529–37.

37. Nademanee K. Sudden unexplained death syndrome in southeast Asia. Am J Cardiol 1997;79(6A):10–1.

38. Miyasaka Y, Tsuji H, Yamada K, et al. Prevalence and mortality of the Brugada-type electrocardiogram in one city in Japan. J Am Coll Cardiol 2001; 38:771–4.

39. Antzelevitch C, Brugada P, Brugada J, et al. Brugada syndrome: 1992–2002. A historical perspective. J Am Coll Cardiol 2003;41:1665–71.

40. Wilde AA, Antzelevitch C, Borggrefe M, et al. Proposed diagnostic criteria for the Brugada syndrome: consensus report. Circulation 2002;106:2514–9.

41. Antzelevitch C, Brugada P, Borggrefe M, et al. Brugada syndrome: report of the second consensus conference: endorsed by the Heart Rhythm Society and the European Heart Rhythm Association. Circulation 2005;111:659–70.

42. Antzelevitch C, Brugada P, Brugada J, et al. Clinical approaches to tachyarrhythmias. The Brugada syndrome. Armonk (NY): Futura Publishing Company; 1999.

43. Belhassen B, Viskin S. Pharmacologic approach to therapy of Brugada syndrome: quinidine as an alternative to ICD therapy? In: Antzelevitch C, Brugada P, Brugada J, et al, editors. The Brugada syndrome: from bench to bedside. Oxford (UK): Blackwell Futura; 2004. p. 202–11.

44. Ohgo T, Okamura H, Noda T, et al. Acute and chronic management in patients with Brugada syndrome associated with electrical storm of ventricular fibrillation. Heart Rhythm 2007;4: 695–700.

45. Antzelevitch C, Brugada P, Brugada J, et al. The Brugada syndrome: from bench to bedside. Oxford (UK): Blackwell Futura; 2005.

46. Probst V, Denjoy I, Meregalli PG, et al. Clinical aspects and prognosis of Brugada syndrome in children. Circulation 2007;115:2042–8.

47. Viskin S. Brugada syndrome in children: don't ask, don't tell? Circulation 2007;115:1970–2.
48. Viskin S, Wilde AA, Tan HL, et al. Empiric quinidine therapy for asymptomatic Brugada syndrome: time for a prospective registry. Heart Rhythm 2009;6:401–4.
49. Kannel WB, Wilson PW, D'Agostino RB, et al. Sudden coronary death in women. Am Heart J 1998;136:205–12.
50. Di Diego JM, Cordeiro JM, Goodrow RJ, et al. Ionic and cellular basis for the predominance of the Brugada syndrome phenotype in males. Circulation 2002;106:2004–11.
51. Mehta SR, Eikelboom JW, Natarajan MK, et al. Impact of right ventricular involvement on mortality and morbidity in patients with inferior myocardial infarction. J Am Coll Cardiol 2001;37:37–43.
52. Di Diego JM, Sun ZQ, Antzelevitch C. I_{to} and action potential notch are smaller in left vs. right canine ventricular epicardium. Am J Physiol 1996;271: H548–61.
53. Volders PG, Sipido KR, Carmeliet E, et al. Repolarizing K+ currents ITO1 and IKs are larger in right than left canine ventricular midmyocardium. Circulation 1999;99:206–10.
54. Shinde R, Shinde S, Makhale C, et al. Occurrence of "J waves" in 12-lead ECG as a marker of acute ischemia and their cellular basis. Pacing Clin Electrophysiol 2007;30:817–9.
55. Jastrzebski M, Kukla P. Ischemic J wave: novel risk marker for ventricular fibrillation? Heart Rhythm 2009;6:829–35.
56. Inoue M, Matsubara T, Yasuda T, et al. Transition of the ST segment from a J wave to a coved-type elevation before ventricular fibrillation induced by coronary vasospasm in the precordial leads. J Electrocardiol 2010;43:418–21.

Mechanisms Underlying Arrhythmogenesis Associated with Heart Failure

David N. Edwards, MD, PhD[a], Andreas S. Barth, MD[b],
Gordon F. Tomaselli, MD[c],*

KEYWORDS

- Ion channels • Action potential • Gene expression
- Heart failure • Remodeling • CRT

Over 5 million Americans suffer from heart failure (HF) and more than 250,000 die annually. The incidence and prevalence has continued to increase with the aging of the United States population, with approximately 600,000 new diagnoses made annually, at a cost of nearly 30 billion dollars annually. Despite remarkable improvements in medical therapy, the prognosis of patients with myocardial failure remains poor with almost 20% of patients dying within 1 year of initial diagnosis and greater than 80% 8-year mortality. Of the deaths in patients with HF, up to 50% are sudden and unexpected; indeed, patients with HF have 6 to 9 times the rate of sudden cardiac death (SCD) of the general population.[1]

Clinically, HF is a systemic syndrome resulting from impaired function of the myocardium, with symptoms arising from inadequate organ perfusion and vascular congestion. Neurohumoral activation is a prominent compensatory mechanism for inadequate myocardial performance that is ultimately maladaptive in its impact on cellular function and structure of the heart. Appropriately, research has focused on HF involving primarily the left side of the heart. Left ventricular (LV) cardiomyopathies can be generally categorized into defects of ventricular filling or a failure of contraction. Restrictive and hypertrophic cardiomyopathies (HCMs) fall into the category of impairment of filling, whereas ischemic and dilated cardiomyopathies primarily result in a failure of contraction. Each of these forms of cardiomyopathy is associated with an increased risk of sudden cardiac death.

Understanding the features of the failing heart that increase the risk of SCD is an unfulfilled goal. In the setting of HCM risk factors include the thickness of the myocardium and age, supporting thought that myocardial disarray and scarring contributes to arrhythmia. Myocardial scarring is also involved in the reentrant arrhythmias associated with ischemic cardiomyopathy. As discussed in the article by Antzelevitch and Burashnikov on basic mechanisms of arrhythmia elsewhere in this issue, macroscopic reentry is a mechanism for arrhythmia that may play a role in multiple forms of HF associated with fibrosis and scarring.

Reentry in scarred myocardium is one of several mechanisms contributing to potentially lethal arrhythmias in HF. Anatomic and functional remodeling of cardiac tissues is a prominent feature in both animal models and human HF. This remodeling involves and alters cardiac

This work was supported by NIH P01 HL077180, R01 HL072488, R33 HL087345 and RC1HL099892 to G.F.T., and NIH T32 HL007227 to A.S.B and D.N.E.
The authors have nothing to disclose.
[a] Division of Cardiology, The Johns Hopkins University, Baltimore, MD, USA
[b] Department of Medicine, The Johns Hopkins Bayview Hospital, Baltimore, MD, USA
[c] The Johns Hopkins University, Baltimore, MD 21205, USA
* Corresponding author.
E-mail address: gtomasel@jhmi.edu

electrophysiology at the tissue and cellular level. Indeed, abnormalities of both atrial and ventricular electrophysiology in the diseased human heart have been recognized for over four decades.[1,2] In this article, we focus on the electrophysiological remodeling of the failing ventricle.

THE CARDIAC ACTION POTENTIAL

Compared with other excitable tissues such as skeletal muscle cells and neurons, a characteristic feature of cardiomyocytes is a long action potential (AP). In the ventricle, the duration of the AP is reflected in the electrocardiographic QT interval. The AP profile and duration vary regionally in the heart and reflect a delicate balance between the activity of depolarizing and repolarizing ionic currents, electrogenic transporters, and exchangers (**Fig. 1**). Depolarizing currents, the inward movement of sodium (Na^+) and calcium (Ca^{2+}), are responsible for the rapid AP upstroke (phase 0) and maintenance of the plateau (phase 2). Repolarizing currents, primarily the outward movement of potassium (K^+), in concert with a reduction in the depolarizing currents are responsible for restoration of the negative resting membrane potential. The transporters and channels responsible for carrying the currents that make up the AP are not uniformly expressed in the ventricular wall; the AP duration and profile

therefore differs across the myocardium in the normal heart.

Prolongation of the Ventricular AP and Cellular Mechanisms of Arrhythmias in HF

The hallmark of cells and tissues isolated from failing hearts independent of the cause is AP prolongation.[3–9] The AP prolongation in the failing heart is not uniform across the ventricular wall, resulting in an exaggeration of the usual physiologic heterogeneity of repolarization.[4,10] For example, in the failing heart with dyssynchronous contraction (see later discussion), the APs of myocytes isolated from the lateral wall of the left ventricle are particularly prolonged.

Downregulation of repolarizing K^+ currents

Downregulation of repolarizing K^+ currents are the most consistent ionic current changes in animal models and human HF.[9,11] K^+ current downregulation may promote arrhythmias either by direct prolongation of AP, predisposing to the development of early afterdepolarizations (EADs), or by heterogeneously reducing repolarization reserve and promoting functional reentry. The detailed changes in currents and channels vary with the model of HF; however, the consistent effect is the generation of heterogeneous prolongation of the AP.

Ionic Basis for Normal and Altered Ventricular AP in Heart Failure

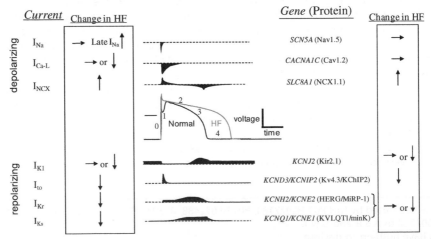

Fig. 1. Inward and outward ionic currents, pumps, and exchangers, which inscribe the mammalian ventricular action potential. The major currents involved in generating the ventricular AP are listed (*left*). A time course of each current is shown (*center*), and the gene product that underlies the current is indicated (*right*). The normal ventricular AP is traced in black at the center of the figure, aligned with the time course of the contributing currents. The AP phases are labeled 0 through 4. The prolonged AP of a failing ventricle is superimposed for comparison, traced in gray. Within the boxes, arrows indicate the relative change in current (*left*) or gene product (*right*) in the setting of HF compared with normal control ventricle.

Transient outward K⁺ current

Although expression of cardiac K^+ channels varies in different species, transient outward potassium current (I_{to}) downregulation is the most consistent ionic current change in failing hearts.[3,5,6,8,12] I_{to} activates shortly following the onset of the AP and is responsible for phase 1 repolarization (see **Fig. 1**) Since I_{to} is an early and transient current, it may have less affect on the longer ventricular action potentials in large mammalian hearts than in rodent ventricles.[13,14]

Interestingly, downregulation of I_{to} in cells isolated from terminally failing human hearts is not associated with a change in its voltage dependence or kinetics.[3] The molecular mechanism of I_{to} downregulation in HF is likely to be multifactorial. I_{to} is tightly regulated by neurohumoral and metabolic factors, which are significantly altered in HF.[15,16] Kv4.3 is the gene that encodes the α subunit responsible for cardiac I_{to} in large mammals.[5] Other accessory subunits may also participate in the formation of native I_{to} channels. For example, Kv4 subunits may form heteromeric complexes with a class of Kv-channel interacting proteins (KChIPs).[17] Reduced steady-state levels of Kv4 mRNA are highly correlated with functional downregulation of I_{to} in human HF.[6,12,18–20] In a canine model, tachycardia downregulates I_{to} expression, with the Ca^{2+}/calmodulin-dependent protein kinase II (CaMKII) and calcineurin/nuclear factor of activated T-cells (NFAT) systems playing roles in rate-dependent I_{to} control.[21,22]

Inward rectifier K⁺ current

The inward rectifier K^+ current (I_{K1}) is encoded by the Kir2 family of genes. I_{K1} maintains the resting membrane potential and contributes to terminal repolarization (phase 3). Reduced inward I_{K1} density in HF[5,23] may contribute to prolongation of AP duration and enhanced susceptibility to spontaneous membrane depolarizations, including delayed afterdepolarizations (DADs).[23,24] Reported changes in I_{K1} functional expression among types of human HF or even within similar experimental HF models are more variable than I_{to}.

In terminal human HF, I_{K1} is significantly reduced at negative voltages,[3] though a differential reduction in I_{K1} was noted between cells isolated from human failing hearts with dilated versus ischemic cardiomyopathy.[25] Within the same animal model of HF induction (eg, pacing-tachycardia), inconsistencies have been observed across species: reduced I_{K1} density in canine[5,10] but no change in rabbit.[23,26] The specific subunits that underlie I_{K1} also vary as a function of species and cardiac chamber. The underlying molecular basis and role of I_{K1} downregulation in HF remains controversial in the absence of consistent changes in the expression of the Kir2 family of genes.

Delayed rectifier K⁺ currents

The delayed rectifier K^+ currents (I_K) play a prominent role in the late phase of repolarization,[27] therefore changes in either the slow (I_{Ks}) or fast (I_{Kr}) activating components of this current could contribute significantly to AP prolongation in HF. Reduced I_K density, slower activation, and faster deactivation kinetics have been observed in hypertrophied feline ventricles.[28] Downregulation of both I_{Kr} and I_{Ks} have been reported in a rabbit model of rapid ventricular pacing HF,[8] whereas I_{Ks} but not I_{Kr} was downregulated in all layers of the LV myocardium in a canine model of tachy-pacing induced HF.[10] Recent measurements of mRNA levels of the genes encoding the α subunits for the rapidly (ERG, Kv11.1) and slowly (KvLQT1, Kv7.1) activating components of I_K in normal and failing canine hearts show a modest but significant reduction in steady state levels.[19] Like I_{K1}, the molecular basis for I_K downregulation in human HF remains controversial.

Ca²⁺ currents and altered Ca²⁺ homeostasis

Altered Ca^{2+} homeostasis underlies abnormalities in excitation-contraction coupling and enhanced arrhythmic risk in HF. Intracellular Ca^{2+} concentration and the AP are intricately linked by a variety of Ca^{2+}-mediated cell surface channels and transporters such as the L-type Ca^{2+} channel, Ca^{2+}-activated chloride and potassium currents, and the sodium-calcium exchanger (NCX).

L-type Ca²⁺ current

L-type Ca^{2+} current (I_{Ca-L}) density is unchanged or reduced in HF, the latter typically occurring in more advanced disease.[9,11,29] Remarkably, in human HF baseline I_{Ca-L} density is consistently unchanged.[30] Single channel studies suggest a reduction in overall channel number in human HF but with a compensatory slowing of channel closure, perhaps due to altered phosphorylation or subunit composition.[31] I_{Ca-L} subunit mRNA transcription in HF varies.[32] Further complexity of molecular basis of Ca^{2+} channel remodeling is highlighted by reports of isoform switching of both α and β subunits of the channel in the failing heart.[33,34]

Sarcoplasmic reticulum

HF is associated with major changes in intracellular and sarcoplasmic reticulum (SR) Ca^{2+} homeostasis.[35] Time-varying changes in intracellular Ca^{2+} concentration generate the cellular calcium transient (CaT). The rate of rise and amplitude of the CaT are governed by release of Ca^{2+} from the SR triggered by Ca^{2+} influx through I_{Ca-L}. The amplitude of the CaT and its rate of decay are reduced in intact preparations and cells isolated from failing ventricles, though systematic comparisons of the CaT profile and dynamics in cells isolated from different regions of the failing heart are limited.[36]

SR Ca^{2+}-ATPase (SERCA2), its inhibitor phospholamban (PLN), and NCX are primary mediators of Ca^{2+} removal from the cytoplasm. In HF, ventricular myocytes exhibit both a greater reliance on NCX for removal of Ca^{2+} from the cytosol and an increase in NCX function,[37] leading to defective SR Ca^{2+} loading.[38] The enhanced NCX function in the failing heart, particularly in the setting of changes in intracellular Na^+ concentration (see later discussion), contribute to augmented transient inward currents (I_{ti}) that underlie arrhythmogenic DADs.[23]

SR Ca^{2+} release is also defective in the failing heart and is associated with dysregulation of the ryanodine receptor (RyR2) function.[39] Hyperphosphorylation of RyR2 by protein kinase A[40] or CaMKII[41] may increase diastolic Ca^{2+} leak and generate spontaneous Ca^{2+} transients underlying triggered arrhythmias in HF. Increased inositol 1,4,5-trisphosphate receptor expression has been suggested to be a general mechanism that underlies remodeling of Ca^{2+} signaling during heart disease, and in particular, in triggering ventricular arrhythmias during hypertrophy.[42] CaMKII may contribute to both the arrhythmic substrate and cardiac decompensation by enhancing RyR2-mediated SR Ca^{2+} leak. Attenuating CaMKII activation can reduce arrhythmias and limit the progression to HF in preliminary studies in animal models.[43] The HF-related alterations in RyR2 function mimic the changes caused by posttranslational modification by reactive oxygen species, thus reduction-oxidation modification of RyR2 may contribute to SR Ca^{2+} leak in chronic HF.[44] The role of RyR2 regulation and gating in altered systolic function and arrhythmic risk in HF remains controversial.[45-47]

Altered Na^+ dynamics and late Na^+ current

Intracellular Na^+ concentration and Ca^{2+} handling are intimately linked and the intracellular Na^+ concentration is increased in failing ventricular myocytes. Increases in intracellular Na^+ may be the result of diminished efflux by reduced Na^+-K^+ ATPase activity or an increase in Na^+ influx via the voltage-gated Na^+ currents (INa) Na^+-H^+ exchanger, NCX, or other Na^+ co-transporters.

Cardiac I_{Na} in HF

Studies of I_{Na} in a canine infarct model of HF revealed a significant downregulation of the overall current, an acceleration of its inactivation properties, and a slowing of its recovery from inactivation in myocytes isolated from the infarct border zone.[48] Normal impulse formation and conduction depend critically on the phase 0 fast inward I_{Na}. Changes in I_{Na} density and kinetics may predispose to arrhythmias by disrupting conduction or by prolonging repolarization.

A prominent increase in late I_{Na} and slowing of overall I_{Na} decay has been described in several models of HF, including that of humans.[49,50] The mechanisms of the increase in late I_{Na} in HF remain uncertain but block of the late current inhibits oxidant-induced early afterdepolarizations and contractile dysfunction.[51] Alterations in CaMKII signaling influence I_{Na} decay and the magnitude of late I_{Na},[52-54] suggesting posttranslational modifications of the Na^+ channel or associated proteins in this complex as a possible mechanism. There are no consistent changes in cardiac Na^+ channel subunit expression in HF; however, aberrant splicing of sodium channel transcripts has been reported in failing human ventricular myocardium.[55]

Na^+-K^+ ATPase

The Na^+-K^+ ATPase, or the Na^+ pump, is responsible for the establishment and maintenance of the Na^+ and K^+ gradients across the cell membrane and belongs to the widely distributed class of ATPases that are responsible for transporting a number of cations. The Na^+-K^+ ATPase hydrolyzes a molecule of ATP to transport K^+ into the cell and Na^+ out with a stoichiometry of 2 to 3 therefore generating an outward current.

The consensus of experimental data reveal that the expression and function of the Na^+-K^+ ATPase are reduced in HF compared with control hearts.[56] Decreased Na^+ pump function in HF may have several consequences relevant to the production of arrhythmias. First, the reduction in the outward repolarizing current could prolong AP duration. Second, reduced pump function reduces Na^+ efflux and may increase intracellular Na^+ concentration. Finally, decreased pump function could increase vulnerability to decreased extracellular K^+ concentrations.

The consequences of increased Na^+ influx or decreased efflux in HF could also result in cytosolic Na^+ loading and subsequent activation of "reverse mode" for NCX, in which excess intracellular Na^+ is exchanged for available extracellular Ca^{2+}. NCX functioning in the reverse mode might be acutely adaptive, promoting an increase influx in activator Ca^{2+}. However, the chronically slowed I_{Na} decay and increased late I_{Na} may also contribute to AP prolongation and more frequent early afterdepolarizations in HF.

Altered currents in HF: increased triggered activity and functional reentry

Congenital and drug-induced AP prolongation create an arrhythmogenic substrate associated with torsades de pointes ventricular tachycardia. The alteration of current densities and kinetics in HF exaggerate the heterogeneity of electrophysiological properties of the ventricular myocardium. In the setting of changes in Ca^{2+} handling and the structural abnormalities of the failing ventricle, lethal arrhythmias, particularly polymorphic ventricular tachycardia are commonplace. The consequences of downregulation of repolarizing K^+ currents, increased late INa and altered Ca^{2+} handling is AP prolongation that is highly variable both spatially in the ventricle and temporally. The long APs seen in HF are susceptible to interruptions in repolarization mediated by I_{Ca-L} reactivation, producing EADs that underlie triggered arrhythmias. The beat-to-beat temporal variability in AP duration is associated with exaggerated QT interval variability and T wave alternans, both of which may predispose to ventricular arrhythmias. The spatial variability of the AP duration in the ventricle underlies heterogeneous electrical recovery of the ventricle that promotes functional reentry. The confluence of triggered activity and functional reentry, mechanisms that are not mutually exclusive, dramatically increase the risk of lethal arrhythmias and SCD in patients with HF.

Network properties of the failing heart: conduction and connexin remodeling in HF

Gap junction channels are intercellular channel proteins that permit electrical and chemical communication between cells. These channels are major mediators of conduction in the heart. Mammalian gap junction channels or connexons are built by the oligomerization of a family of closely related genes encoding connexins (Cx).[57] Three different Cx have been identified in the mammalian heart: Cx40, Cx43, and Cx45, named for their respective molecular masses.

Slowed intraventricular conduction is a prominent feature of HF. There are a number of mechanisms by which conduction is slowed in HF, including fibrosis and scarring in ischemic and other forms of cardiomyopathy, changes in I_{Na} density in failing myocytes and alteration in gap junction structure and function. It likely that all three mechanisms are involved in the maladaptive remodeling of conduction in the failing heart. HF is associated with a reduction in the density, altered distribution and posttranslational modification of the major cardiac gap junction protein (Cx43).[58] In both hypertrophied and ischemic human ventricular myocardium, Cx43 is downregulated and redistributed from the intercalated disk to the entire cell border (lateralization),[59] a pattern observed in early cardiac development. Downregulation and lateralization of Cx43 in tachy-pacing induced HF is progressive[60] and associated with conduction slowing. The mechanism of Cx43 downregulation is not completely understood but may involve altered renin-angiotensin-aldosterone system signaling, changes in binding partners or defective trafficking.[61] In tachy-pacing HF, Cx43 downregulation is associated with a reduction in Cx43 mRNA and may be regulated by microRNAs (eg, miR-1).[62]

Arrhythmogenesis in HF: Role of Altered Metabolism

Myocardial energy metabolism and electrical activity are intricately related.[63] All ion transport processes are driven directly or indirectly by the free energy released from hydrolysis of high-energy phosphates. Under physiologic conditions, ATP is mainly supplied by mitochondrial oxidative phosphorylation and to a lesser degree by glycolysis. The critical dependence of the ion homeostasis on sufficient energy supply becomes evident in several circumstances including myocardial ischemia and HF, where a mismatch in ATP supply and ATP use may lead to electrical instability. For instance, downregulation of SERCA2, which transports Ca^{2+} from the cytosol of the cell to the lumen of the SR at the expense of ATP hydrolysis during muscle relaxation, is considered to be a hallmark of abnormal Ca^{2+} homeostasis and electrical remodeling in HF. We have previously demonstrated that downregulation of SERCA2 is tightly linked to prolongation of AP duration and altered expression of metabolic transcripts. About half of the transcripts associated with SERCA2 expression (18 out of 37) were linked to oxidative phosphorylation, ATP synthesis, fatty acid β-oxidation, and the tricarboxylic acid (TCA) cycle in a genome-wide transcription study in a canine nonischemic HF model,[64] suggesting a coordinate dysregulation shared by SERCA2 and energetic pathways in HF. A recent study demonstrating that the mitochondrial transcription factors Tfam and Tfb2m bind to the SERCA2 promoter and regulate SERCA2 transcript levels, provide first mechanistic insights into the coordinate regulation of mitochondrial ATP production and expenditure in mammalian myocardium.[65]

In addition to SERCA2, the expression of other Ca^{2+}-handling genes ($\alpha 1$ subunit of I_{Ca-L} [CACNA1C] and calsequestrin [CASQ2]) as well as transcripts responsible for impulse propagation (I_{Na} α subunit SCN5A encoding Nav1.5 and GJA1 encoding Cx43) and repolarization (KCND4, KCHN2, and KCNQ1: the genes encoding Kv4, Kv11.1, and Kv7.1 channel α subunits) are closely correlated with mitochondrial bioenergetic pathways at the transcriptional level. There is a growing body of literature indicating that HF is characterized by transcriptional downregulation of mitochondrial bioenergetic pathways in human HF and a wide range of experimental HF models.[66–68] The tight transcriptional co-expression of metabolic and ion channel transcripts in myocardium suggests that downregulation of metabolic pathways, as observed in the failing myocardium, is strongly associated with lower abundance of a wide variety of ion channel transcripts and thus, possibly electrical instability in failing myocardium.

Life-threatening ventricular tachyarrhythmias are prevalent in virtually every cardiovascular condition associated with structural or functional abnormalities. Although the combination of electrophysiological and molecular techniques has resulted in significant advances in our understanding of the molecular processes associated with ion channel function, pharmacologic therapies modulating only the electrical activity have proven ineffective to prevent arrhythmias in the long-term. For instance, clinical trials such as the Cardiac Arrhythmia Suppression Trial (CAST)[69] and Survival With Oral d-Sotalol (SWORD)[70] revealed that, at least in postinfarction patients, antiarrhythmic therapy may lead to increased rather than reduced mortality. In contrast, significant advances have been achieved with pharmacologic therapies that affect regulatory pathways that impinge upon ion channels, for instance β-blockers, statins, angiotensin-converting enzymes, and aldosterone inhibitors, highlighting that the electrical activity has to be viewed in the larger context of the cellular milieu. Given the proarrhythmic risk associated with conventional, ion channel-targeted antiarrhythmic drug therapies, a new approach to arrhythmias, based on a better understanding of the interrelated pathophysiological processes leading to maladaptive ion channel remodeling, is urgently needed. In this respect, correction of the cellular bioenergetic deficit associated with structural heart disease, either pharmacologically or by the use of devices, represents a novel and promising antiarrhythmic strategy.

Special Case: Dyssynchronous Contraction in HF and the Effect of Cardiac Resynchronization Therapy on the Arrhythmic and Metabolic Substrates

Dyssynchronous contraction resulting from an intraventricular conduction delay is present in ~30% of patients with HF[71] and has been identified as an independent predictor of mortality in HF patients.[72–74] A left bundle branch block (LBBB) decreases regional loading, contractile work, myocardial blood flow, and oxygen consumption in the early-activated anterior myocardium, while these parameters are increased in the late-activated lateral LV.[75,76] Furthermore, dyssynchronous LV activation in patients with dilated cardiomyopathy and LBBB leads to reduced septal glucose metabolism, as measured by uptake of (18)F-fluorodeoxyglucose (FDG) with positron emission tomography: in dyssynchronous HF (DHF), baseline FDG uptake has been shown to be regionally heterogeneous, with lowest uptake in the septal region and highest uptake in the lateral region. During biventricular pacing employed in cardiac resynchronization therapy (CRT)—septal and anterior uptake of FDG increases while lateral uptake decreases, resulting in restoration of homogeneous myocardial glucose metabolism.[77] To examine the underlying molecular mechanisms contributing to regional disparities in DHF, we used a global gene expression profiling approach in a recently developed canine model of DHF and CRT. We found that in DHF changes in gene expression were primarily observed in the anterior LV, most prominently downregulation of metabolic transcripts, whereas only minor changes were observed in the lateral LV in DHF. Thus, DHF induced an increased regional heterogeneity of gene expression within the LV (Fig. 2). Importantly, CRT corrected the alterations in gene expression in the anterior wall, supporting a global effect of biventricular pacing on the ventricular transcriptome that extends beyond the pacing site in the lateral wall.[77,78]

As DHF significantly increased the heterogeneity of gene expression between early- and late-activated LV wall regions, it is tempting to speculate that this increased heterogeneity within the LV wall also reflects regionally heterogeneous remodeling of ion channels that exists in this HF model. CRT uniquely and significantly shortened the AP in lateral myocytes, reduced the regional heterogeneity in AP duration within the LV, and lowered the frequency of EADs in cells isolated from both the anterior and lateral LV.[19]

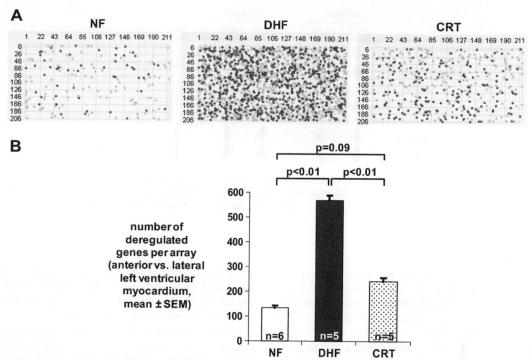

Fig. 2. Dyssynchrony leads to increased regional heterogeneity in gene expression that is partially reduced with CRT. (*A*) Pseudo-images of representative microarrays from non-failing (NF), DHF, and CRT hearts with 211 columns and 206 rows (44 K array). RNA from the anterior and lateral regions was labeled with different fluorescent dyes, Cy3 and Cy5, and hybridized in a two-color design onto one array. Light and dark gray dots represent statistically significant differentially expressed transcripts between anterior and lateral wall, respectively. (*B*) A bar plot of the number of deregulated genes comparing the anterior and lateral regions in NF, DHF, and CRT hearts. In DHF, the number of differentially expressed transcripts between anterior and lateral wall increases 4-fold, while it is greatly reduced by CRT. (*Reproduced* from Barth AS, Aiba T, Halperin V, et al. Cardiac resynchronization therapy corrects dyssynchrony-induced regional gene expression changes on a genomic level. Circ Cardiovasc Genet 2009;2(4):371–8; with permission.)

CRT restores specific ion currents and handling

K^+ current changes associated with CRT are variable. The downregulation of I_{to} is regionally uniform in the left ventricle in DHF and is unique among regulated K^+ currents in HF in that it is not reversed by CRT; Kv4.3 and KChIP2 mRNA and protein expression remain downregulated. However, CRT partially restores I_{K1} density and decreases membrane resistance even in the setting of continued HF. With the improved Ca^{2+} handling in CRT described below, restoration of I_{K1} may reduce the frequency of arrhythmogenic DADs. CRT also partially restores DHF-induced downregulation of I_K density in both anterior and lateral LV myocytes (**Fig. 3**).[19]

Though alterations in net I_{Ca-L} are minimal or compensated in human HF, in DHF there are exaggerated intraventricular regional heterogeneities in I_{Ca-L} and these changes are partially restored by CRT. DHF produced a reduction of peak I_{Ca-L} density and slowed current decay in myocytes isolated from the late-activated lateral LV wall. In contrast, peak I_{Ca-L} density in anterior myocytes was increased compared with nonfailing controls, thus DHF produced regional heterogeneity of Ca^{2+} current density and kinetics. CRT restored the peak current density but did not alter the I_{Ca-L} decay in the lateral cells, eliminating the anterior-lateral I_{Ca-L} density gradient. Neither DHF nor CRT exhibit consistent changes in Ca^{2+} channel subunit mRNA or protein levels.[19]

In canine pacing DHF, CaT amplitudes are depressed and kinetics slowed particularly in cells isolated from the late-activated lateral LV myocardium. These changes are also partially restored by CRT (**Fig. 4**). In DHF, mRNA and protein levels of SERCA2, PLN, and RyR2 were downregulated and NCX upregulated without a change in CRT. There were also no regional differences in mRNA and protein expression in any of these mediators of Ca^{2+} handling when comparing DHF and CRT, suggesting that the global and regional differences of Ca^{2+} handling function in DHF and its restoration by CRT are posttranslational.[19]

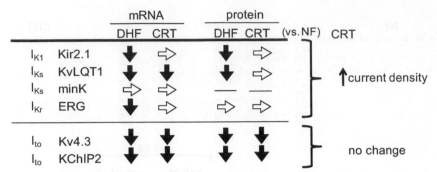

Fig. 3. CRT partially reverses DHF-induced downregulation of IK1 and IK but not Ito. DHF reduces the inward rectifier I_{K1}, the delayed rectifier (I_K) and transient outward K$^+$ currents (I_{to}) in ventricular cells. CRT partially restores the DHF-induced reduction of I_{K1} and I_K but not I_{to}, consistent with changes in steady state K$^+$ channel mRNA subunit and protein expression.

The mechanisms underlying the differences in regional remodeling of K$^+$ currents and Ca^{2+} handling in DHF remain obscure. At the molecular level, tumor necrosis factor-α (TNF-α) and CaMKII were increased in DHF prominently in the lateral wall. TNF-α is known to decrease I_{to} and prolong the AP duration in rat ventricular myocytes.[79] CaMKII influences Ca^{2+} current, SR function,[80,81] and increases persistent Na$^+$ current,[54,82]

resulting in prolongation of AP duration.[83] The functional upregulation of TNF-α and CaMKII in the lateral compared with the anterior wall of the left ventricle were eliminated by CRT.[84]

In some models of DHF, β-adrenergic blockade mitigated the slower decay of I_{Ca-L} inactivation.[85] These findings suggest that DHF-induced changes of I_{Ca-L} inactivation kinetics might be mediated by regionally heterogeneous uncoupling

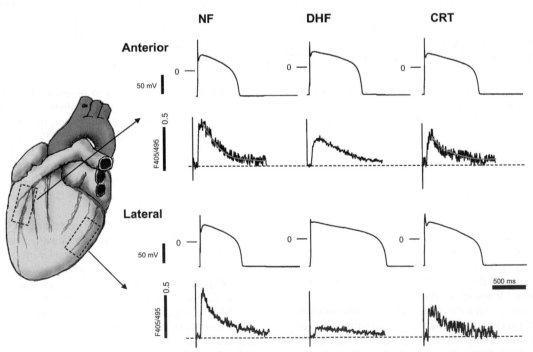

Fig. 4. Regional heterogeneity of AP and CaT in DHF and its restoration by CRT. CRT abbreviates DHF-induced prolongation of the AP and restores amplitude and decay of CaT in the lateral cells, thus reducing regional heterogeneity of repolarization and Ca handling. (*From* Aiba T, Tomaselli GF. Electrical remodeling in the failing heart. Curr Opinions in Cardiol 2009;25:29–36; with permission.)

of β-adrenergic receptor signaling. Consistent with this hypothesis, the Ca^{2+}-handling proteins are functionally regulated by phosphorylation, prominently by the intracellular enzymes protein kinase A and CaMKII,[80,81,86] and a variety of phosphatases that may be regionally regulated.[84] Aberrant β-adrenergic signaling, with alterations in receptor density and uncoupling of receptor activation from downstream effectors, is a key feature of HF. CRT restores the DHF-induced baseline reduction of I_{Ca-L} and the blunted response to β-adrenergic (β1 >> β2) receptor stimulation. Moreover, CRT improves baseline Ca^{2+} handling and its adrenergic responsiveness, which may contribute to improvement in contractility and altered arrhythmia susceptibility.[87,88]

Finally, HF increases late I_{Na} and slows I_{Na} decay. CRT partially restores DHF-induced altered I_{Na} gating kinetics. I_{Na} blockers have a notorious history in the treatment of cardiac arrhythmias with substantial proarrhythmic liability. Strategies that target the late current may have more promise.

Partial normalization of the electrical phenotype as demonstrated in experimental CRT models (shortening of AP duration, reversal of DHF-induced downregulation of K^+ currents, improved Na^+ channel gating, and Ca^{2+} homeostasis, as well as restoration of the DHF-induced blunted β-adrenergic receptor responsiveness) may provide an explanation for the reduced risk for arrhythmias and better overall prognosis after CRT. The features of DHF and its reversibility by CRT offer a unique opportunity to explore additional therapeutic targets that may help to further advance treatment of patients presenting with congestive HF and arrhythmias.

REFERENCES

1. Rosamond W, Flegal K, Furie K, et al. Heart disease and stroke statistics—2008 update: a report from the American Heart Association Statistics Committee and Stroke Statistics Subcommittee. Circulation 2008;117(4):e25—146.

2. Trautwein W, Kassebaum DG, Nelsol RM, et al. Electrophysiological study of human heart muscle. Circ Res 1962;10:306—12.

3. Beuckelmann DJ, Nabauer M, Erdmann E. Alterations of K+ currents in isolated human ventricular myocytes from patients with terminal heart failure. Circ Res 1993;73(2):379—85.

4. Akar FG, Rosenbaum DS. Transmural electrophysiological heterogeneities underlying arrhythmogenesis in heart failure. Circ Res 2003;93(7):638—45.

5. Kaab S, Nuss HB, Chiamvimonvat N, et al. Ionic mechanism of action potential prolongation in ventricular myocytes from dogs with pacing-induced heart failure. Circ Res 1996;78(2):262—73.

6. Kaab S, Dixon J, Duc J, et al. Molecular basis of transient outward potassium current downregulation in human heart failure: a decrease in Kv4.3 mRNA correlates with a reduction in current density. Circulation 1998;98(14):1383—93.

7. Rose J, Armoundas AA, Tian Y, et al. Molecular correlates of altered expression of potassium currents in failing rabbit myocardium. Am J Physiol Heart Circ Physiol 2005;288(5):H2077—87.

8. Tsuji Y, Zicha S, Qi XY, et al. Potassium channel subunit remodeling in rabbits exposed to long-term bradycardia or tachycardia: discrete arrhythmogenic consequences related to differential delayed-rectifier changes. Circulation 2006;113(3):345—55.

9. Nattel S, Maguy A, Le Bouter S, et al. Arrhythmogenic ion-channel remodeling in the heart: heart failure, myocardial infarction, and atrial fibrillation. Physiol Rev 2007;87(2):425—56.

10. Li GR, Lau CP, Ducharme A, et al. Transmural action potential and ionic current remodeling in ventricles of failing canine hearts. Am J Physiol Heart Circ Physiol 2002;283(3):H1031—41.

11. Tomaselli GF, Marban E. Electrophysiological remodeling in hypertrophy and heart failure. Cardiovasc Res 1999;42(2):270—83.

12. Nabauer M, Beuckelmann DJ, Erdmann E. Characteristics of transient outward current in human ventricular myocytes from patients with terminal heart failure. Circ Res 1993;73(2):386—94.

13. Greenstein JL, Wu R, Po S, et al. Role of the calcium-independent transient outward current i(to1) in shaping action potential morphology and duration. Circ Res 2000;87(11):1026—33.

14. Nerbonne JM. Molecular basis of functional voltage-gated K+ channel diversity in the mammalian myocardium. J Physiol 2000;525(Pt 2):285—98.

15. Li X, Tang K, Xie B, et al. Regulation of Kv4 channel expression in failing rat heart by the thioredoxin system. Am J Physiol Heart Circ Physiol 2008;295(1):H416—24.

16. Rozanski GJ, Xu Z. A metabolic mechanism for cardiac K+ channel remodelling. Clin Exp Pharmacol Physiol 2002;29(1—2):132—7.

17. An WF, Bowlby MR, Betty M, et al. Modulation of A-type potassium channels by a family of calcium sensors. Nature 2000;403(6769):553—6.

18. Zicha S, Xiao L, Stafford S, et al. Transmural expression of transient outward potassium current subunits in normal and failing canine and human hearts. J Physiol 2004;561(Pt 3):735—48.

19. Aiba T, Hesketh GG, Barth AS, et al. Electrophysiological consequences of dyssynchronous heart failure and its restoration by resynchronization therapy. Circulation 2009;119(9):1220—30.

20. Akar FG, Wu RC, Juang GJ, et al. Molecular mechanisms underlying K+ current downregulation in canine tachycardia-induced heart failure. Am J Physiol Heart Circ Physiol 2005;288(6):H2887–96.

21. Xiao L, Coutu P, Villeneuve LR, et al. Mechanisms underlying rate-dependent remodeling of transient outward potassium current in canine ventricular myocytes. Circ Res 2008;103:733–42.

22. Wagner S, Hacker E, Grandi E, et al. Ca/Calmodulin Kinase II differentially modulates potassium currents. Circ Arrhythm Electrophysiol 2009;2(3):285–94.

23. Pogwizd SM, Schlotthauer K, Li L, et al. Arrhythmogenesis and contractile dysfunction in heart failure: roles of sodium-calcium exchange, inward rectifier potassium current, and residual beta-adrenergic responsiveness. Circ Res 2001;88(11):1159–67.

24. Nuss HB, Kaab S, Kass DA, et al. Cellular basis of ventricular arrhythmias and abnormal automaticity in heart failure. Am J Physiol 1999;277(1 Pt 2):H80–91.

25. Koumi S, Backer CL, Arentzen CE. Characterization of inwardly rectifying K+ channel in human cardiac myocytes. Alterations in channel behavior in myocytes isolated from patients with idiopathic dilated cardiomyopathy. Circulation 1995;92(2):164–74.

26. Rozanski GJ, Xu Z, Whitney RT, et al. Electrophysiology of rabbit ventricular myocytes following sustained rapid ventricular pacing. J Mol Cell Cardiol 1997;29(2):721–32.

27. Liu DW, Antzelevitch C. Characteristics of the delayed rectifier current (IKr and IKs) in canine ventricular epicardial, midmyocardial, and endocardial myocytes. A weaker IKs contributes to the longer action potential of the M cell. Circ Res 1995;76(3):351–65.

28. Furukawa T, Bassett AL, Furukawa N, et al. The ionic mechanism of reperfusion-induced early afterdepolarizations in feline left ventricular hypertrophy. J Clin Invest 1993;91(4):1521–31.

29. Pitt GS, Dun W, Boyden PA. Remodeled cardiac calcium channels. J Mol Cell Cardiol 2006;41(3):373–88.

30. Chen X, Piacentino V 3rd, Furukawa S, et al. L-type Ca2+ channel density and regulation are altered in failing human ventricular myocytes and recover after support with mechanical assist devices. Circ Res 2002;91(6):517–24.

31. Schroder F, Handrock R, Beuckelmann DJ, et al. Increased availability and open probability of single L-type calcium channels from failing compared with nonfailing human ventricle. Circulation 1998;98(10):969–76.

32. Takahashi T, Allen PD, Lacro RV, et al. Expression of dihydropyridine receptor (Ca2+ channel) and calsequestrin genes in the myocardium of patients with end stage heart failure. J Clin Invest 1992;90(3):927–35.

33. Yang Y, Chen X, Margulies K, et al. L-type Ca2+ channel alpha 1c subunit isoform switching in failing human ventricular myocardium. J Mol Cell Cardiol 2000;32(6):973–84.

34. Hullin R, Khan IF, Wirtz S, et al. Cardiac L-type calcium channel beta-subunits expressed in human heart have differential effects on single channel characteristics. J Biol Chem 2003;278(24):21623–30.

35. Bers DM. Altered cardiac myocyte Ca regulation in heart failure. Physiology (Bethesda) 2006;21:380–7.

36. O'Rourke B, Kass DA, Tomaselli GF, et al. Mechanisms of altered excitation-contraction coupling in canine tachycardia-induced heart failure, I: experimental studies. Circ Res 1999;84(5):562–70.

37. Hobai IA, O'Rourke B. Enhanced Ca(2+)-activated Na(+)-Ca(2+) exchange activity in canine pacing-induced heart failure. Circ Res 2000;87(8):690–8.

38. Hobai IA, O'Rourke B. Decreased sarcoplasmic reticulum calcium content is responsible for defective excitation-contraction coupling in canine heart failure. Circulation 2001;103(11):1577–84.

39. Reiken S, Gaburjakova M, Guatimosim S, et al. Protein kinase A phosphorylation of the cardiac calcium release channel (ryanodine receptor) in normal and failing hearts. Role of phosphatases and response to isoproterenol. J Biol Chem 2003;278(1):444–53.

40. Marx SO, Reiken S, Hisamatsu Y, et al. PKA phosphorylation dissociates FKBP12.6 from the calcium release channel (ryanodine receptor): defective regulation in failing hearts. Cell 2000;101(4):365–76.

41. Curran J, Hinton MJ, Rios E, et al. Beta-adrenergic enhancement of sarcoplasmic reticulum calcium leak in cardiac myocytes is mediated by calcium/calmodulin-dependent protein kinase. Circ Res 2007;100(3):391–8.

42. Harzheim D, Movassagh M, Foo RS, et al. Increased InsP3Rs in the junctional sarcoplasmic reticulum augment Ca2+ transients and arrhythmias associated with cardiac hypertrophy. Proc Natl Acad Sci U S A 2009;106(27):11406–11.

43. Ling H, Zhang T, Pereira L, et al. Requirement for Ca2+/calmodulin-dependent kinase II in the transition from pressure overload-induced cardiac hypertrophy to heart failure in mice. J Clin Invest 2009;119(5):1230–40.

44. Terentyev D, Gyorke I, Belevych AE, et al. Redox modification of ryanodine receptors contributes to sarcoplasmic reticulum Ca2+ leak in chronic heart failure. Circ Res 2008;103(12):1466–72.

45. Jiang MT, Lokuta AJ, Farrell EF, et al. Abnormal Ca2+ release, but normal ryanodine receptors, in canine and human heart failure. Circ Res 2002;91(11):1015–22.

46. Xiao B, Jiang MT, Zhao M, et al. Characterization of a novel PKA phosphorylation site, serine-2030, reveals no PKA hyperphosphorylation of the cardiac ryanodine receptor in canine heart failure. Circ Res 2005;96(8):847–55.

47. MacDonnell SM, Garcia-Rivas G, Scherman JA, et al. Adrenergic regulation of cardiac contractility does not involve phosphorylation of the cardiac ryanodine receptor at serine 2808. Circ Res 2008; 102(8):e65–72.

48. Pu J, Boyden PA. Alterations of Na+ currents in myocytes from epicardial border zone of the infarcted heart. A possible ionic mechanism for reduced excitability and postrepolarization refractoriness. Circ Res 1997;81(1):110–9.

49. Undrovinas AI, Maltsev VA, Sabbah HN. Repolarization abnormalities in cardiomyocytes of dogs with chronic heart failure: role of sustained inward current. Cell Mol Life Sci 1999;55(3):494–505.

50. Valdivia CR, Chu WW, Pu J, et al. Increased late sodium current in myocytes from a canine heart failure model and from failing human heart. J Mol Cell Cardiol 2005;38(3):475–83.

51. Song Y, Shryock JC, Wagner S, et al. Blocking late sodium current reduces hydrogen peroxide-induced arrhythmogenic activity and contractile dysfunction. J Pharmacol Exp Ther 2006;318(1): 214–22.

52. Aiba T, Hesketh GG, Liu T, et al. Na+ channel regulation by Ca2+/calmodulin and Ca2+/calmodulin-dependent protein kinase II in guinea-pig ventricular myocytes. Cardiovasc Res 2010;85:454–63.

53. Deschenes I, Neyroud N, DiSilvestre D, et al. Isoform-specific modulation of voltage-gated Na(+) channels by calmodulin. Circ Res 2002;90(4):E49–57.

54. Wagner S, Dybkova N, Rasenack EC, et al. Ca2+/calmodulin-dependent protein kinase II regulates cardiac Na+ channels. J Clin Invest 2006;116(12): 3127–38.

55. Shang LL, Pfahnl AE, Sanyal S, et al. Human heart failure is associated with abnormal C-terminal splicing variants in the cardiac sodium channel. Circ Res 2007;101(11):1146–54.

56. Erdmann E, Schwinger R, Bohm M. Beta-blocking agents and positive inotropic agents in the therapy of chronic heart failure. J Cardiovasc Pharmacol 1990;16(Suppl 5):S138–44.

57. Saffitz JE, Schuessler RB, Yamada KA. Mechanisms of remodeling of gap junction distributions and the development of anatomic substrates of arrhythmias. Cardiovasc Res 1999;42(2):309–17.

58. Akar FG, Spragg DD, Tunin RS, et al. Mechanisms underlying conduction slowing and arrhythmogenesis in nonischemic dilated cardiomyopathy. Circ Res 2004;95(7):717–25.

59. Peters NS, Green CR, Poole-Wilson PA, et al. Reduced content of connexin43 gap junctions in ventricular myocardium from hypertrophied and ischemic human hearts. Circulation 1993;88(3): 864–75.

60. Akar FG, Nass RD, Hahn S, et al. Dynamic changes in conduction velocity and gap junction properties during development of pacing-induced heart failure. Am J Physiol Heart Circ Physiol 2007;293(2): H1223–30.

61. Hesketh GG, Shah MH, Halperin VL, et al. Ultra-structure and regulation of lateralized connexin43 in the failing heart. Circ Res 2010;106(6):1153–63.

62. Yang B, Lin H, Xiao J, et al. The muscle-specific microRNA miR-1 regulates cardiac arrhythmogenic potential by targeting GJA1 and KCNJ2. Nat Med 2007;13(4):486–91.

63. Barth AS, Tomaselli GF. Cardiac metabolism and arrhythmias. Circ Arrhythm Electrophysiol 2009; 2(3):327–35.

64. Gao Z, Barth AS, DiSilvestre D, et al. Key pathways associated with heart failure development revealed by gene networks correlated with cardiac remodeling. Physiol Genomics 2008;35(3):222–30.

65. Watanabe A, Arai M, Ohyama Y, et al. Mitochondrial transcription factors, Tfam and Tfb2m regulate the SERCA2 gene transcription - a novel mechanism of the coordinate regulation of energy production and expenditure. Circulation 2008;118(18):S517.

66. Akavia UD, Benayahu D. Meta-analysis and profiling of cardiac expression modules. Physiol Genomics 2008;35(3):305–15.

67. Gao Z, Xu H, DiSilvestre D, et al. Transcriptomic profiling of the canine tachycardia-induced heart failure model: global comparison to human and murine heart failure. J Mol Cell Cardiol 2006;40(1): 76–86.

68. Sharma UC, Pokharel S, Evelo CT, et al. A systematic review of large scale and heterogeneous gene array data in heart failure. J Mol Cell Cardiol 2005;38(3):425–32.

69. Preliminary report: effect of encainide and flecainide on mortality in a randomized trial of arrhythmia suppression after myocardial infarction. The Cardiac Arrhythmia Suppression Trial (CAST) Investigators. N Engl J Med 1989;321(6):406–12.

70. Waldo AL, Camm AJ, deRuyter H, et al. Effect of d-sotalol on mortality in patients with left ventricular dysfunction after recent and remote myocardial infarction. The SWORD Investigators. Survival With Oral d-Sotalol. Lancet 1996;348(9019):7–12.

71. Baldasseroni S, Opasich C, Gorini M, et al. Left bundle-branch block is associated with increased 1-year sudden and total mortality rate in 5517 outpatients with congestive heart failure: a report from the Italian network on congestive heart failure. Am Heart J 2002;143(3):398–405.

72. Bader H, Garrigue S, Lafitte S, et al. Intra-left ventricular electromechanical asynchrony. A new

independent predictor of severe cardiac events in heart failure patients. J Am Coll Cardiol 2004; 43(2):248–56.

73. Kass DA, Chen CH, Curry C, et al. Improved left ventricular mechanics from acute VDD pacing in patients with dilated cardiomyopathy and ventricular conduction delay. Circulation 1999;99(12): 1567–73.

74. Spragg DD, Kass DA. Pathobiology of left ventricular dyssynchrony and resynchronization. Prog Cardiovasc Dis 2006;49(1):26–41.

75. van Oosterhout MF, Prinzen FW, Arts T, et al. Asynchronous electrical activation induces asymmetrical hypertrophy of the left ventricular wall. Circulation 1998;98(6):588–95.

76. Vernooy K, Verbeek XA, Peschar M, et al. Left bundle branch block induces ventricular remodelling and functional septal hypoperfusion. Eur Heart J 2005; 26(1):91–8.

77. Nowak B, Sinha AM, Schaefer WM, et al. Cardiac resynchronization therapy homogenizes myocardial glucose metabolism and perfusion in dilated cardiomyopathy and left bundle branch block. J Am Coll Cardiol 2003;41(9):1523–8.

78. Barth AS, Aiba T, Halperin V, et al. Cardiac resynchronization therapy corrects dyssynchrony-induced regional gene expression changes on a genomic level. Circ Cardiovasc Genet 2009;2(4):371–8.

79. Fernandez-Velasco M, Ruiz-Hurtado G, Hurtado O, et al. TNF-alpha downregulates transient outward potassium current in rat ventricular myocytes through iNOS overexpression and oxidant species generation. Am J Physiol Heart Circ Physiol 2007; 293(1):H238–45.

80. Kohlhaas M, Zhang T, Seidler T, et al. Increased sarcoplasmic reticulum calcium leak but unaltered contractility by acute CaMKII overexpression in isolated rabbit cardiac myocytes. Circ Res 2006; 98(2):235–44.

81. Maier LS, Zhang T, Chen L, et al. Transgenic CaMKIIdeltaC overexpression uniquely alters cardiac myocyte Ca2+ handling: reduced SR Ca2+ load and activated SR Ca2+ release. Circ Res 2003;92(8):904–11.

82. Maltsev VA, Reznikov V, Undrovinas NA, et al. Modulation of late sodium current by Ca2+, calmodulin, and CaMKII in normal and failing dog cardiomyocytes: similarities and differences. Am J Physiol Heart Circ Physiol 2008;294(4):H1597–608.

83. Wu Y, Temple J, Zhang R, et al. Calmodulin kinase II and arrhythmias in a mouse model of cardiac hypertrophy. Circulation 2002;106(10):1288–93.

84. Chakir K, Daya SK, Tunin RS, et al. Reversal of global apoptosis and regional stress kinase activation by cardiac resynchronization. Circulation 2008; 117(11):1369–77.

85. Plotnikov AN, Yu H, Geller JC, et al. Role of L-type calcium channels in pacing-induced short-term and long-term cardiac memory in canine heart. Circulation 2003;107(22):2844–9.

86. Ai X, Curran JW, Shannon TR, et al. Ca2+/calmodulin-dependent protein kinase modulates cardiac ryanodine receptor phosphorylation and sarcoplasmic reticulum Ca2+ leak in heart failure. Circ Res 2005;97(12):1314–22.

87. Aiba T, Barth AS, Liu T, et al. Cardiac resynchronization therapy restores alpha-adrenergic reserve of Ca2+ homeostasis in a canine model of dyssynchronous heart failure. Circulation 2008;118(Suppl): 523–4.

88. Chakir K, Daya SK, Aiba T, et al. Mechanisms of enhanced beta-adrenergic reserve from cardiac resynchronization therapy. Circulation 2009;119(9): 1231–40.

Biologic Pacemakers: Past, Present, and Future

Ira S. Cohen, MD, PhD[a,b,*], Lior Gepstein, MD, PhD[c]

KEYWORDS

- Biological pacemaker • Embryonic stem cell
- HCN genes • Human mesenchymal stem cell
- Autonomic responsiveness

ELECTRONIC PACEMAKERS—HISTORY, INDICATIONS, ADVANTAGES, AND SHORTCOMINGS

Cardiac pacemakers are one of the most important medical innovations of our era. The term, *pacemaker*, was coined by Albert Hymen, who described in 1932 an electromechanical instrument, powered by a spring-wound hand-cranked motor, which could provide electric shocks.[1] In 1952, Paul Zoll developed transcutaneous pacing devices using large rechargeable batteries as power supplies.[2] In 1957, engineer Earl Bakken, the founder of Medtronic, produced the first wearable external pacemaker for a patient of Dr C. Walton Lillehei. The transistorized pacemaker, housed in a small plastic box, had controls to permit adjustment of pacing rate and output voltage and was connected to electrodes leads that passed through the skin of a patient to terminate in electrodes attached to the surface of the myocardium.

In 1958, transvenous endocardial pacing was first demonstrated by Seymour Furman, during which a catheter electrode was inserted via a patient's basilic vein.[3] The first clinical implantation into a human of a fully implantable pacemaker took place in October 1958 at the Karolinska

Institute in Solna, Sweden, using a pacemaker designed by Rune Elmquist and surgeon Ake Senning.[4] The pacemaker was connected to electrodes attached to the myocardium by thoracotomy. The device failed after 3 hours. A second device was then implanted, which lasted for 3 days. The patient, Arne Larsson, who became the first world's first pacemaker patient, went on to receive 26 different pacemakers during his lifetime and died in 2001 at the age of 86.

Since these initial pioneering attempts, cardiac pacing has become a permanent fixture in clinical practice. Traditional indications for cardiac pacing include symptomatic slow heart rate (bradycardia) due to either abnormalities in the initiation of the electric impulse in the atria (sick sinus syndrome, which accounts for approximately 50% of cases) or in its conduction to the ventricle (atrioventricular [AV] block).[5] Other indications include tachycardia-bradycardia syndrome, alternating bundle branch block, neuromuscular disease with or without AV block, long QT syndrome, carotid sinus hypersensitivity, and more recently also left ventricular dyssynchrony in the setting of heart failure.[5]

In recent years, the role of implantable pacing devices has expanded dramatically beyond the aforementioned traditional indications. This was

This work was supported by grants HL67101 and HL094410 from the NIH (ISC) and in part by the Nahum Guzik research fund (LG).

[a] Department of Physiology and Biophysics, Health Sciences Center, Stony Brook University, Stony Brook, NY 11794-8661, USA
[b] Institute for Molecular Cardiology, Stony Brook University, Stony Brook, NY 11794-8661, USA
[c] The Sohnis Family Research Laboratory for Cardiac Electrophysiology and Regenerative Medicine, The Bruce Rappaport Faculty of Medicine, Technion-Israel Institute of Technology, PO Box 9649, Haifa 31096, Israel
* Corresponding author. Department of Physiology and Biophysics, Health Sciences Center, Stony Brook University, Stony Brook, NY 11794-8661.
E-mail address: ira.cohen@stonybrook.edu

Card Electrophysiol Clin 3 (2011) 69–76
doi:10.1016/j.ccep.2010.10.007

coupled with significant advances in the design and properties of these devices. Modern pacemakers' functions include various modes of dual-chamber pacing, rate-response algorithms with dual sensors for optimum physiologic response, cardiac resynchronization therapy, arrhythmia-prevention algorithms, antitachycardia pacing, and hemodynamic monitoring. Current pacemaker design also offers physiologic pacing algorithms that minimize ventricular pacing and reduce the incidence of atrial fibrillation significantly.

Although serving as the treatment of choice for bradyarrhythmias for more than 5 decades, electronic pacemakers are not without limitations. These include (1) the need for a surgical procedure with its associated small but existing risks, such as vascular complications, bleeding, pneuomothorax, and infection (especially during pacemaker changes); (2) the requirement for repeated procedures for battery replacement and at times electrode extraction; (3) occasional technical failures of the device or the implanted electrodes; (4) problems in the pediatric population due to the inability to adequately adapt equipment to the growth and development of the child; and (5) the inability to adjust heart rate and the resulting electric activation sequence with the same effectiveness as the native pacemaker (sinoatrial [SA] node) and cardiac conduction system. This inability is exemplified by the deterioration of left ventricular performance during traditional right ventricular apical pacing because of the resulting left ventricular dyssynchrony.

ADVANTAGES OF BIOLOGIC PACING

Given the success of electronic pacemakers, it is reasonable to ask why a biologic alternative should be created. The simple answer is that it has the potential to function better. Although electronic pacemakers require maintenance and/or battery replacement, a biologic pacemaker could function indefinitely maintenance-free. Although improved programming has made electronic devices simulate autonomic responsiveness more effectively, a true biologic pacemaker would be autonomically responsive. Although electronic pacemakers have limited placement options, catheter delivery of a biologic pacemaker provides greater options to optimize mechanical responses individualized to each patient. Deployment of the electronic pacemaker usually results in substantial tissue damage, leading to fibrosis; anatomic damage is unlikely with delivery of a biologic pacemaker. Ultimately, a successful biologic pacemaker can be designed to produce optimal basal rate, autonomic responsiveness, and mechanical response imparting minimal tissue damage during implantation, an impossibility with current electronic pacemaker technology.

GENERAL PRINCIPLES OF BIOLOGIC PACEMAKER DESIGN

In the sinus node, a small net inward current during diastole generates the spontaneous pacemaker depolarization, whereas in the ventricle and much of the atrium there is no net current flow (and thus no change in membrane potential) between action potentials. The challenge in creating a biologic pacemaker is to convert a diastolic interval with zero net current flow into a period of small net inward current.

STRATEGIES FOR THE DEVELOPMENT OF BIOLOGIC PACEMAKERS
Gene Therapy

Beginning in 1998,[6] multiple approaches have been used to either enhance the spontaneous rate of existing secondary pacemakers or initiate pacemaker activity in quiescent tissue. These approaches require a delivery system and an approach to create or enhance net inward current. The delivery system can be a naked plasmid,[6] a virus,[7,8] or a cell.[9,10] The approach to enhance net inward current can be a receptor gene,[6] a channel gene[9,10] delivered by any of those three approaches, or alternatively a naturally pacing cell[10] capable of initiating pacing in the region of implantation.

Overexpression of the β_2-adrenergic receptor
The first biologic pacemaker was created by delivery of the β_2-adrenergic receptor to the murine right atrium.[6,11] Expression of this receptor increased pacemaker rate by 40%. This report made biologic pacing a reality.[6] The approach had several disadvantages, however. First, in the initial study, the naked plasmid delivery system limited both the uptake and duration of the effect. Second, the chosen protein, the β_2-adrenergic receptor, activated myriad ion channels/transporters as well as other cellular functions regulated by cyclic adenosine monophosphate (cAMP). Their studies using the β_2-adrenergic receptor demonstrated biologic pacing was possible but because of its lack of specificity and the potential for arrhythmogenic outcomes this approach has not been pursued.

Reducing a background outward potassium current initiates pacemaker activity in quiescent myocytes
I_{K1} is a dominant membrane conductance in the diastolic voltage range in atrial and ventricular myocytes. Reducing this outward current in normally

quiescent tissue should result in a depolarization. If the reduction is of the right magnitude, a net inward current generating a pacemaker-like membrane depolarization toward threshold can occur. Miake and colleagues[8] reduced I_{K1} by delivering via adenovirus a nonfunctional dominant negative construct of KiR2.1 (one of the molecular correlates of the I_{K1} channel, which combines with native KiR2.1 subunits to create nonfunctional channels) in vivo to the guinea pig ventricle. This resulted in a reduction in the magnitude of I_{K1}. A major disadvantage of such an approach is that I_{K1} contributes to final repolarization of the ventricular action potential. Thus, not surprisingly, besides inducing pacemaker activity, delivery of this dominant negative form of I_{K1} prolonged the action potential and the QT interval.[12] It is not sufficient just to create pacemaker activity; it is also important that the target protein that is delivered not be proarrhythmic by altering channels that have key functions during phases of the action potential other than pacemaker depolarization. Nevertheless, this result was an important advance because it was the first study to specifically target ion channels as a potential means to create biologic pacemakers.

Adding inward pacemaker current also creates pacemaker activity

If net inward current is required for pacemaker activity, the obvious alternative approach to reducing outward current is to add an inward current. The channel that carries the major inward current during the pacemaker potential in the sinus node is called I_F.[13] This channel is present but not normally activated at diastolic potentials in quiescent atrium or ventricle. The alpha subunit of this channel is encoded by the hyperpolarization-activated cyclic nucleotide-gated (HCN) gene family.[14,15] It provides inward current (activates) when the action potential repolarizes to diastolic membrane potentials.[13,16] It rapidly closes on depolarization, limiting its action to the diastolic time period. This last property avoids the problems of action potential prolongation associated with down-regulation of I_{K1} (discussed previously). Another advantage of this approach is that the HCN channels have a cyclic nucleotide binding site in the cytoplasm leading to the opening of more I_F channels when cAMP is elevated by sympathetic stimulation.[17,18] Thus, this channel's presence automatically creates autonomic responsiveness in the biologic pacemaker. The authors began their investigation of this approach with the HCN2 gene (one member of this multigene family) delivered by adenovirus to the canine left atrium or left bundle branch[7,19] by adenovirus

where it created (atrium) or enhanced (left bundle branch) native pacemaker function. With this approach, the virus infected the myocytes and the myocytes expressed the HCN2 channels and a pacemaker current sufficient to generate (left atrium) or enhance (left bundle branch) pacemaker activity. Although native genes demonstrated both acceptable basal rates (approximately 60 beats per minute) and some increase in rate in response to catecholamines, neither was optimal.

Modified HCN genes

If the native pacemaker genes are not optimal, improved HCN channels could be created. For the HCN gene family, the portions of the channel responsible for its voltage dependence, its kinetics, and its cAMP binding were defined.[20] To increase pacemaker rate, more I_F channels must open during diastole. Shifting the activation voltage dependence to more positive potentials or speeding the kinetics of channel opening generates more inward current. The authors chose a mutant HCN channel with a more positive voltage dependence but it expressed more poorly in myocytes than the native channel.[21] There was no increase in basal pacemaker rate although there was enhanced catecholamine sensitivity. Tse and colleagues[22] used a mutated form of the most rapidly activating HCN isoform, HCN1, whose voltage dependence favored channel opening. They were able to achieve physiologic rates in the atrium with some autonomic responsiveness where there is a smaller I_{K1}. If adding more I_F speeds pacemaker rate, is there any limit to this approach? The theoretic answer is yes, because I_F is an inward current it can cause a steady depolarization making cells inexcitable. The same group produced larger magnitudes of i_F with the same HCN1 mutant and demonstrated that too much pacemaker current can lead to termination of pacemaker function.[23] The other approach to increase I_F is to accelerate the kinetics of channel opening. A chimeric channel formed from HCN1 and HCN2 has more rapid activation kinetics. HCN1 has faster kinetics than HCN2 whereas HCN2 has better cAMP sensitivity than HCN1. Thus, the chimeric HCN1/HCN2 channel had rapid kinetics and autonomic responsiveness.[24] This channel was delivered by adenovirus to the canine left bundle branch where it generated a ventricular tachycardia.[25] The inward current added must be titrated against the outward current present in the delivery location to achieve the optimal pacemaker rate. HCN channels have taught the authors that a persistent pacemaker function at acceptable rates with autonomic responsiveness can be accomplished. It is possible to change the basal rate or autonomic responsiveness by genetic engineering; however, the ideal HCN channel has yet to be created by genetic engineering. This ideal channel is likely to differ depending on implantation location and a risk of excessive rates does exist; however, HCN-induced pacemaker function can be terminated by ivabridine, an HCN channel blocker, which should cause induced arrhythmias to cease.[25]

Cell Therapy

An alternative strategy that can theoretically overcome some of the limitations of the gene therapy strategies (discussed previously), such as the general risks associated with the use of viral vectors; the inability to achieve long-term transgene expression; and the inability to adequately control the level of transgene expression within the cells, the number of transfected myocytes, and their spatial distribution, may be the use of cell therapy to establish a biologic pacemaker in vivo. To achieve this goal, using either unmodified or genetically modified cells was proposed. In the latter case, a desired cell population is initially genetically modified ex vivo and then grafted into the heart.[9] This may allow precise characterization and engineering of the modified cells before cell grafting, improved localization of the therapeutic effect to the site of cell transplantation, and potential for long-term expression of the transgene within the heart.

Two distinct cell therapy paradigms were suggested for the creation of biologic pacemakers. The first strategy proposes to ex vivo engineer a noncardiomyocyte to display some or all of the required pacemaker properties by overexpressing cardiac-specific pacemaking currents.[9] The alternative approach seeks to take advantage of recent developments in cardiac stem cell biology to direct the differentiation of stem cells, ex vivo, to generate the appropriate pacemaking cells.[10] In both strategies, the generated cells are then grafted into the heart and are expected to form electrotonic connections with host cardiac tissue, thereby forming a biologic pacemaker unit that should now drive the electric activity of the heart.

Human mesenchymal stem cells transfected with the HCN gene

Because adenoviruses are not persistent, the authors looked for an alternative approach to create more long-lasting pacemaker function. Given the uncertain safety of more persistent viral vectors, they decided to pursue an altogether different approach, choosing human mesenchymal stem cells (hMSCs,) an immunoprivileged readily available autologous or allogenic cell type, as the delivery platform, used electroporation to insert the HCN2 gene into the hMSCs, and demonstrated that the hMSC expressed a large I_F.[9] An additional problem, however, was faced: how would the hMSCs and the myocytes that were hoped to be stimulated interact? Current is delivered from one cell to another in the heart via local circuit currents that require gap junctions between the myocytes. The authors needed to determine whether or not hMSCs expressed connexins (the building blocks of gap junction channels) and if they would couple to adult canine ventricular cardiac myocytes. Both expression and coupling were confirmed[9,26] and more recently the authors demonstrated that a single hMSC expressing the HCN2 gene induces pacing when coupled to an adult canine ventricular myocyte.[27] Persistent biologic pacemaker function was demonstrated for 6 weeks when at least 700,000 hMSCs (approximately half carrying the HCN2 gene) were delivered to the canine left ventricular free wall.[28] The hMSCs carrying the gene showed no evidence of humoral or cellular rejection and the rhythm was catecholamine sensitive. The absence of hMSC rejection in this xenograft was not a complete surprise because these cells are known to possess some immune privilege.

Cells with a complete complement of genes

In the alternative cell therapy approach, cardiomyocytes with inherent pacemaker properties (ie, expressing a complete set of genes required for this task) are used for transplantation. Initial feasibility studies proposed evaluating the use of fetal SA nodal cells for this purpose. These studies demonstrated the ability of fetal atrial tissue (containing nodal cells) to pace the canine left ventricle.[29] Because engraftment of fetal tissue for this task seems clinically impractical because of technical and ethical limitations, efforts have shifted in recent years to identifying alternatives, such as coaxing the differentiation of stem cells to derive the necessary cardiac pacemaking cells.

To demonstrate the feasibility of this concept, the authors recently assessed the ability of human embryonic stem cell (hESC)–derived cardiomyocytes (hESC-CMs) to serve as a biologic pacemaker in the swine complete AV block mode.[10] hESCs are pluripotent stem cell lines, derived from human blastocytes, which can be propagated in the undifferentiated state in culture while retaining the capability to differentiate into cell derivatives of all three germ layers,[30] including bona fide cardiomyocytes.[31–33] More recently, the authors demonstrated that this system is not limited to the generation of isolated cardiomyocytes; rather, a functional cardiomyocyte syncytium is generated with spontaneous pacemaking activity and action potential propagation.[34] Electrophysiologic studies revealed the presence of typical action potentials and ionic transients.[33,35,36] These studies also provided mechanistic insights for the basis for spontaneous automaticity and excitability in these cells, namely, the presence of large Na^{2+} and I_f currents in face of a low-density Ik_1 current.[35]

To assess the ability of the hESC-CMs to serve as a biologic pacemaker in vivo, the authors established a swine model of slow heart rate by ablating the AV node.[10] This resulted in complete dissociation between the atrial and ventricular electric activities, mimicking the clinical scenario of patients suffering from complete AV block. A few days after transplantation of the hESC-CMs (as beating clusters because dispersed donor cells are less likely to capture the heart due to sink-source mismatches) into the pig's left ventricular myocardium, the authors could detect episodes of a new ectopic ventricular rhythm in some of the animals studied. Electrophysiologic mapping pinpointed the source of this new ventricular activity to the site of cell grafting, and histologic examination confirmed the presence of the hESC-CMs and the formation of gap junctions with host myocytes. The new ventricular pacemaker was sensitive to adrenergic stimulation because the pacing rate increased after infusion with isoproterenol. More recently, a similar conceptual study demonstrated similar results by showing the ability of enhanced green fluorescent protein-expressing hESC-CMs to pace the isolated guinea pig heart.[37]

Although the aforementioned studies provided proof-of-concept evidence for the ability to use stem cell–CMs for biologic pacemaking, they also pointed to several shortcomings. The first problem relates to the phenotype of the transplanted cells, which is thought to represent a mixture of nodal-, atrial-, and ventricular-like cells. Moreover, it is possible that with time the engrafted hESC-CMs, which display pacemaker characteristics initially, may lose this property after in vivo maturation. To this end, efforts are made to identify potential signals that may drive the cardiomyocytes differentiation of the hESC-CMs into specific subtypes. A recent study reported that that inhibition of NRG-1β/ErbB signaling greatly enhanced the proportion of hESC-CMs showing the nodal phenotype.[38] The investigators conclude that targeted manipulation of this signaling pathway may allow investigators to generate preparations of enriched working-type myocytes for infarct repair, or, conversely, nodal cells for potential use in a biologic pacemaker.

The second problem lies in the allogeneic nature of hESC-CMs transplantation. Although hESC derivatives are considered less immunogenic than adult organs, they are still expected to be rejected. Given the success of electronic pacemakers, administration of immunosupression to allow the biologic alternatives would probably be inadequate. A potential solution to this problem may lie in the recent groundbreaking induced pluripotent stem cell (iPS) technology.

In 2006, Takahashi and Yamanaka reported on their ability to reprogram mouse fibroblasts by retroviral overexpression of 4 transcription factors (Oct4, Sox2, c-Myc, and Klf4), yielding cells with characteristics similar to those of embryonic stem cells.[39] Since this initial breakthrough, the field has advanced at an amazing pace. Several groups have reproduced Yamanaka's results and also demonstrated the ability to generate iPS lines from other somatic cell types, using different sets of reprogramming factors and small molecules.[40] More recently, the ability to produce iPSCs without c-Myc, with reduced number of retroviral integration sites or even without the use of retroviruses,[41] was reported. In 2007, the first human iPSC (hiPSC) lines were described.[42,43] This was soon followed by the generation of patient-specific hiPSC lines.[44] More recently, the ability to induce differentiation of the hiPSCs into the cardiac lineage was reported by the authors' group[45] and others, yielding cardiomyocytes with the appropriate molecular, structural, and functional properties.[45–47] The ability to generate patient-specific cardiomyocytes using the iPS technology may provide a potential solution to the immunogenic hurdle associated with the clinical use of hESC-CMs for biologic pacemaking. Nevertheless, other concerns may limit the use of the iPS technology in the near future, namely, the potential risk for malignant transformation and the strict regulatory issues that may be impractical for generation of patient-specific treatments.

BIOLOGIC PACEMAKERS—NOW AND IN THE FUTURE
Current Accomplishments

The results (discussed previously) for both gene and cell approaches have demonstrated that a biologic pacemaker can be created that can achieve physiologic function for some period of time. Thus, proof of principle for biologic pacing exists. Important questions remain, however. In examining what has been achieved, there is a major difference between normal pacemaker function originating in the SA node and biologic pacing generated elsewhere. Whatever the approach taken, the anatomic structure of the SA node has not been reproduced nor has its spatial relationship and coupling to the atrium. Success should be judged not on creating a new sinus node but on replicating as closely as possible its function. In that regard, basal rates and autonomic responsiveness have been achieved that approach those generated by the SA node but, given mechanistic differences in biologic pacemaker function, several questions and challenges remain.

Future Challenges to Creating a Viable Product

The challenges fall into two categories, those related to gene therapies and cell therapies generated without a full complement of pacemaker channels and those generated by fully functional pacemaker cells.

Gene/cell therapies without a full complement of pacemaker channels

There are number of differences between the SA node and these gene and cell therapies that must be acknowledged and investigated. (1) The SA node upstroke is generated by L-type calcium current; biologic pacemaker upstroke in all gene/cell therapies in this category employ a sodium current-dependent upstroke.[48] This means that high-frequency stimulation of these pacemakers results in a substantial sodium load with the possible associated problem of sustained overdrive suppression of pacemaker function. (2) The cells generating the pacemaker function possess an I_{K1} generating a maximum diastolic potential that is more negative than that observed for SA node myocytes. I_{K1} conductance increases approximately as the square root of the external [K].[49] Pacing rate in the SA node is largely independent of external [K] because of the absence of I_{K1}; however, the pacing rate of a biologic pacemaker may depend too steeply on the plasma [K]. (3) When gene delivery employs a cellular platform, as with hMSCs, then gap junctional coupling is essential.[27] This coupling is known to be dependent on internal pH, raising the question of whether or not such a biologic pacemaker can be made that is largely insensitive to local ischemia. (4) hMSC-based delivery runs the risk of loss of function over time because these cells are known to wander from the site of implantation.

Gene/cell therapies with a full complement of pacemaker channels

With the exception of autologous SA node cells, other cellular approachs require the differentiation of pluripotent stem cells (either embryonic or iPSs). (1) These populations tend to heterogeneous and it is unclear whether or not further differentiation will occur that alters pacemaker function. (2) If embryonic stem cells are used, they are likely to provoke an immune response requiring immunosuppresion. Given the success of electronic pacemakers it is unclear that this would be an acceptable risk. (3) Both embryonic stem cells and IPS cells incur a significant risk of neoplasm if all nondifferentiated cells are not excluded. Selection procedures are not yet sufficiently developed to guarantee safety. (4) Like hMSC-based biologic pacemakers (discussed previously), the embryonic and IPS-CMs require successful gap junctional coupling to the myocytes in the neighborhood of their implantation. And it is unclear that regional ischemia that reduces gap junctional coupling would not affect their function.

REFERENCES

1. Hyman AS. Resuscitation of the stopped heart by intracardial therapy. Arch Intrn Med 1932;50:283.
2. Zoll PM. Resuscitation of the heart in ventricular standstill by external electric stimulation. N Engl J Med 1952;247:768–71.
3. Furman S, Schwedel JB. An intracardiac pacemaker for Stokes-Adams seizures. N Engl J Med 1959;261: 943–8.
4. Elmquist R, Senning A. Implantable pacemaker for the heart. In: Smyth CN, editor. Medical electronics. Springfield (IL): Thomas; 1960. p. 253.
5. Epstein AE, DiMarco JP, Ellenbogen KA, et al. ACC/AHA/HRS 2008 Guidelines for Device-Based Therapy of Cardiac Rhythm Abnormalities: a report of the American College of Cardiology/American Heart Association Task Force on Practice Guidelines (Writing Committee to Revise the ACC/AHA/NASPE 2002 Guideline Update for Implantation of Cardiac Pacemakers and Antiarrhythmia Devices): developed in collaboration with the American Association for Thoracic Surgery and Society of Thoracic Surgeons. Circulation 2008;117:e350–408.
6. Edelberg JM, Aird WC, Rosenberg RD. Enhancement of murine cardiac chronotropy by the molecular transfer of the human beta2 adrenergic receptor cDNA. J Clin Invest 1998;101:337–43.
7. Plotnikov AN, Sosunov EA, Qu J, et al. Biological pacemaker implanted in canine left bundle branch provides ventricular escape rhythms that have physiologically acceptable rates. Circulation 2004;109: 506–12.
8. Miake J, Marban E, Nuss HB. Biological pacemaker created by gene transfer. Nature 2002;419:132–3.
9. Potapova I, Plotnikov A, Lu Z, et al. Human mesenchymal stem cells as a gene delivery system to create cardiac pacemakers. Circ Res 2004;94: 952–9.

10. Kehat I, Khimovich L, Caspi O, et al. Electromechanical integration of cardiomyocytes derived from human embryonic stem cells. Nat Biotechnol 2004; 22:1282–9.

11. Edelberg JM, Huang DT, Josephson ME, et al. Molecular enhancement of porcine cardiac chronotropy. Heart 2001;86:559–62.

12. Miake J, Marban E, Nuss HB. Functional role of inward rectifier current in heart probed by Kir2.1 overexpression and dominant-negative suppression. J Clin Invest 2003;111:1529–36.

13. DiFrancesco D. The contribution of the 'pacemaker' current (if) to generation of spontaneous activity in rabbit sino-atrial node myocytes. J Physiol 1991; 434:23–40.

14. Santoro B, Liu DT, Yao H, et al. Identification of a gene encoding a hyperpolarization-activated pacemaker channel of brain. Cell 1998;93:717–29.

15. Ludwig A, Zong X, Jeglitsch M, et al. A family of hyperpolarization-activated mammalian cation channels. Nature 1998;393:587–91.

16. DiFrancesco D. A new interpretation of the pacemaker current in calf Purkinje fibres. J Physiol 1981;314:359–76.

17. DiFrancesco D, Tortora P. Direct activation of cardiac pacemaker channels by intracellular cyclic AMP. Nature 1991;351:145–7.

18. Wainger BJ, DeGennaro M, Santoro B, et al. Molecular mechanism of cAMP modulation of HCN pacemaker channels. Nature 2001;411:805–10.

19. Qu J, Plotnikov AN, Danilo P Jr, et al. Expression and function of a biological pacemaker in canine heart. Circulation 2003;107:1106–9.

20. Biel M, Schneider A, Wahl C. Cardiac HCN channels: structure, function, and modulation. Trends Cardiovasc Med 2002;12:206–12.

21. Bucchi A, Plotnikov AN, Shlapakova I, et al. Wild-type and mutant HCN channels in a tandem biological-electronic cardiac pacemaker. Circulation 2006;114:992–9.

22. Tse HF, Xue T, Lau CP, et al. Bioartificial sinus node constructed via in vivo gene transfer of an engineered pacemaker HCN Channel reduces the dependence on electronic pacemaker in a sick-sinus syndrome model. Circulation 2006;114: 1000–11.

23. Lieu DK, Chan YC, Lau CP, et al. Overexpression of HCN-encoded pacemaker current silences bioartificial pacemakers. Heart Rhythm 2008;5:1310–7.

24. Wang J, Chen S, Siegelbaum SA. Regulation of hyperpolarization-activated HCN channel gating and cAMP modulation due to interactions of COOH terminus and core transmembrane regions. J Gen Physiol 2001;118:237–50.

25. Plotnikov AN, Bucchi A, Shlapakova I, et al. HCN212-channel biological pacemakers manifesting ventricular tachyarrhythmias are responsive to treatment with I(f) blockade. Heart Rhythm 2008;5: 282–8.

26. Valiunas V, Doronin S, Valiuniene L, et al. Human mesenchymal stem cells make cardiac connexins and form functional gap junctions. J Physiol 2004; 555:617–26.

27. Valiunas V, Kanaporis G, Valiuniene L, et al. Coupling an HCN2-expressing cell top a myocyte creates a two-cell pacing unit. J Physiol 2009; 587(21):5211–26.

28. Plotnikov AN, Shlapakova I, Szabolcs MJ, et al. Xenografted adult human mesenchymal stem cells provide a platform for sustained biological pacemaker function in canine heart. Circulation 2007; 116:706–13.

29. Ruhparwar A, Tebbenjohanns J, Niehaus M, et al. Transplanted fetal cardiomyocytes as cardiac pacemaker. Eur J Cardiothorac Surg 2002;21: 853–7.

30. Thomson JA, Itskovitz-Eldor J, Shapiro SS, et al. Embryonic stem cell lines derived from human blastocysts. Science 1998;282:1145–7.

31. Kehat I, Kenyagin-Karsenti D, Snir M, et al. Human embryonic stem cells can differentiate into myocytes with structural and functional properties of cardiomyocytes. J Clin Invest 2001;108:407–14.

32. Mummery C, Ward-van Oostwaard D, Doevendans P, et al. Differentiation of human embryonic stem cells to cardiomyocytes: role of coculture with visceral endoderm-like cells. Circulation 2003;107:2733–40.

33. Xu C, Police S, Rao N, et al. Characterization and enrichment of cardiomyocytes derived from human embryonic stem cells. Circ Res 2002;91: 501–8.

34. Kehat I, Gepstein A, Spira A, et al. High-resolution electrophysiological assessment of human embryonic stem cell-derived cardiomyocytes: a novel in vitro model for the study of conduction. Circ Res 2002; 91:659–61.

35. Satin J, Kehat I, Caspi O, et al. Mechanism of spontaneous excitability in human embryonic stem cell derived cardiomyocytes. J Physiol 2004;559: 479–96.

36. He JQ, Ma Y, Lee Y, et al. Human embryonic stem cells develop into multiple types of cardiac myocytes: action potential characterization. Circ Res 2003;93:32–9.

37. Xue T, Cho HC, Akar FG, et al. Functional integration of electrically active cardiac derivatives from genetically engineered human embryonic stem cells with quiescent recipient ventricular cardiomyocytes: insights into the development of cell-based pacemakers. Circulation 2005;111:11–20.

38. Zhu WZ, Xie Y, Moyes KW, et al. Neuregulin/ErbB signaling regulates cardiac subtype specification in differentiating human embryonic stem cells. Circ Res 2010;107(6):776–86.

39. Takahashi K, Yamanaka S. Induction of pluripotent stem cells from mouse embryonic and adult fibroblast cultures by defined factors. Cell 2006;126: 663–76.

40. Huangfu D, Maehr R, Guo W, et al. Induction of pluripotent stem cells by defined factors is greatly improved by small-molecule compounds. Nat Biotechnol 2008;26:795–7.

41. Stadtfeld M, Nagaya M, Utikal J, et al. Induced pluripotent stem cells generated without viral integration. Science 2008;322:945–9.

42. Takahashi K, Tanabe K, Ohnuki M, et al. Induction of pluripotent stem cells from adult human fibroblasts by defined factors. Cell 2007;131:861–72.

43. Yu J, Vodyanik MA, Smuga-Otto K, et al. Induced pluripotent stem cell lines derived from human somatic cells. Science 2007;318:1917–20.

44. Park IH, Arora N, Huo H, et al. Disease-specific induced pluripotent stem cells. Cell 2008;134:877–86.

45. Zwi L, Caspi O, Arbel G, et al. Cardiomyocyte differentiation of human induced pluripotent stem cells. Circulation 2009;120:1513–23.

46. Haase A, Olmer R, Schwanke K, et al. Generation of induced pluripotent stem cells from human cord blood. Cell Stem Cell 2009;5:434–41.

47. Zhang J, Wilson GF, Soerens AG, et al. Functional cardiomyocytes derived from human induced pluripotent stem cells. Circ Res 2009;104:e30–41.

48. Noble D. Initiation of the heart beat. 2nd edition. Oxford (UK): Clarendon Press; 1979.

49. Sakmann B, Trube G. Conductance properties of single inwardly rectifying potassium channels in ventricular cells from guinea-pig heart. J Physiol 1984;347:641–57.

Mechanisms and Implications for Cardiac Memory

David S. Rosenbaum, MD[a],*, Darwin Jeyaraj, MD[a],
Michael R. Rosen, MD[b]

KEYWORDS

- Cardiac memory • Ventricular remodeling • T-wave
- Signaling pathway

The electrocardiographic T-wave is a summation of repolarization gradients in the ventricle. Although the QT interval provides an index of the duration of repolarization, changes in T-wave polarity reflect a physiologically or pathologically altered repolarization state. Myocardial ischemia is a common clinical cause of T-wave changes. However, there are various causes for changes in T-wave polarity. Classical electrocardiographers defined 2 general types of T-wave change. Secondary T-wave changes were rigorously dependent on an altered QRS complex in various settings, including myocardial infarction, heart failure, or hypertrophy. All these involved an altered activation pattern of the ventricle resulting from what is now called structural remodeling. In contrast, primary T-wave changes occurred independently of a change in the QRS complex and in the absence of overt structural remodeling (eg, an ion channelopathy that represents another type of remodeling, in this case, of myocardial repolarization).

In 1982, Mauricio Rosenbaum and colleagues[1] described an additional form of T-wave change: here, the T-wave took on vectorial characteristics determined by altered QRS complexes, but, the T-wave changes persisted long after the QRS complex had returned to its prior baseline. In keeping with the terminology of the time, Rosenbaum referred to the T-wave change as "pseudoprimary," suggesting that it might derive from altered electrotonus among cardiac cells. He coined the term "cardiac memory," because the T-wave seemed to "remember" the preceding QRS complex (**Fig. 1**).[1] In his initial descriptions, cardiac memory could last for long intervals and was considered a benign electrocardiographic (ECG) change, albeit one that could be confused with signs of ischemia. A far greater complexity has been discovered in the ensuing years.

The complexity can begin to be resolved if one accepts that in normal hearts of all species studied, there is great plasticity of repolarization throughout life. This derives from developmental changes in ion channels and receptor systems that influence the inward and outward currents occurring during the action potential and that are the building blocks of the T-wave. If one considers the T-wave and its underlying currents at birth to be a reference point for the evolution of repolarization, then there is modeling throughout subsequent life. Such modeling has generally (and unfortunately) been referred to as remodeling, "unfortunately" because it removes specificity from the word "remodeling." Remodeling implies that modeling has already occurred. Moreover, in various settings, remodeling represents a return to a fetal or neonatal electrophysiologic program.

This study was supported by National Institutes of Health grants KO8-HL094660 (Darwin Jeyaraj), RO1-HL54807 (David S. Rosenbaum), and RO1-HL067101 and HL094410 (Michael R. Rosen).
a The Heart and Vascular Center, MetroHealth Campus of Case Western Reserve University, 2500 MetroHealth Drive, Hamman Building, Room H330, Cleveland, OH 44109, USA
b Center for Molecular Therapeutics, Columbia University Medical Center, 630 West 168 Street, PH 7W-321, New York, NY 10032, USA
* Corresponding author.
E-mail address: drosenbaum@metrohealth.org

Card Electrophysiol Clin 3 (2011) 77–85
doi:10.1016/j.ccep.2010.10.015

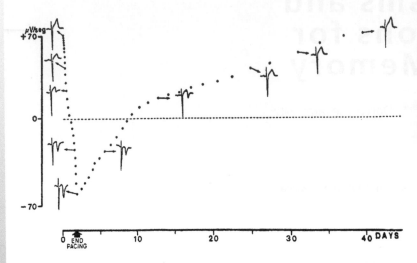

Fig. 1. Time course of evolution and resolution of T-wave memory. There is persistent change in the polarity of the T-wave after ventricular pacing. The T-wave returns to its normal shape after several weeks. (*Adapted from* Rosenbaum MB, Blanco HH, Elizari MV, et al. Electrotonic modulation of the T-wave and cardiac memory. Am J Cardiol 1982; 50(2):213–22; with permission.)

As generically described, remodeling can derive from physiologic events, such as growth and development, or pathologic events, as in hypertrophy or infarction. In the latter context, remodeling of cardiac repolarization persists after the perturbation that induced it has stabilized. Within the universe of remodeling, cardiac memory fills a specific and narrow niche; it is still defined per Rosenbaum's terminology; the T-wave change must follow that of an abnormal QRS and must persist even after the QRS has reverted to normal. However, based on information that follows, cardiac memory probably occupies an interface between physiologic and pathologic change. If it can be understood and defined adequately as a signal, it may be understood to be a harbinger of change, which might require reversing and might be found more readily reversible than that of the more overt remodeling accompanying clinically apparent disease.

In this article, the physiologic/pathophysiologic factors triggering the remodeling of cardiac repolarization that characterizes cardiac memory are considered. The authors discuss the ionic/molecular signaling mechanisms that transduce triggering stimuli to functional changes in ion channels, which influence repolarization. Finally, clinical implications of cardiac memory are considered. Because the field is an evolving one, clear conclusions have not been reached in certain areas—not based on experimental data, because the authors share the belief that the experiment is always right, but on interpretation of the meaning of these data. Much more fruitful research is needed if the end of this story is to be reached.

TRIGGERING MECHANISMS FOR INDUCING CARDIAC MEMORY

In querying the mechanisms responsible for cardiac memory, one encounters a complex sequence of events. Using ventricular or AV sequential electrical pacing as a simple means to induce memory, the input signal is the paced impulse causing an alteration in activation pathway and the output signal is the altered T-wave, which persists in its anomalous pattern for variable intervals after activation has normalized. The next level of complexity arises from the understanding that the altered myocardial contraction induced by the abnormal activation pathway is critical to initiating the remodeling events of cardiac memory.

Broadly, 2 types of cardiac memory come to clinical attention based on the duration of the perturbation: short-term and long-term. In his classic study of cardiac memory, Mauricio Rosenbaum and colleagues[1] found a direct correlation between duration of altered activation and persistence of cardiac memory in human subjects. Even brief periods of altered activation are sufficient to induce memory. Inciting events commonly include transient left bundle branch block, brief episodes of tachyarrhythmias, temporary cardiac pacing, or, in patients with Wolff-Parkinson-White (WPW) syndrome, intermittent pre-excitation. After these transient events, the duration of memory is also brief and hence termed "short-term memory." In contrast, in patients with persistent pre-excitation, chronic pacing, or prolonged tachycardia, the memory changes are evident for days to months and are referred to as "long-term memory."

Two triggering mechanisms have been found to modulate myocardial repolarization in response to altered activation. One is related to electrotonic current flow generated by the activating impulse, such that after a focal pacemaker discharge, current flow from myocyte to myocyte moving downstream from the pacing electrode results in shortening of action potential duration (APD) in the direction of propagation. For example, in isolated rabbit hearts, prolongation of APD occurs in regions adjacent to site of pacing, whereas shortening in the direction of propagation is seen within minutes of onset of altered activation.[2] These findings are also observed in the isolated canine ventricular myocardium, in which action potential prolongation occurs in regions adjacent to the pacing site.[3] Although these changes begin within minutes to hours, they persist even after a normal activation sequence is restored and represent a trigger for inducing ventricular electrical remodeling.[4,5] This form of remodeling alters regional and transmural gradients of repolarization in isolated myocardial tissues.[5,6] Further, the characteristic action potential remodeling in memory incorporates attenuation of the epicardial phase1 notch, because of reduced expression of the transient outward current (I_{to}).[4] Changes in electrotonic load also play an important role in the remodeling of I_{to}.[7] Consequently, myocytes adjacent to the source of altered activation exhibit attenuation of the epicardial phase1 notch and prolongation of the APD.

A second triggering mechanism impacting on cardiac memory derives from the impact of altered myocardial stress-strain relationships on downstream signaling processes. Jeyaraj and colleagues[8] recently explored this mechanism after long-term pacing of the canine ventricle. This model manifests a persistent and progressive inversion of the T-wave polarity after pacing from the anterior left ventricle (LV; **Fig. 2**). After the induction of memory, 2 distinct patterns of action potential remodeling are seen using optical imaging of action potentials from multiple LV segments. The segment proximal to the pacing site, that is, the early-activated anterior region, exhibits significant attenuation of the epicardial phase1 notch with modest action potential prolongation (**Fig. 3**). In contrast, the region distal to the site of altered activation, that is, the late-activated posterior region, shows marked APD prolongation with minimal changes in action potential morphology (see **Fig. 3**). Clearly, remodeling in the late-activated region cannot be explained by an electrotonic mechanism, which would predict progressive shortening of the APD in the direction of propagation.

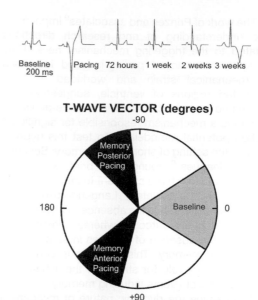

Fig. 2. Cardiac memory from a canine model of pacing (A) ECG after cessation of pacing illustrates progressive change in T-wave polarity during normal sinus activation. (B) Note that the T-wave vector changes after anterior or posterior LV pacing are distinct, indicating underlying regional remodeling that depends on the anatomic origin of altered activation. (*Adapted from* Jeyaraj D, Wilson LD, Zhong J, et al. Mechanoelectrical feedback as novel mechanism of cardiac electrical remodeling. Circulation 2007; 115(25):3145–55; with permission.)

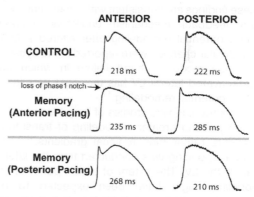

Fig. 3. Action potential remodeling in cardiac memory. Optically measured epicardial action potentials from the early and late-activated regions after 4 weeks of LV pacing from the anterior LV. There was significant attenuation of the epicardial phase1 notch and action potential prolongation in the early-activated anterior LV. In the late-activated posterior LV region, APD was markedly prolonged. The converse was noted when memory was induced from the posterior LV. (*Adapted from* Jeyaraj D, Wilson LD, Zhong J, et al. Mechanoelectrical feedback as novel mechanism of cardiac electrical remodeling. Circulation 2007;115(25):3145–55; with permission.)

The work of Prinzen and associates[9] impacts on the understanding of and research directions related to the triggering mechanism here. They described ventricular pacing-induced increases in mechanical strain and workload in late-activated regions of ventricle, suggesting that enhanced mechanical strain in the late-activated region is a mechanism responsible for significant action potential remodeling. To test this hypothesis, in the setting of short-term memory, Sosunov and colleagues[10] found that brief periods of myocardial stretch are sufficient to induce cardiac memory in the isolated, Langendorff-perfused rabbit heart. Stretch in the absence of altered activation affects this outcome, whereas altering activation in the absence of changes in stretch does not induce memory. This outcome is consistent with a primary role for stretch in the initiation of the cascade of events inducing memory.

To examine the dynamic nature of myocardial strain in triggering remodeling, Jeyaraj and colleagues[8] induced memory by pacing the posterior wall of the canine LV. In this case, a unique change in the T-wave vector of the heart in situ (see **Fig. 2**) is accompanied by marked action potential prolongation in the late activated anterior regions studied as an isolated preparation (see **Fig. 3**). An important consequence of the marked prolongation of regional APD is a significant increase in regional repolarization gradients, which was interpreted as responsible for the marked T-wave inversions characteristic of cardiac memory. These findings are consistent with a mechanoelectrical feedback mechanism underlying regional action potential remodeling after altered activation. Similar changes were reported in the dyssynchronous model of heart failure in which the late-activated lateral LV has the most prominent action potential remodeling.[11]

In contrast, in vivo studies of long-term cardiac memory found greater remodeling of transmural gradients rather than regional gradients.[12,13] In this case, pacing was conducted from the lateral wall of the LV. The extent of action potential remodeling might have been expected to be maximal in the septal region but was not measured. Studies using the same techniques in the setting of short-term memory demonstrated the major gradient change to be apicobasal rather than transmural.[14] All these studies demonstrate that (1) changes in mechanical contraction patterns of the myocardium are central to triggering the action potential remodeling that occurs following altered activation and (2) changes in transmural and regional gradients of myocardial repolarization reflect the reality of memory accumulation and the pacing protocol,

the species of animal, and the experimental method used.

SIGNALING AND IONIC MECHANISMS UNDERLYING CARDIAC MEMORY

This section examines mechanisms through which the aforementioned biophysical and mechanical processes converge to modulate expression and function of repolarizing ion channels. At this point, a rich network of cellular processes are engaged that combine to result in a T-wave change that reflects remodeling. As explained earlier, specific myocardial regions exhibit remodeling based on the proximity to the source of altered activation. The molecular and signaling mechanisms have largely been studied in the early-activated region. Remodeling of the late-activated region remains poorly understood and is an area of active investigation in the authors' and other laboratories. The cellular events that occur in cardiac memory are summarized in **Fig. 4**, where they are subdivided into short-term processes involving trafficking of ion channels and long-term processes involving gene transcription.

Short-Term Memory

As reviewed earlier, a key factor in engaging memory is the change in stretch on myocytes. Memory seems to be induced even in the absence of altered activation if stretch is changed during the cardiac cycle.[10] This has been shown to alter the T-wave and activate the immediate early gene program.[15] One result of altered stretch is an increase in synthesis and release of angiotensin II (see **Fig. 4**), initially demonstrated in cells in culture, in which the source of the angiotensin II is the myocytes and/or fibroblasts present.[16] Later, assays of tissue angiotensin II levels in the hearts of dogs paced for 2 hours have similarly shown an increase in angiotensin II levels.[17] Moreover, preadministration of angiotensin-converting enzyme (ACE) inhibitors or angiotensin II receptor blockers prevent the short-term evolution of the T-wave changes and delays (but does not ultimately prevent) the long-term changes in repolarization induced by pacing.[18] That the angiotensin II derives from myocardial tissue synthesis and release is supported by the observation that chymostatin, a tissue protease inhibitor, also suppresses the short-term evolution of the T-wave changes.[18] Because myocardial tissue chymase is active in angiotensin II synthesis, the suppression of memory by chymostatin argues against circulating angiotensin II and in favor of the locally synthesized hormone in the initiation

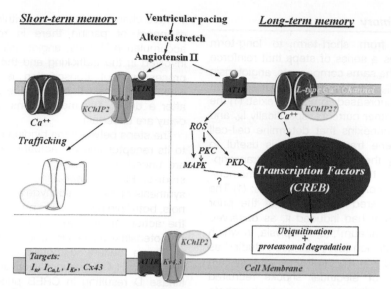

Fig. 4. Overview of signaling and molecular mechanisms in cardiac memory. See text for description. (*Modified from* Ozgen N, Rosen MR. Cardiac memory: a work in progress. Heart Rhythm 2009;6(4):564–70; with permission.)

of cardiac memory. Also important in these early changes of cardiac memory is the role of calcium (see **Fig. 4**): indeed, L-type calcium (Ca) channel blockade, like angiotensin II receptor blockade, ACE inhibition, or chymostatin administration, prevents the onset of short-term memory.[19]

If we accept the need for angiotensin II in the short-term evolution of memory, does repolarization change and what changes in repolarizing currents are engaged? Repolarization is altered creating an apicobasal gradient in the epicardium of intact dogs paced for 2 hours from the LV epicardium, which has been shown in situ using monophasic action potential (MAP) recordings.[14] The basis for reducing the action potential notch in these experiments seems to involve angiotensin II and the transient outward current, I_{to} (see **Fig. 4**).[20] Experiments performed in cell lines have demonstrated that the angiotensin II type 1 (AT-1) receptor forms a macromolecular complex with Kv4.3 and K+ channel interacting protein 2 (KChIP2), respectively, the pore-forming unit and an accessory protein that combine to generate I_{to}.[21] The tight association of these 3 components has been demonstrated in coimmunoprecipitation experiments in the myocardium as well as via fluorescence resonance emission tomography.[20] Although the macromolecular complex resides in the cell membrane under basal conditions, exposure to angiotensin II results in its internalization. With this internalization, there is a loss of I_{to}, which would alter the voltage-time course of repolarization. Studies of epicardial myocytes disaggregated from the canine heart and

incubated with angiotensin II have demonstrated a loss of I_{to} and the action potential notch.[21] Endocardial myocytes have little to no I_{to} and are unresponsive to angiotensin II incubation.[21] However, incubation with the AT-1 receptor blocker, losartan, results in the appearance of an action potential notch.[21] This suggests the presence of high native angiotensin II levels near the endocardium and low levels epicardially. Supporting the existence of such a gradient are preliminary data showing a transmural gradient for angiotensinogen (Ira S. Cohen, unpublished data). The primacy of I_{to} in the initiation of short-term memory is seen in the observation that memory is not inducible in neonatal dogs in which there is no I_{to}.[22] With maturation and the appearance of I_{to}, the ability to induce memory evolves.

The changes in I_{to} induced by angiotensin II are not associated with alterations in messenger RNA (mRNA) for Kv4.3. This supports the concept that the altered repolarization is the outcome of a translational process, with the occurrence of trafficking, as described earlier. Further support is provided by observations referable to the tubulin network, an important thoroughfare for trafficking. Although still in preliminary form, it seems that colchicine, which inhibits tubulin polymerization, prevents the evolution of the T-wave changes in short-term cardiac memory.[23] More needs be done to understand the spectrum of events involved in short-term memory; whether other ion channels play a role, and if so, in what way remains to be determined.

Long-Term Memory

The transition from short-term to long-term memory involves a series of steps that reinforce the loss of I_{to}. The same components, angiotensin II, calcium, and I_{to}, are involved at the outset, but at least 2 levels of increased complexity exist: (1) the involvement of other currents, specifically I_{Kr} and $I_{Ca,L}$ and the connexins that determine cell-cell coupling; (2) gene transcription. It is useful to understand why the search began for transcriptional changes in the setting of cardiac memory. This was the outcome of 2 observations: (1) The T-wave "remembered" the vector of the prior QRS complex that had induced it, as observed by Mauricio Rosenbaum[1]; (2) In Aplysia, in which long-term potentiation (LTP) has been studied as a form of memory in the central nervous system (CNS), delivery of electrical shocks recruited synthesis of the cyclic adenosine monophosphate (cAMP) response element binding protein (CREB), an important transcription factor, as observed by Kandel.[24] It was hypothesized that if there were a commonality of mechanism between memory in the CNS and that in muscle, then CREB might also be important in the latter. The interest in a role for CREB was heightened by the knowledge that there is a cAMP response element binding site near the promoter regions of Kv4.3 and KChIP2.[25] However, this is where the association between memory in the CNS and that in the heart breaks down. Specifically, with electrical shock and the increase in LTP seen in Aplysia, there is an increase in CREB synthesis and a strengthening of protein-protein associations in neural synaptic regions.[24] In contrast, pacing the heart results in reduction in CREB levels and with this, a reduction in the ion channel proteins of interest (with KChIP2 having been the one most studied).[25] The CREB reduction begins rapidly after the onset of pacing, and by 2 hours, it is clearly demonstrable, as is reduction in KChIP2 protein levels.[25]

The primacy of CREB here is best seen in experiments designed to test whether the CREB reduction and the loss of I_{to} are epiphenomena resulting from pacing and/or altered stretch. Experiments in which the canine myocardium was injected with a CREB antisense virus, in situ, showed that they are not epiphenomena. Four days later, MAP recordings of epicardial action potentials in injected regions showed no notches, and myocytes disaggregated from the injected region showed no I_{to}.[26] In contrast, noninjected regions show normal CREB levels, action potential notches, and robust I_{to}. Although 2 hours after onset of pacing, angiotensin II receptor blockade or L-type Ca channel blockade prevents the CREB reduction and the

T-wave changes of memory, within 1 to 2 weeks of onset of pacing there is robust memory accumulation.[19] Thus, angiotensin II and Ca are involved in the trafficking and the transcriptional processes, but transcription is initiated even when angiotensin II and Ca are blocked, albeit after a delay. The mechanisms involved in this delay are uncertain.

The steps between the binding of angiotensin II to its receptor and the actual reduction in CREB are uncertain but have been clarified in recent studies. Pacing the canine heart results in the synthesis of malondialdehyde and 4-hydroxyalkenols, both lipid peroxidation products derived from the action of reactive oxygen species (ROS).[17] Angiotensin II initiates ROS synthesis, and studies in tissue culture demonstrate that hydrogen peroxide (H_2O_2) induces activation of protein kinase D resulting in CREB phosphorylation at serine 133 and the downregulation of CREB.[27] Adenoviral delivery of a small interfering RNA that decreases PKD1 expression prevents the CREB decrease, emphasizing that PKD1 is critical to the process. A general pathway for CREB removal is its ubiquitination and proteasomal degradation. Studies of the canine heart have demonstrated that the ubiquitination of CREB and the proteasomal inhibitor, lactacystin, prevent the CREB reduction induced by H_2O_2 in culture as well as that induced by pacing the heart in situ.[28]

The impact of CREB reduction on I_{to} in the setting of long-term memory is profound, with changes being seen in the kinetics and the magnitude of the current. These changes occur nonuniformly in the myocardium. With LV free wall epicardial pacing, epicardial I_{to} density is reduced, while activation occurs at more positive potentials and recovery from inactivation is slower than in control myocytes.[4] The outcome in the setting of long-term memory is an action potential notch that is reduced in amplitude and that, in effect, alters the "set point" of the depolarizing ($I_{Ca,L}$) and repolarizing (I_{Kr} and I_{Ks}) currents that follow.[19,29] The action potential in this setting manifests a higher plateau and a longer duration than normal.[4] Changes are marked near the pacing site, and MAP mapping experiments in situ demonstrate a variable distribution at more distant sites that may reflect regions in which strain has been altered (as discussed earlier). In this setting as well, there is the appearance of a transmural gradient for repolarization, with epicardium becoming longer than endocardium.[13]

In long-term memory, epicardial and endocardial action potentials show elevated plateaus and prolonged APD near the pacing site, highlighting that channels other than I_{to} contribute to the action potential changes. Given that the endocardium has little or no I_{to}, the importance of other ion currents, such as I_{CaL}[19] and I_{Kr},[29] become apparent. Of interest in considering these other ion channel changes is the impact of one of the protein subunits responsible for I_{to}, KChIP2, on L-type calcium current. $I_{Ca,L}$ shows no change in density in long-term memory; but its activation is more positive and its time constants of inactivation are longer in memory than in control hearts.[19] These types of changes can well contribute to increased plateau height. A recent study has demonstrated that KChIP2 is an accessory protein influencing $I_{Ca,L}$.[30] Although performed in KChIP2 knockout mice and not canine hearts, the implications of the effect of KChIP2 for other mammalian species are clear.[30] Current density in the KChIP2 knockout mice is reduced, and molecular studies indicate that KChIP2 binds to the N-terminal inhibitory module of the CaV1.2 α-1C subunit to augment $I_{Ca,L}$ density. This occurs with no increase in CaV1.2 protein expression or trafficking to the cell membrane. Clearly, the change in $I_{Ca,l}$ density in the mouse is at odds with the change in kinetics in the dog; however, this may reflect a species difference in the protein subunit interactions that occur. KChIP2 has an accessory protein function for I_{Na}.[31] However, this current has not been studied in cardiac memory, so the implications of the association are uncertain.

Changes in the delayed rectifier current (I_{Kr}) also have been shown in long-term memory.[29] In noninstrumented, control dogs and sham-instrumented, atrially paced dogs, I_{Kr} density as well as the mRNA and protein of its α subunit, ERG, manifest a transmural gradient with current density and ERG expression in epicardium greater than endocardium.[29] In the setting of long-term memory, the transmural gradients of I_{Kr}, message, and protein are reversed.[29,32] Also, I_{Kr}-blocking drugs attenuate cardiac memory induction. Because ERG does not have a cAMP response element, other transcription pathways have been sought here. A promising factor in preliminary studies is activator protein-1, (AP-1; N Ozgen, M Rosen, preliminary data), which incorporates either a Jun-Jun homodimer or Jun-Fos heterodimer. Preliminary studies show transmural gradients (epicardium>endocardium) for c-Jun and c-Fos mRNA in canine LV free wall. These gradients are lost during ventricular pacing.

Finally, the gap junctional protein, connexin43 (C×43), shows major changes in the setting of cardiac memory. C×43 distribution becomes lateralized and C×43 density is reduced in long-term memory. The greatest changes occur in the region of the pacing electrode.[33] These changes might indicate some alteration in electrotonic coupling in cardiac memory. Although coupling has not been studied directly in this setting, in his initial considerations regarding the causes of memory, Mauricio Rosenbaum hypothesized altered coupling to be of paramount importance.[1]

CLINICAL IMPLICATIONS

Elucidation of cardiac memory based on a history of altered activation due to pacing or tachyarrhythmia was initially used to exclude ischemia as a cause of inverted ECG T-waves. However, in the last 2 decades, this view of memory as an epiphenomenon has started to change, arising from a greater understanding of the biophysical, cellular, and molecular remodeling of myocytes during altered activation, as described in the earlier sections. Chatterjee and colleagues[34] first noted that the disposition of cardiac memory on the surface ECG depends on the source of the altered activation. As described earlier, there are at least two distinct triggers, electrotonic effects and mechanical strain, that are operative in different regions of the heart during altered activation. An interplay of these 2 mechanisms probably underlies the regional remodeling of repolarization in cardiac memory. This is also evident after ablation of an accessory pathway in WPW syndrome, in which the ECG leads with the most prominent T-wave changes can be correlated with the anatomic position of the accessory pathway.[35] In summary, these observations reaffirm the regional nature of the remodeling response that is mediated by distinct triggers that modulate myocardial repolarization.

Recent clinical studies have provided a better appreciation of the clinical time course of the onset and resolution of memory. Wecke and colleagues[36] found that significant memory was induced in human subjects within one week of onset of ventricular pacing, resolving within a month after cessation of pacing. Memory was also associated with significant changes in noninvasive indices of myocardial repolarization, eg, Tpeak-end.[37] An objective method of distinguishing cardiac memory from myocardial ischemia would be of great clinical value. Shvilkin and colleagues[38] identified T-wave vector changes that could be used to discriminate repolarization patterns of cardiac memory from those induced by myocardial ischemia. The remodeling processes initiated by alteration of electrical activation sequence, as in ventricular pacing, may play a significant role in the deleterious effects of cardiac pacing. Conversely, restoration of normal ventricular activation by cardiac resynchronization therapy may reverse ventricular electrical remodeling and partially explain some of the beneficial effects of this therapy.

SUMMARY

In this article, the authors summarize their understanding of the electrophysiological basis for the form of ventricular electrical remodeling, often manifest clinically as cardiac memory. Further, they have outlined initiating mechanisms, signaling pathways, and transcription factors that play a role in cardiac memory. The evidence highlights the considerable plasticity of cardiac muscle in response to various physiologic stimuli. However, several aspects of ventricular electrical remodeling remain to be explored. The mechanisms through which the myocyte transduces altered activation would be key to understanding the potential signaling pathways. Although the angiotensin II pathway has an important role, the other pathways or transcription factors involved in memory remain to be identified. The authors have also provided insights into the highly regional nature of ventricular remodeling. Elucidation of the ionic, molecular, and signaling pathways operative in specific regions will enhance development of pharmacologic, biologic, and device therapies to ameliorate cardiac remodeling or possibly induce reverse remodeling where therapeutically beneficial.

REFERENCES

1. Rosenbaum MB, Blanco HH, Elizari MV, et al. Electrotonic modulation of the T wave and cardiac memory. Am J Cardiol 1982;50(2):213–22.
2. Costard-Jackle A, Goetsch B, Antz M, et al. Slow and long-lasting modulation of myocardial repolarization produced by ectopic activation in isolated rabbit hearts. Evidence for cardiac "memory". Circulation 1989;80(5):1412–20.
3. Geller JC, Rosen MR. Persistent T-wave changes after alteration of the ventricular activation sequence. New insights into cellular mechanisms of 'cardiac memory'. Circulation 1993;88(4 Pt 1):1811–9.
4. Yu H, McKinnon D, Dixon JE, et al. Transient outward current, Ito1, is altered in cardiac memory. Circulation 1999;99(14):1898–905.
5. Libbus I, Rosenbaum DS. Transmural action potential changes underlying ventricular electrical remodeling. J Cardiovasc Electrophysiol 2003;14(4):394–402.
6. Shvilkin A, Danilo P Jr, Wang J, et al. Evolution and resolution of long term cardiac memory. Circulation 1998;97(18):1810–7.
7. Libbus I, Wan X, Rosenbaum DS. Electrotonic load triggers remodeling of repolarizing current Ito in ventricle. Am J Physiol Heart Circ Physiol 2004;286(5):H1901–9.
8. Jeyaraj D, Wilson LD, Zhong J, et al. Mechanoelectrical feedback as novel mechanism of cardiac electrical remodeling. Circulation 2007;115(25):3145–55.
9. Prinzen FW, Hunter WC, Wyman BT, et al. Mapping of regional myocardial strain and work during ventricular pacing: experimental study using magnetic resonance imaging tagging. J Am Coll Cardiol 1999;33(6):1735–42.
10. Sosunov EA, Anyukhovsky EP, Rosen MR. Altered ventricular stretch contributes to initiation of cardiac memory. Heart Rhythm 2008;5(1):106–13.
11. Aiba T, Hesketh GG, Barth AS, et al. Electrophysiological consequences of dyssynchronous heart failure and its restoration by resynchronization therapy. Circulation 2009;119(9):1220–30.
12. Opthof T, Coronel R, Wilms-Schopman FJ, et al. Dispersion of repolarization in canine ventricle and the electrocardiographic T wave: Tp-e interval does not reflect transmural dispersion. Heart Rhythm 2007;4(3):341–8.
13. Coronel R, Opthof T, Plotnikov AN, et al. Long-term cardiac memory in canine heart is associated with the evolution of a transmural repolarization gradient. Cardiovasc Res 2007;74(3):416–25.
14. Janse MJ, Sosunov EA, Coronel R, et al. Repolarization gradients in the canine left ventricle before and after induction of short-term cardiac memory. Circulation 2005;112(12):1711–8.
15. Meghji P, Nazir SA, Dick DJ, et al. Regional workload induced changes in electrophysiology and immediate early gene expression in intact in situ porcine heart. J Mol Cell Cardiol 1997;29(11):3147–55.
16. Sadoshima J, Xu Y, Slayter HS, et al. Autocrine release of angiotensin II mediates stretch-induced hypertrophy of cardiac myocytes in vitro. Cell 1993;75(5):977–84.
17. Ozgen N, Lau DH, Shlapakova IN, et al. Determinants of CREB degradation and KChIP2 gene transcription in cardiac memory. Heart Rhythm 2010;7(7):964–70.
18. Ricard P, Danilo P Jr, Cohen IS, et al. A role for the renin-angiotensin system in the evolution of cardiac memory. J Cardiovasc Electrophysiol 1999;10(4):545–51.
19. Plotnikov AN, Yu H, Geller JC, et al. Role of L-type calcium channels in pacing-induced short-term and long-term cardiac memory in canine heart. Circulation 2003;107(22):2844–9.
20. Doronin SV, Potapova IA, Lu Z, et al. Angiotensin receptor type 1 forms a complex with the transient outward potassium channel Kv4.3 and regulates its

gating properties and intracellular localization. J Biol Chem 2004;279(46):48231—7.

21. Yu H, Gao J, Wang H, et al. Effects of the renin-angiotensin system on the current I(to) in epicardial and endocardial ventricular myocytes from the canine heart. Circ Res 2000;86(10):1062—8.

22. Plotnikov AN, Sosunov EA, Patberg KW, et al. Cardiac memory evolves with age in association with development of the transient outward current. Circulation 2004;110(5):489—95.

23. Ozgen NLD, Shlapakova IN, Danilo P Jr, et al. Ventricular pacing regionally reduces KChIP2 in intact cardiomyocyte membranes, and this is reduced by angiotensin II receptor blockade or disruption of microtubular polymerization. Heart Rhythm 2010;7:S411.

24. Kandel ER. The molecular biology of memory storage: a dialogue between genes and synapses. Science 2001;294(5544):1030—8.

25. Patberg KW, Rosen MR. On the role of the cAMP response element binding protein in long-term cardiac memory. Circ Res 2003;93(9):e87.

26. Patberg KW, Obreztchikova MN, Giardina SF, et al. The cAMP response element binding protein modulates expression of the transient outward current: implications for cardiac memory. Cardiovasc Res 2005;68(2):259—67.

27. Ozgen N, Guo J, Gertsberg Z, et al. Reactive oxygen species decrease cAMP response element binding protein expression in cardiomyocytes via a protein kinase D1-dependent mechanism that does not require Ser133 phosphorylation. Mol Pharmacol 2009;76(4):896—902.

28. Ozgen NLD, Shlapakova IN, Sherman W, et al. The decreased CREB level determining K channel transcription in cardiac memory results from its ubiquitination and subsequent proteasomal degradation. Heart Rhythm 2008;5:S358.

29. Obreztchikova MN, Patberg KW, Plotnikov AN, et al. I(Kr) contributes to the altered ventricular repolarization that determines long-term cardiac memory. Cardiovasc Res 2006;71(1):88—96.

30. Thomsen MB, Wang C, Ozgen N, et al. Accessory subunit KChIP2 modulates the cardiac L-type calcium current. Circ Res 2009;104(12):1382—9.

31. Deschenes I, Armoundas AA, Jones SP, et al. Post-transcriptional gene silencing of KChIP2 and Navbeta1 in neonatal rat cardiac myocytes reveals a functional association between Na and Ito currents. J Mol Cell Cardiol 2008;45(3):336—46.

32. Obreztchikova MN, Sosunov EA, Plotnikov A, et al. Developmental changes in IKr and IKs contribute to age-related expression of dofetilide effects on repolarization and proarrhythmia. Cardiovasc Res 2003;59(2):339—50.

33. Patel PM, Plotnikov A, Kanagaratnam P, et al. Altering ventricular activation remodels gap junction distribution in canine heart. J Cardiovasc Electrophysiol 2001;12(5):570—7.

34. Chatterjee K, Harris AM, Davies JG, et al. T-wave changes after artificial pacing. Lancet 1969;1(7598):759—60.

35. Geller JC, Carlson MD, Goette A, et al. Persistent T-wave changes after radiofrequency catheter ablation of an accessory connection (Wolff-parkinson-white syndrome) are caused by "cardiac memory". Am Heart J 1999;138(5 Pt 1):987—93.

36. Wecke L, Gadler F, Linde C, et al. Temporal characteristics of cardiac memory in humans: vectorcardiographic quantification in a model of cardiac pacing. Heart Rhythm 2005;2(1):28—34.

37. Wecke L, Rubulis A, Lundahl G, et al. Right ventricular pacing-induced electrophysiological remodeling in the human heart and its relationship to cardiac memory. Heart Rhythm 2007;4(12):1477—86.

38. Shvilkin A, Ho KK, Rosen MR, et al. T-vector direction differentiates postpacing from ischemic T-wave inversion in precordial leads. Circulation 2005;111(8):969—74.

Calcium Channel Dysfunction in Inherited Cardiac Arrhythmia Syndromes

Martin Tristani-Firouzi, MD[a],*, Susan P. Etheridge, MD[b]

KEYWORDS

- Channelopathy • Long QT syndrome • Autism • Arrhythmia
- Sudden death

The first case of Timothy syndrome (TS) was reported in 1992 in a German report describing an infant with a 2:1 atrioventricular (AV) block, prolonged QT interval, syndactyly, and subsequent sudden death.[1] The association between severe long QT syndrome and syndactyly was then defined in a small cohort of 3 patients, 2 of whom died of ventricular fibrillation.[2] Mutations in the known long QT (LQT) syndrome genes and in the coding sequence of the cardiac L-type calcium channel $Ca_v1.2$ were excluded in this population. Subsequently, novel alternatively spliced $Ca_v1.2$ isoforms were described, and a mutation in a splice variant was identified in a cohort of patients with TS.[3]

THE MOLECULAR PHYSIOLOGY OF L-TYPE CALCIUM CHANNELS

L-type voltage-gated calcium channels are heteromeric protein complexes composed of $\alpha1$, $\alpha2/\delta$, β, and, in some tissues, γ subunits. The primary subunit $\alpha1$ forms the voltage-sensitive functional pore structure[4,5] and is composed of 4 homologous domains (I–IV), each of which contains 6 putative transmembrane segments (S1–S6). CACNA1C encodes the α_{1C} subunit ($Ca_v1.2$),

which is widely expressed in a variety of tissues, including the heart and brain. CACNA1C spans 640 kb and comprises 50 exons.[6] CACNA1C undergoes extensive alternative splicing, thereby imparting tissue-specific and physiologically distinct calcium current properties.[6,7] In the heart, CACNA1C undergoes mutually exclusive splicing of exon 8. Both exons 8 and 8a encode the S6 segment in domain I, which is 1 of the 4 transmembrane segments that line the channel pore (**Fig. 1**). Approximately 23% of L-type calcium channels in the heart are encoded by the exon 8a variant, with 77% encoded by exon 8.[3] This differential expression has implications for the severity of TS symptoms, as is discussed later.

L-type calcium channels are critical for normal excitation-contraction coupling by providing the initial calcium influx that triggers a secondary release of calcium from the sarcoplasmic reticulum (ie, calcium-induced calcium release). This initial calcium influx also provides depolarizing current during the plateau phase of the ventricular action potential, and thus, changes in the L-type calcium current can ultimately affect the duration of the QT interval. For example, gain-of-function mutations in genes encoding the L-type calcium channel

The authors have nothing to disclose.
[a] Division of Pediatric Cardiology and the Nora Eccles Harrison Cardiovascular Research and Training Institute, University of Utah School of Medicine, Pediatric Cardiology Suite 1500 PCMC, 100 North Medical Drive, Salt Lake City, UT 84113, USA
[b] Division of Pediatric Cardiology and the Nora Eccles Harrison, University of Utah School of Medicine, Pediatric Cardiology Suite 1500 PCMC, 100 North Medical Drive, Salt Lake City, UT 84113, USA
* Corresponding author.
E-mail address: mfirouzi@cvrti.utah.edu

Card Electrophysiol Clin 3 (2011) 87–92
doi:10.1016/j.ccep.2010.11.002
1877-9182/11/$ – see front matter © 2011 Elsevier Inc. All rights reserved.

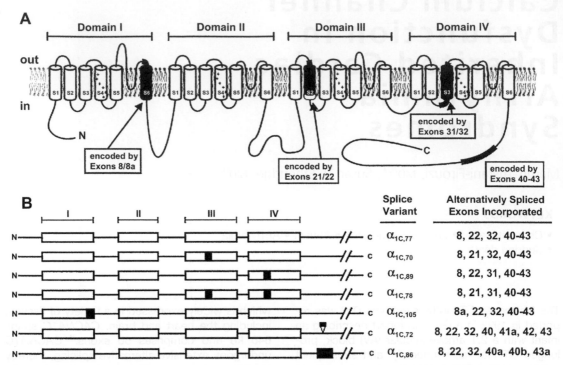

Fig. 1. Schematic representation of the L-type calcium α_{1C} subunit and its isoforms. (*A*) The human α_{1C} subunit is characterized by 4 homologous domains (I–IV), each containing 6 transmembrane segments (S1–S6). Segments encoded by alternatively spliced exons are indicated. (*B*) The complementary DNA constructs with alternatively spliced exons are schematically presented, with the respective exon combinations indicated in the right column. Exons 8 and 8a, 21 and 22, as well as 31 and 32 are pairs of mutually exclusive homologous exons. (*From* Zuhlke RD, Bouron A, Soldatov NM, et al. Ca2+ channel sensitivity towards the blocker isradipine is affected by alternative splicing of the human alpha1C subunit gene. FEBS Lett 1998;427:220–4; with permission.)

subunits would prolong the QT interval, whereas loss-of-function mutations would cause shortening. In the heart, the α_{1C} subunit coassembles with the auxiliary subunits $Ca_V\beta2b$ and $Ca_V\alpha2\delta1$. The $Ca_V\beta2b$ subunits, encoded by the gene *CACNB2b*, facilitate cell surface expression of the heteromultimeric channel and modulate channel inactivation.[8] The $Ca_V\alpha2\delta1$ subunits also promote cell surface expression and alter channel gating but to a lesser extent than the β subunits.[8]

Because calcium is a key signaling factor and excessive calcium levels are cytotoxic, several mechanisms that tightly regulate the open probability of L-type calcium channels exist. One such mechanism is inactivation, an intrinsic channel process that eliminates conductance at depolarized potentials. L-type calcium channels display 2 forms of inactivation: calcium-dependent and voltage-dependent mechanisms. Voltage-dependent inactivation is assessed under conditions in which calcium is substituted with barium as the charge carrier. In the presence of calcium, an additional component of inactivation is induced. In addition to the negative-feedback mechanisms (eg, inactivation), the open probability of L-type calcium

channels is also positively modulated by β-adrenergic stimulation and intracellular regulators, such as calmodulin and calmodulin-dependent kinase II (CaMKII).[8] For example, calcium influx activates CaMKII, which increases the open probability of L-type calcium channels and facilitates calcium release from the sarcoplasmic reticulum. These regulatory mechanisms participate in the pathophysiology of TS and contribute to the substrate for ventricular arrhythmias.

CLINICAL MANIFESTATIONS OF TS

TS is a rare primarily sporadic disorder that affects the development of many organ systems. Although originally described as severe LQT syndrome and syndactyly,[2] the ascertainment of more patients revealed a more complex clinical constellation, including congenital heart disease, developmental delay (including autism), abnormal dentition, and facial dysmorphic features (**Fig. 2**).[3] All patients with TS1 display QT prolongation, syndactyly, baldness at birth, and small teeth.[3] The vast majority of the patients display a 2:1 AV block in the neonatal period as

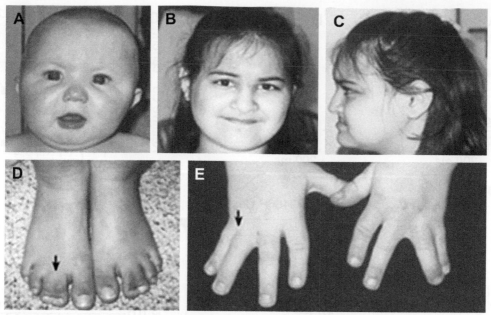

Fig. 2. Typical dysmorphic features in patients with TS. (*A–C*) Dysmorphic facial features, including round face, flat nasal bridge, receding upper jaw, and thin upper lip. (*D, E*) Webbing of the toes and fingers (syndactyly). (*From* Splawski I, Timothy KW, Sharpe LM, et al. Ca(V)1.2 calcium channel dysfunction causes a multisystem disorder including arrhythmia and autism. Cell 2004;119:19–31; with permission.)

a consequence of severe LQT syndrome. Because the sinus rate decreases with increase in age, a 1:1 AV conduction ensues. Consistent with the severe degree of QT prolongation, these individuals are at a high risk for sudden cardiac death. The pleiotropic manifestations of this disease are a consequence of the wide expression pattern of the alternatively spliced variant of *CACNA1C*, including in the heart, brain, gastrointestinal system, lungs, immune system, and smooth muscle.[3] Two cases of atypical TS were subsequently described (TS2), notable for the absence of the cardinal feature of syndactyly. As discussed later, mutations in the primary *CACNA1C* transcript were identified in this subset of patients.[9]

MOLECULAR AND CELLULAR BASIS OF TS

CACNA1C was initially screened as a candidate gene for TS, but no mutations were found in 47 of the 50 exons studied. Once the alternatively spliced exon 8a was described, *CACNA1C* was reconsidered as a candidate gene, and patients were discovered to harbor a mutation in the alternative isoform.[3] A remarkable feature of TS is its molecular homogeneity; all the original cases (TS1) occurred as a result of the identical missense mutation in exon 8a (G406R). In the heart, approximately 23% of calcium channels are encoded by the exon 8a variant, with 77% encoded by

exon 8.[3] In the heterozygote state, only 11.5% of Ca_v1.2 channels carry the G406R mutation; however, this mutation causes sufficient calcium channel dysfunction to produce severe QT prolongation and other clinical manifestations. The de novo predilection for the G406R exon 8a mutation is likely related to the high incidence of infant mortality, making its inheritance rare. In TS2, which is characterized by the absence of syndactyly, 2 mutations in the dominant splice variant exon 8 were identified: G402S and G406R.[9] All TS mutations are localized to the most terminal portion of the S6 transmembrane domain in domain I.

Expression of TS mutant Ca_v1.2 channels in heterologous expression systems revealed that mutant channels displayed near-complete loss of voltage-dependent inactivation, while maintaining the calcium-dependent component of inactivation (**Fig. 3**).[3,9] Initial computer simulations of the effect of reduced Ca_v1.2 voltage-dependent inactivation in the heterozygous state revealed marked prolongation of the action potential duration and the development of delayed afterdepolarizations (DADs).[3,9] These general findings were corroborated in subsequent more-detailed in silico analyses.[10,11] Further analysis of TS1 mutants was performed in virally transfected adult rat ventricular myocytes. This model not only confirmed a defect in voltage-dependent inactivation but

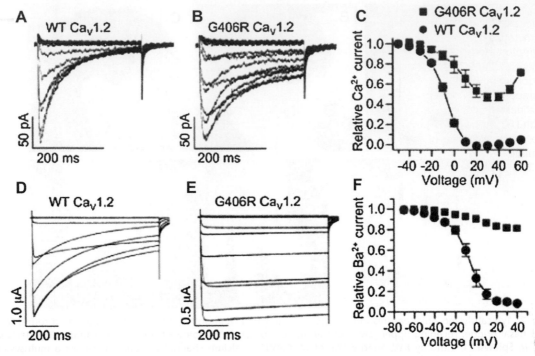

Fig. 3. TS mutation reduces Ca$_V$1.2 channel inactivation. Wild-type (*A*) and G406R (*B*) Ca$_V$1.2 channel currents recorded from Chinese hamster ovary cells in response to voltage pulses applied in 10-mV increments from −40 to +60 mV. Note that both wild-type and mutant channels display decreased current with time, consistent with intact calcium-dependent inactivation. (*C*) Voltage dependence of Ca^{2+} current inactivation. (*D, E*) Wild-type (*A*) and G406R (*B*) Ca$_V$1.2 channel currents recorded with the voltage protocol described earlier but using Ba^{2+} as the charge carrier to abolish calcium-dependent inactivation. Note that the mutant current does not decline, consistent with voltage-dependent inactivation. (*F*) Voltage dependence of Ba^{2+} current inactivation. (*From* Splawski I, Timothy KW, Sharpe LM, et al. Ca(V)1.2 calcium channel dysfunction causes a multisystem disorder including arrhythmia and autism. Cell 2004;119:19–31; with permission.)

also implicated increased activity of CaMKII in promoting excessive calcium release from the sarcoplasmic reticulum.[12] Calcium overload resulted in an increased activity of the sodium-calcium exchanger, with secondary development of DADs. Thus, the cellular basis of arrhythmia in TS is reduced voltage-dependent Ca$_V$1.2 inactivation, leading to sustained inward calcium current during the plateau phase of the cardiac action potential, marked prolongation of the action potential duration, and subsequent QT prolongation. The sustained inward calcium current leads to secondary DADs, ventricular arrhythmias, and sudden death, facilitated by an increased activity of CaMKII.

Studies on TS mutations may help in the understanding of the fundamental biophysical gating processes of L-type calcium channels. The molecular mechanisms underlying voltage- and calcium-dependent inactivation in L-type calcium channels are not completely understood; however, distinct regions of the channel seem to differentially regulate each process. The cytoplasmic linker between

domains I and II (I–II linker) likely represents an important structural determinant of voltage-dependent inactivation.[13] The I–II linker may function as a lid or an inactivating blocking particle that occludes the inner mouth of the channel pore. The TS mutation G406R is located in the S6 C-terminal region of domain I and likely influences the ability of the adjacent I–II linker to participate in channel inactivation. Substitution of the glycine at position 406 with charged, polar, or hydrophobic residues also impairs channel inactivation, implying that glycine is an absolute requirement for voltage-dependent inactivation.[9] Glycine is a flexible amino acid and functions as a hinge in other ion channels. G406 may function as a hinge that allows proper bending of the intracellular inactivation gate.

Although mutant Ca$_V$1.2 channels do not inactivate properly, they remain sensitive to L-type calcium channel blockers with potencies in nanomolar concentrations,[3] which suggests that calcium channel blockers may prove to be useful therapeutic strategies for TS. Indeed, in a recent case report, Jacobs and colleagues[14] described a patient with TS2 (G402S) in whom verapamil successfully reduced the incidence of ventricular arrhythmias. Over time, the patient developed symptomatic atrial fibrillation that responded favorably to treatment with the nonspecific ion channel blocker ranolazine.[15] In a subsequent report, verapamil did not reduce but, in fact, increased the incidence of ventricular arrhythmias in a patient with TS1.[16] The differential effects of verapamil may be a consequence of the distinct location of the mutation or an isoform-specific effect.

The initial reports of TS described a severely affected cohort with a high incidence of sudden cardiac death and developmental defects. More recently, a less-severe phenotype was described in patients mosaic for the TS1 mutation.[16] Mosaicism refers to the presence of genetically distinct populations of somatic and germline tissues, with tissue-to-tissue variations that may not follow the mendelian rules of inheritance. This observation raises the possibility that the TS phenotype may not be as dismal as previously reported. In addition, some of the previously described de novo TS mutations may represent cases of parental mosaicism and warrant careful genotyping of tissues other than the peripheral blood lymphocytes.

LOSS-OF-FUNCTION MUTATIONS IN THE L-TYPE CALCIUM CHANNEL SUBUNIT GENES CAUSE DISEASE

Recently, an association between loss-of-function mutations in genes encoding the cardiac L-type calcium channel subunits and a clinical entity with combined phenotype of Brugada syndrome and shorter-than-normal QT interval was described.[17] Three patients in a Brugada syndrome registry were identified to harbor a mutation in the genes encoding $\alpha1$ and β subunits. These individuals manifested the classic ST-segment elevation in precordial leads V_1 and V_2 and a corrected QT interval of 360 milliseconds or less. In 1 family, 6 genotype-positive individuals were ascertained, who also manifested the Brugada phenotype. Functional characterization revealed that mutations in CACNA1C (A39V and G490R) and CACNB2b (S481L) markedly decrease the L-type calcium current magnitude (**Fig. 4**).[17] The association between the L-type calcium channel subunits and the disease was further expanded to include mutations in genes encoding the $\alpha1$, β, and $\alpha2/\delta$ subunits in patients with Brugada syndrome, idiopathic ventricular fibrillation, and early repolarization syndrome.[18] However, the small families and

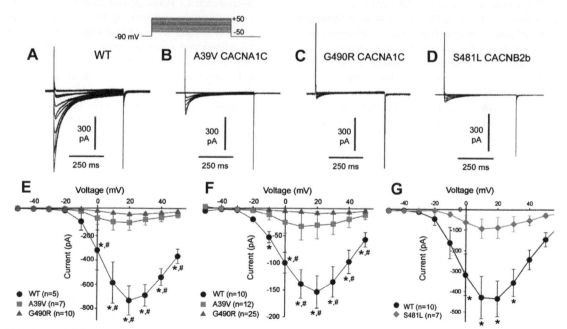

Fig. 4. Loss-of-function mutations in the L-type calcium channel subunit genes cause disease. (A–D) L-type calcium currents recorded in Chinese hamster ovary cells heterologously expressing wild-type, A39V, and G490R CACNA1C or S481L CACNB2b elicited by indicated voltage protocol (inset). The listed mutations markedly reduce the magnitude of calcium current. (E, F, G) Current-voltage relationships for the wild-type and mutant L-type calcium subunits as measured in (A–D). (From Antzelevitch C, Pollevick GD, Cordeiro JM, et al. Loss-of-function mutations in the cardiac calcium channel underlie a new clinical entity characterized by ST-segment elevation, short QT intervals, and sudden cardiac death. Circulation 2007;115:442–9; with permission.)

incomplete functional characterization of the genetic variants limit the interpretation of causality between the variants and the clinical disease. With time, the connection (or absence of connection) will be defined with certainty.

REFERENCES

1. Reichenbach H, Meister EM, Theile H. [The heart-hand syndrome. A new variant of disorders of heart conduction and syndactylia including osseous changes in hands and feet]. Kinderarztl Prax 1992; 60:54–6 [in German].

2. Marks ML, Whisler SL, Clericuzio C, et al. A new form of long QT syndrome associated with syndactyly. J Am Coll Cardiol 1995;25:59–64.

3. Splawski I, Timothy KW, Sharpe LM, et al. Ca(V)1.2 calcium channel dysfunction causes a multisystem disorder including arrhythmia and autism. Cell 2004;119:19–31.

4. Catterall WA. Functional subunit structure of voltage-gated calcium channels. Science 1991; 253:1499–500.

5. Hofmann F, Biel M, Flockerzi V. Molecular basis for Ca2+ channel diversity. Annu Rev Neurosci 1994; 17:399–418.

6. Soldatov NM. Genomic structure of human L-type Ca2+ channel. Genomics 1994;22:77–87.

7. Soldatov NM, Zuhlke RD, Bouron A, et al. Molecular structures involved in L-type calcium channel inactivation. Role of the carboxyl-terminal region encoded by exons 40-42 in alpha1C subunit in the kinetics and Ca2+ dependence of inactivation. J Biol Chem 1997;272:3560–6.

8. Catterall WA. Structure and regulation of voltage-gated Ca2+ channels. Annu Rev Cell Dev Biol 2000;16:521–55.

9. Splawski I, Timothy KW, Decher N, et al. Severe arrhythmia disorder caused by cardiac L-type calcium channel mutations. Proc Natl Acad Sci U S A 2005;102:8089–96 [discussion: 8086–8].

10. Faber GM, Silva J, Livshitz L, et al. Kinetic properties of the cardiac L-type Ca2+ channel and its role in myocyte electrophysiology: a theoretical investigation. Biophys J 2007;92:1522–43.

11. Zhu ZI, Clancy CE. L-type Ca2+ channel mutations and T-wave alternans: a model study. Am J Physiol Heart Circ Physiol 2007;293:H3480–9.

12. Thiel WH, Chen B, Hund TJ, et al. Proarrhythmic defects in Timothy syndrome require calmodulin kinase II. Circulation 2008;118:2225–34.

13. Adams B, Tanabe T. Structural regions of the cardiac Ca channel alpha subunit involved in Ca-dependent inactivation. J Gen Physiol 1997;110:379–89.

14. Jacobs A, Knight BP, McDonald KT, et al. Verapamil decreases ventricular tachyarrhythmias in a patient with Timothy syndrome (LQT8). Heart Rhythm 2006;3:967–70.

15. Shah DP, Baez-Escudero JL, Weisberg IL, et al. Ranolazine safely decreases ventricular and atrial fibrillation in Timothy syndrome (LQT8). Pacing Clin Electrophysiol 2010. [Epub ahead of print].

16. Etheridge SP, Bowles N, Arrington C, et al. Somatic mosaicism contributes to phenotypic variation in Timothy syndrome. 2010, in press.

17. Antzelevitch C, Pollevick GD, Cordeiro JM, et al. Loss-of-function mutations in the cardiac calcium channel underlie a new clinical entity characterized by ST-segment elevation, short QT intervals, and sudden cardiac death. Circulation 2007;115:442–9.

18. Burashnikov E, Pfeiffer R, Barajas-Martinez H, et al. Mutations in the cardiac L-type calcium channel associated with inherited J wave syndromes and sudden cardiac death. Heart Rhythm 2010;7(12): 1872–82.

Inherited Cardiac Arrhythmia Syndromes: Role of the Sodium Channel

Roos F.J. Marsman, MSc, PhD, Arthur A.M. Wilde, MD, PhD,
Connie R. Bezzina, PhD*

KEYWORDS

- Arrhythmia • Sudden death • Sodium channel
- Brugada syndrome • Long QT syndrome

Voltage-gated sodium channels, located in the sarcolemma of excitable cells, are essential for the initiation and propagation of the action potential. The rapid inward sodium current conducted by the cardiac sodium channel is responsible for the fast depolarization of cardiomyocytes and is thereby responsible for rapid conduction of the electrical impulse through the heart.

A considerable amount of research has been conducted on the cardiac sodium channel, as hundreds of genetic variants have been identified in *SCN5A*, the gene encoding the pore-forming (alpha) subunit of this channel. Mutations in *SCN5A* have been associated with various cardiac arrhythmia syndromes referred to as *sodium channelopathies*. These mutations can impact in many different ways on sodium channel function, in gross terms leading to either loss or gain of function, which in turn gives rise to various phenotypes, including the Brugada syndrome, the long QT syndrome (LQTS), cardiac conduction disease, and sick sinus syndrome.[1] In addition to the rare inherited arrhythmia syndromes, subclinical expression of *SCN5A* mutations may also manifest as drug-induced arrhythmias and increased arrhythmia risk in specific populations.[2,3]

STRUCTURE, FUNCTION, AND MODULATION

The *SCN5A* gene encoding the alpha subunit of the cardiac sodium channel (Nav1.5) maps to the short arm of chromosome 3 (3p21) and contains 28 exons spanning approximately 80 kilobases.[4,5] At the molecular level, the glycosylated alpha subunit is a 2016–amino acid protein that consists of four structurally homologous hydrophobic domains (DI–DIV), connected by hydrophilic cytoplasmic linkers, that are arranged around a central ion-conducting pore. In turn, each domain contains six transmembrane segments (S1–S6), linked by intracellular and extracellular loops, with the amino- and the carboxy-terminal domains located intracellularly (**Fig. 1**). Besides the alpha subunit, the channel protein complex is also comprised of beta accessory subunits.

Highly conserved residues, located within the S5–S6 linkers lining the ion-conducting pore are required for permeation and ion selectivity.[6] The positively charged S4 segments serve as the major voltage sensors. The highly conserved linker between domain III and IV, the intracellular S4–S5 linkers of DIII and DIV and the docking sites on S6 of DIV, are responsible for fast inactivation. Moreover, the intracellular carboxyl terminus stabilizes inactivation by formation of a molecular complex with the DIII–IV linker.[7]

Upon changes in the membrane potential, sodium channels transit among three conformational states: activated (open), inactivated, and closed (resting); a process known as *gating*.[8] In response to membrane depolarization, the voltage sensors (S4 segments) move concertedly in an

Heart Failure Research Center, Department of Clinical and Experimental Cardiology, Academic Medical Center, Meibergdreef 15, 1105 AZ Amsterdam, The Netherlands
* Corresponding author.
E-mail address: c.r.bezzina@amc.uva.nl

Card Electrophysiol Clin 3 (2011) 93–112
doi:10.1016/j.ccep.2010.10.004

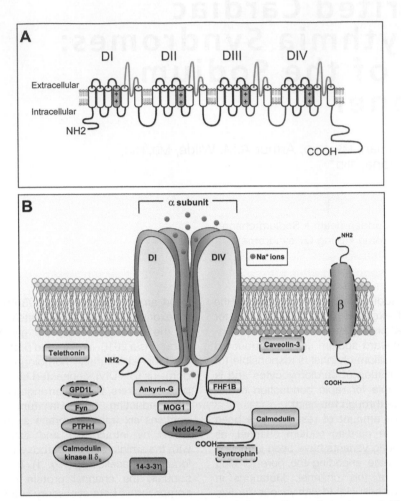

Fig. 1. (*A*) Transmembrane topology of the alpha subunit of the cardiac sodium channel. The four domains (DI–DIV), each consisting of six membrane-spanning segments, are connected by intracellular linkers. The residues between S5 and S6 of each domain, responsible for ion selectivity and permeation, are depicted in *green*. The positively charged S4 segments of each domain act as voltage sensors and are depicted in *blue*. Residues on the cytoplasmic linker between DIII and DIV, the S4/S5 linkers of DIII and DIV, and the carboxy-terminal region, depicted in *red*, are responsible for inactivation. (*B*) Schematic depiction of the cardiac sodium channel macromolecular complex. The proteins are classified in four groups based on function: (1) targeting proteins involved in trafficking and ubiquitination (*dark gray*); (2) proteins involved in posttranslational modifications (*pink*); (3) cytoskeletal proteins (*turquoise*); and (4) proteins that regulate expression or alter biophysical properties of the channel in a yet-unknown manner. Enzymes are shown as ovals. Dashed lines represent proteins that are mutated in patients with inherited arrhythmia disorders.

outward direction, causing the channel to open (*activation*) from its closed resting state. This process allows for passage of sodium ions, producing the rapid upstroke of the action potential. Within tens of milliseconds, the channel enters a nonconducting state (*fast inactivation*), a distinct gating form from which transition into the open state does not occur as channels undergo recovery from inactivation. In addition, channels may gradually enter a separate kinetic state referred to as *slow inactivation* during prolonged depolarization.[9] Furthermore, a unique characteristic intrinsic to sodium channels is a process termed *closed-state inactivation*, in which a small but significant fraction of channels inactivate from a closed state without prior opening.[10]

Posttranslational modification (eg, [de]phosphorylation, glycosylation) and protein–protein interactions modulate abundance, distribution, and gating characteristics of the channel. Besides beta subunits, proteins known to be associated with the sodium channel may be categorized as (1) targeting proteins involved in trafficking and ubiquitylation (14-3-3η, Nedd4-2 like); (2) enzymes involved in post-translational modifications (CAM-KII, PTPH1); and (3) structural proteins involved in anchoring at the sarcolemma (ankyrin-G, syntrophin). Mutations affecting these proteins or sodium channel mutations that disrupt interaction with these proteins can impair the sodium current, resulting in a clinical phenotype (**Table 1**).

LONG QT SYNDROME

The inherited LQTS is a repolarization disorder characterized by prolongation of the QT interval on the electrocardiogram (ECG) (**Fig. 2**). It is a well-described genetically heterogeneous disorder, with 13 genetic subtypes reported to date.[22] The syndrome is estimated to affect 1 in 2200 individuals[23] and is typically inherited as an autosomal dominant trait (Romano-Ward syndrome).[24] The most common genetic forms of LQTS are caused by mutations in *KCNQ1* (chromosome 11p15.5) underlying LQTS type 1, which accounts for 42% to 54% of cases, and *KCNH2* (7q35-q36) underlying LQTS type 2, which accounts for 35% to 42% of cases. These genes encode cardiac potassium channel subunits responsible for outward repolarizing currents (I_{ks} and I_{kr}). *SCN5A* mutations occur in 1.7% to 10% of LQTS cases.[25,26] More than 700 mutations have been described for LQTS, with more than 80 distinct sequence changes in the *SCN5A* gene associated with LQTS type 3 (LQT3) (Inherited Arrhythmia Database; http://fsm.it/cardmoc).

Repolarization occurs when net outward current exceeds net inward current. The common pathophysiologic mechanism underlying delayed repolarization and action potential prolongation in LQTS results from either a decrease in repolarizing outward potassium currents (loss-of-function) or an increase in inward (sodium or calcium) current during the action potential plateau phase (gain-of-function) (**Fig. 3**). Numerous studies have characterized the biophysical mechanisms underlying LQT3 mutations. In most cases, mutant channels exhibit disrupted (fast) inactivation associated with abnormal sustained (persistent) inward sodium current (I_{sus}), and in accordance, 65% of *SCN5A* mutations are located in exons 20 through 28 encoding the DII/DIII intracellular linker through to the carboxy-terminal end, all of which constitute channel domains important for inactivation.[27]

A functionally well-characterized LQT3 mutation is the p.1505—1507del mutation in the DIII—DIV linker, commonly referred to as *delKPQ* or *ΔKPQ*. ΔKPQ channels fail to inactivate completely and exhibit intermittent reopenings

after fast inactivation, resulting in sustained current.[28] Accordingly, the transgenic ΔKPQ mouse model displays prolonged QT interval, ventricular tachycardia (VT), and ventricular fibrillation (VF) (**Table 2**).[31] An increase in sustained sodium current is considered the prototypical sodium channel defect leading to LQT3, although other biophysical defects can also cause LQT3.[33,34]

Delayed repolarization predisposes to ventricular arrhythmias through increasing dispersion of refractoriness (the substrate) and the occurrence of early-after-depolarizations (the trigger), which involves reactivation of L-type calcium channels. These two processes precipitate conditions required for reentry arrhythmias, allowing an electrical impulse from depolarized tissue to prematurely re-excite (ie, trigger spontaneous action potentials) adjacent tissue that has already repolarized. A distinct type of polymorphic VT, torsades de pointes, is associated with LQTS, with a typical twisting of QRS complexes around the isoelectric baseline.

Several studies have focused on the identification of distinguishing features between the most common LQTS subtypes (LQT1—3), showing gene-specific ECG characteristics and triggers of arrhythmia. On the ECG, the LQT3 pattern typically exhibits a long isoelectric ST segment (delayed onset of the T-wave) with a narrow peaked T-wave.[35,36] The onset of torsades de pointes in patients with LQT3 is usually bradycardia dependent, and is most likely to occur during rest or sleep, in contrast to patients with LQT1 and LQT2, in whom exercise and emotional stress, respectively, induce events.[37] In several families with LQT3, sinus bradycardia, pauses, and arrest in addition to QT prolongation have been described and may contribute to disease-related mortality.[34,38]

Accordingly, gene-based risk stratification, and disease management have been introduced in clinical practice. Current risk stratification in LQTS is largely based on previous cardiac events,[39,40] the degree of QTc prolongation,[39] patient characteristics[41] and genotype. Patients with LQT3 have a lower frequency of cardiac events but potentially higher lethality than those with LQT1 and -2.[42] Risk and prognosis cannot be predicted through QTc prolongation in patients with LQT3; however, male sex seems to be a risk factor,[39] and mutation-specific risk has also been observed.[43]

The major therapeutic options for LQTS are pharmacologic agents in the form of ß-blockers and implantable devices (implantable cardioverter defibrillator [ICD]). Some debate exists on the use

Table 1
Mutations affecting sodium channel–interacting proteins

Gene	Protein	Locus	Clinical Phenotype	Proposed Molecular Mechanism
SCN1B[11,12]	Sodium channel subunit beta-1	19q13.1	Brugada syndrome and/or conduction disease; atrial fibrillation	Subunit noncovalently linked to Nav1.5. Loss of SCN1B function results in decreased I_{NA}
SCN2B[12]	Sodium channel subunit beta-2	11q23	Atrial fibrillation	Subunit disulfide-linked to Nav1.5. Loss of SCN2B function results in decreased I_{NA}
SCN3B[13,14]	Sodium channel subunit beta-3	11q23.3	Brugada syndrome; sudden infant death syndrome	Subunit noncovalently linked to Nav1.5. Loss of SCN3B membrane expression/function disrupts trafficking of Nav1.5 to the membrane
SCN4B[13,15]	Sodium channel subunit beta-4	11q23.3	Long QT syndrome 10; sudden infant death syndrome	Subunit disulfide-linked to Nav1.5. Loss of SCN4B function results in persistent I_{NA}
CAV3[16,17]	Caveolin-3	3p25	Long QT syndrome 9; sudden infant death syndrome	Caveolin-3 is an integrated membrane protein, hypothesized to regulate Nav1.5 phosphorylation
SNTA1[18,19]	Alpha-1 syntrophin	20q11.2	Long QT syndrome 12; sudden infant death syndrome	SNTA1 connects Nav1.5 to the nNOS–PMCA complex. Loss of interaction between SNTA1 and PMCA results in an increase in Nav1.5 nitrosylation and increase in I_{NA}
GPD1L[20,21]	Glycerol 3 phosphate dehydrogenase 1–like	3p22.3	Brugada syndrome; sudden infant death syndrome	GPD1L catalyzes the conversion of G3P into DHAP. Loss of GPD1L results in G3P PKC-dependent phosphorylation of Nav1.5. PKC phosphorylation decreases I_{NA}

Abbreviations: DHAP, dihydroxyacetone phosphate; G3P, glycerol-3-phosphate; nNOS, neuronal nitric oxide synthase; PKC, protein kinase C; PMCA, plasma membrane Ca-ATPase.

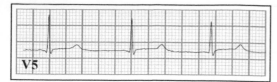

Fig. 2. Prolonged QT interval of a patient with LQT3. The QTc interval exceeds 480 ms.

of β-adrenergic blockade in patients with LQT3, because of the high risk of bradycardia-dependent ventricular arrhythmias.[44] However, ß-blockade is not contraindicated in LQT3. Beneficial effects of β-adrenergic blockade have been reported in subgroups of patients with LQT3,[45] although monitoring before and after initiation of treatment is recommended.[46] Patients with LQT3 represent only approximately 10% of the LQTS population, and consequently LQT3 sample sizes in studies investigating gene-specific effects on disease characteristics are small, necessitating

caution in the interpretation of findings. Sodium channel blockade normalizes the QTc interval in patients with LQT3[47,48]; however, in patients with overlapping Brugada syndrome or conduction disease it may theoretically also increase the probability of cardiac events,[49] and additionally the response to the drugs may be mutation-specific.[33] QT-prolonging drugs should be avoided (see www.qtdrugs.org). The placement of an ICD can be considered in high-risk patients with LQT3 (survivors of cardiac arrest) and individuals with a QTc longer than 500 ms,[50] and may be reasonable in asymptomatic patients with excessively abnormal ECGs and a strong family history of sudden cardiac death. The presence of an SCN5A mutation alone may not necessarily indicate ICD implantation.

BRUGADA SYNDROME

The Brugada syndrome was first introduced as a distinct clinical entity in 1992.[51] It is characterized

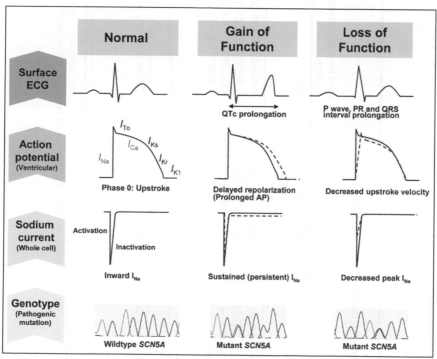

Fig. 3. Pathophysiologic mechanisms of SCN5A mutations leading to gain- or loss-of-function. A genetic abnormality, in the sequence chromatograms represented by a double-peak pattern, causes a molecular phenotype of sustained (gain-of-function; *red dashed line, middle*) or reduced sodium current (loss-of-function; *red dashed line, right*). The sustained current causes a cellular phenotype of prolonged action potential duration (*red dashed line, middle*). The reduced (*peak*) sodium current decreases the upstroke velocity of the action potential (*red dashed line, right*). Prolonged action potential duration may produce QT-interval prolongation on the surface ECG (*schematic ECG representation, upper middle*). A decrease in upstroke velocity may lead to conduction slowing, associated with prolongation of the PR and QRS intervals (*upper right*). I_{Ca}, calcium current; I_{K1}, inward rectifier potassium current; I_{Kr}, rapid delayed rectifier potassium current; I_{Ks}, slow delayed rectifier potassium current; I_{NA}, sodium current; I_{To}, transient outward current.

Table 2
Genetically engineered mouse models of sodium channelopathies

Mouse Genotype	Human Disease	Phenotype	Electrocardiographic Defects	Effect on I_{NA}	Reference
Scn5a −/−	NA	Intra-uterine lethality at E11.5; severe defects in ventricular morphogenesis	NA	NA	Papadatos et al[29]
Scn5a ±	Progressive cardiac conduction disease	Inducible ventricular arrhythmias; fibrosis	P-wave, PR and QRS prolongation; AVB	Decreased current (~50%)	Papadatos et al[29]
Scn5a 1798insD	Long QT syndrome, Brugada syndrome, PCCD	Sinus bradycardia; conduction slowing; inducible ventricular arrhythmias; cardiac fibrosis	PR-, QRS-, and QT-interval prolongation	Persistent current (slow rates); decreased current (fast rates; ~50%)	Remme et al[30]
Scn5a delKPQ	Long QT syndrome	Spontaneous ventricular arrhythmias	QT-interval prolongation	Persistent current	Nuyens et al[31]
Scn5a N1325S	Long QT syndrome	Spontaneous ventricular arrhythmias cardiac fibrosis; contractile dysfunction; cardiomyocyte apoptosis	QT-interval prolongation	Persistent current	Tian et al[32]

Abbreviations: AVB, atrioventricular block; NA, not applicable; PCCD, progressive cardiac conduction disease.
Data from Charpentier F, Bourgé A, Mérot J. Mouse models of SCN5A-related cardiac arrhythmias. Prog Biophys Mol Biol 2008;98(2–3):230–7.

by ECG features that include ST-segment elevation in the right precordial leads (V1–V3) and conduction delay at different cardiac levels, in association with sudden cardiac death from polymorphic VT or VF. The characteristic ST-segment elevation may be present at baseline or is unmasked (or exacerbated) through administration of sodium channel–blocking drugs. Brugada syndrome is oftentimes familial, displaying an autosomal dominant pattern of inheritance.

The first clinical symptoms, which may be sudden death, manifest during adulthood, with an average age of 40 years; however, arrhythmic events have been described over a wide range of ages (range, 2 days to 84 years).[52,53] The exact worldwide incidence of Brugada syndrome is unknown, although it is considered to be more common in Asian populations.[54] One prospective study performed on a large Japanese population-based cohort identified a prevalence of 0.27% for type I Brugada syndrome ECG.[55] Differences in incidence may reflect the lack of consensus on the diagnosis of Brugada syndrome, and the dynamic and frequently concealed Brugada ECG sign at baseline conditions. Male predominance is a common feature of Brugada syndrome, with a male-to-female ratio of 8:1, independent of *SCN5A* mutation carriership.

The (first) clinical presentation of Brugada syndrome is broad, and varies from absence of any clinical (ECG) abnormalities to sudden death. Symptoms include syncope, seizures, and sleep disturbance in the case of self-terminating arrhythmia episodes, and sudden death in the case of sustained ventricular arrhythmias. Asymptomatic individuals may present with an abnormal ECG during routine examination, or during screening of relatives of patients known to have Brugada syndrome. The FINGER (France, Italy, Netherlands, Germany) Brugada registry recently showed that asymptomatic patients with a normal baseline ECG are at low risk for arrhythmic events.[56]

The most important clinical characteristic of the Brugada syndrome, which is required for diagnosis, is the type 1 Brugada ECG pattern characterized by coved-type ST-segment elevation of 2 mm or greater in more than one right precordial lead (V1–V3), followed by a negative or biphasic T-wave. Two other distinct ST-segment patterns have been described; type 2, which is characterized by an elevated J point (≥ 2 mm) with a gradually descending ST segment that remains at least 1 mm above the isoelectric line followed by a biphasic or positive T-wave ("saddleback" ST–T configuration), and type 3, which is similar to the type 1 or type 2 morphology, but with a smaller (≤ 1 mm) ST-segment elevation. Type 2 and 3 ECG patterns are not considered diagnostic. They may, however, be dynamic and change over time or in the presence of sodium channel blockade to a coved type 1 pattern (**Fig. 4**).[57] Sodium channel blockers, such as flecainide, ajmaline, and procainamide, may be used to accentuate or evoke the Brugada ECG sign. Current guidelines do not take into account whether a diagnostic coved-type ECG is spontaneous or drug-induced, although spontaneous coved-type pattern ECG indicates a worse prognosis than only drug-induced type 1 ECG.[58]

Several predisposing factors have been reported to induce the type 1 Brugada ECG and ventricular arrhythmias, including parasympathetic activity, body temperature (fever), and (antiarrhythmic) drugs. Most arrhythmias occur at rest or during sleep and may be triggered postprandially. The role of parasympathetic activity is further supported by the effect of acetylcholine, which accentuates ST-segment elevation, and ß-receptor stimulation (isoproterenol), which attenuates ST elevation in affected subjects.[59,60]

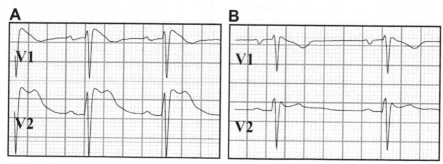

Fig. 4. Precordial leads V1 and V2 showing the three Brugada ECG patterns. (*A*) Lead V1 shows a type 1 (coved) ECG, lead V2 shows a type 2 (saddle-back). (*B*) In lead V2, significant J point elevation and a saddle-back ECG pattern (type 3) is shown.

Moreover, fever has been reported to unmask or exacerbate type 1 Brugada ECG and increase the risk for ventricular arrhythmias.[61] Furthermore, many drugs are reported to induce the Brugada sign and arrhythmias in affected individuals (www.brugadadrugs.org).[62]

The finding that sodium channel blockade could provoke the distinct coved-type Brugada ECG led to the hypothesis that sodium channel dysfunction (ie, genetic defects in SCN5A) could lead to the phenotype. In 1998, Chen and colleagues[63] described the first mutations in the SCN5A gene, predicted to decrease sodium current, associated with Brugada syndrome. To date, almost 100 different SCN5A mutations have been associated with Brugada syndrome, though only an estimated 15% to 30% of patients carry a mutation in SCN5A.[64] Furthermore, mutations in six other genes, encoding proteins that directly or indirectly contribute to action potential morphology, have been associated with Brugada syndrome, however the prevalence of these mutations remains low (see **Table 1**).

Although the pathophysiologic basis of Brugada syndrome has received a lot of attention in the past years, the mechanisms underlying the disorder remain incompletely understood. Several electrophysiologic studies have been performed in patients[65,66] and many Brugada syndrome—associated mutations have been characterized functionally in vitro. All studied mutations have been reported to exhibit loss-of-function effects through either decreased cell surface expression or changes in functional properties; however, the pathophysiologic mechanism by which reduced sodium channel function underlies the characteristic Brugada syndrome ST-segment elevation remains controversial.

Two alternative theories have been proposed to explain the mechanism of ST elevation and the strong link between Brugada syndrome and VT/VF.[67] The repolarization disorder hypothesis rests on the fact that the transient outward current (I_{to}), responsible for early repolarization, is expressed more abundantly in the outer layer (epicardium) than in the inner layer (endocardium) of myocardial muscle.[68] Decreased sodium current (through a genetic defect or pharmacologically) in combination with the prominent epicardial repolarizing current (ie, I_{to}) contribute to the loss of the characteristic action potential dome and shortening of action potentials in the epicardium but not in the endocardium. The transmural voltage gradient that ensues inscribes the ST-segment elevation on the ECG. Dispersion of repolarization provides a substrate for reentry arrhythmias.[69] This model has been validated using right ventricular wedge preparations of dogs and computational methods.

The depolarization disorder hypothesis, however, is based on electrophysiologic heterogeneities between the right ventricle and the right ventricular outflow tract, and proposes that delayed activation of the right ventricular outflow tract drives a potential gradient, giving rise to ST elevations, and that subsequent unidirectional block may facilitate reentrant arrhythmias.[66]

The contribution of loss of sodium channel function in Brugada syndrome remains complex, because within families with SCN5A-related Brugada syndrome, type 1 ECGs have been found in individuals that did not carry the familial SCN5A mutation.[70] Experts have proposed that the inconsistent association between Brugada syndrome genotype and phenotype may (partly) be explained by other genetic factors such as genetic modifiers. A complex interaction between (common) variants, not necessarily directly related to the sodium channel, may affect the penetrance and severity of the disease. The influence of genetic background is further evidenced in a transgenic mice model expressing the Scn5a-1798insD mutation that exhibit differences in cardiac phenotype in a strain-dependent manner.[71]

Defining risk factors relating to the prognosis of Brugada syndrome is controversial. Most studies agree that a history of syncope and the occurrence of a spontaneous type 1 ECG are risk factors; however, the predictive value of the induction of VT/VF during programmed electrical stimulation is debated.[56,58,64,72] Gender, family history of sudden cardiac death, and the presence of an SCN5A mutations have not been found to be risk markers.[56,73]

For high-risk patients with Brugada syndrome (ie, with a history of syncope or cardiac arrest), the only therapy with proven efficacy is the implantation of an ICD.[74] However, controversy exists regarding the primary prevention of malignant arrhythmias in asymptomatic patients, because the rate of spontaneous VF in these patients with electrophysiologically induced arrhythmias seems to be only 1% per year, whereas 28% develop complications related to ICD implantation.[75] Currently no proven pharmacotherapy exists for Brugada syndrome, although data suggest benefit from quinidine, a blocker of I_{to}, with evidence supporting prevention of inducible and spontaneous ventricular arrhythmias.[76] Currently, patients are recruited for a prospective trial to determine whether quinidine therapy will reduce the long-term risk of arrhythmic events in asymptomatic patients (see http://clinicaltrials.gov/ct2/show/NCT00789165?term_brugada&rank_2).[77]

PROGRESSIVE CARDIAC CONDUCTION DEFECT

Progressive cardiac conduction defect (PCCD), also referred to as *Lev's* or *Lenegre's disease*, is a relatively common cardiac conduction disorder characterized by an age-dependent progressive delay in the propagation of the cardiac impulse through the His-Purkinje system with right or left bundle branch block and widening of the QRS complex, eventually resulting in complete atrio-ventricular block, syncope, and sudden death (**Fig. 5**).

SCN5A is the first gene associated with PCCD. In 1999, Schott and colleagues[78] described a splice-site mutation that segregated with PCCD in an autosomal dominant fashion in a large French kindred. None of the affected family members exhibited ECG feature character-istic of LQTS or Brugada syndrome, indicating an isolated conduction defect phenotype. Recently, mutations in *SCN1B* encoding the beta-1 subunit of the sodium channel have been identified in families with conduction disease or Brugada syndrome.[11]

As for Brugada syndrome, *SCN5A* mutations causing PCCD lead to loss of sodium channel function. A decrease in sodium current density reduces the action potential upstroke velocity, which will lead to conduction slowing (conduction failure) and electrical inexcitability. However, the reason why loss of sodium channel function leads to conduction disease in some individuals and Brugada syndrome in others remains unknown. The frontier between these two clinical syndromes is therefore unclear, and even in the same family the same *SCN5A* mutation can lead to either Bru-gada syndrome or isolated conduction defects.[79] Gender and genetic modifiers are suspected to play a role.[79] Heterozygous *Scn5a* knock-out mice, carrying only one functional *Scn5a* allele, recapitulate the clinical PCCD phenotype, including progressive impairment of atrial and ventricular conduction with aging in association with fibrosis.[29,80] This finding supports the hypoth-esis that *SCN5A*-related inherited conduction disease is the result of combined reduced sodium current (manifested by haploinsufficiency) and an age-related increase in fibrosis.[80,81] Evidence

exists that fibrosis in these cases could even be mediated by the sodium channelopathy itself.[82]

Currently, pacemaker devices are the most effective treatment for conduction disease, although they are suboptimal, particularly in the pediatric population. In patients in whom conduc-tion disease is associated with malignant ventric-ular arrhythmias, ICDs may be implanted.

CONGENITAL SICK SINUS SYNDROME

Congenital sick sinus syndrome (SSS) is defined by ECG criteria and characterized by abnormali-ties in sinus node impulse formation and propaga-tion, including sinus bradycardia, sinoatrial exit block, sinus arrest, or atrial standstill in the absence of underlying acquired conditions (ischemia, cardiomyopathy, or degenerative, infectious, or postoperative disease). SSS is also associated with conduction disease and supra-ventricular tachyarrhythmias (also referred to as the *brady-tachy syndrome*[83]).

In 2003, Benson and colleagues[84] identified compound heterozygous *SCN5A* mutations segregating with congenital SSS in three families in whom all heterozygous mutation carriers were asymptomatic without ECG abnormalities, recog-nizing the first recessive form of cardiac sodium channelopathy. Merely 14 *SCN5A* mutations have been associated with the disease, including mutations associated with other phenotypes such as Brugada syndrome and PCCD (overlap-ping syndromes[85]). Most of these mutant channels have been studied in expression systems and consistently showed loss-of-function effects through altered channel kinetics (gating defects) or impaired cell surface expression (maturation/trafficking deficiencies).[86] More than 100 distinct possible Brugada syndrome– or PCCD-asso-ciated *SCN5A* loss-of-function mutations have been identified[87]; however, *SCN5A*-related SSS is a rare observation, the expression of which seems to be modulated by yet-unknown (genetic) factors acting alongside the sodium current reduc-tion and aging.

Specific mechanisms through which sodium channel mutations cause sinus node dysfunction remain uncertain, partly because the contribution of Nav1.5 to pacemaker activity is still

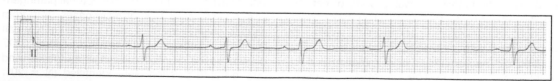

Fig. 5. Sinus bradycardia and conduction defects (prolonged PR interval with a broad QRS complex) in an individual with progressive cardiac conduction disease.

controversial because these channels are expressed in the peripheral sinoatrial node cells but not in central sinoatrial node cells (which mainly control the cardiac rhythm).[88] Experimental and computational (tissue simulation) analyses have shown that (loss-of-function) SCN5A mutations not only slowed down pacemaking (in addition, simulated vagal activity amplified the bradycardiac effects of the mutations) but also compromised coupling between the sinoatrial node and adjacent atrial tissue, recapitulating sinoatrial node exit block and sinus arrest, which are the majors features of SSS.[89,90] Additional evidence for the role of the sodium channel in sinus node dysfunction has come from heterozygous Scn5a+/− mice that showed (sinus) bradycardia, slowed sinoatrial conduction, and persistent sinoatrial block.[29,90]

Gain-of-function mutations in SCN5A have also been related to sinus node dysfunction (most prominently sinus bradycardia and arrest), although always in concurrence with a LQTS phenotype.[91,92] Using sinoatrial node action potential models, Veldkamp and colleagues[34] showed that gain-of-function effects of the 1795insD mutation, consisting of persistent inward current and a negative shift in voltage-dependence of inactivation, cause a reduction in sinus rate. A persistent inward sodium current therefore not only underlies QT prolongation but also may contribute to sinus bradycardia and sinus pauses.

ATRIAL STANDSTILL

Congenital atrial standstill is a rare arrhythmogenic condition characterized by the absence of electrical (ie, the absence of P waves on the ECG) and mechanical activity in the atria. Atrial standstill is mostly found as a complication of myocarditis, amyloidosis, or muscular dystrophy. In 2003, in a family with primary atrial standstill (ie, in the absence of structural heart disease or systemic disease), a loss-of-function SCN5A mutation (D1275 N) was identified that cosegregated with two rare connexin40 polymorphisms.[93] Connexin40 is an atrium-specific gap junction protein encoded by the Cx40 (alias GJA5) gene. These polymorphisms, located in the proximal promoter region of this gene, caused a reduction in connexin40 expression in vitro. It was proposed that the additive effect of decreased coupling as a consequence of decreased connexin40 levels, in combination with a decrease in atrial excitability caused by the sodium channel mutation, led to a progressive phenotype of atrial standstill, because the individuals that carried only one of the variants were clinically unaffected. This study was the first to show the action of a modifier gene modulating the phenotype in sodium channelopathy.

FAMILIAL ATRIAL FIBRILLATION

Atrial fibrillation, the most common sustained arrhythmia in clinical practice, is characterized by rapid electrical activation of the atrial myocardium, resulting in loss of contractility. Its prevalence in the population increases with age, however atrial fibrillation can develop in younger subjects (<65 years) in the absence of known risk factors (hypertension, structural heart disease, congestive heart failure), a condition known as lone atrial fibrillation, which is responsible for 10% to 30% of atrial fibrillation. A familial form of the disease has long been recognized, and several genetic loci and genes related to the disorder have been reported.[94] Mutations in SCN5A have been discovered in patients with lone atrial fibrillation,[95,96] and some of these have been investigated functionally. Diverse functional effects have been described, with some mutations displaying gain-of-function effects potentially associated with enhanced atrial excitability,[96,97] and others displaying loss of sodium channel function.[98] Similarly, atrial fibrillation–associated mutations in the sodium channel beta-subunit genes SCN1B, SCN2B, and SCN3B reduced sodium currents (when coexpressed with SCN5A); the mutations in SCN1B and SCN2B also altered channel gating.[12] Some mutations lead to atrial fibrillation in combination with other phenotypes (eg, 15%−20% of patients with Brugada syndrome also manifest atrial fibrillation).[99] Clarification on the mechanisms of SCN5A-related atrial fibrillation requires further investigation.

SUDDEN INFANT DEATH SYNDROME

Sudden infant death syndrome (SIDS) is defined as the sudden unexpected death of an infant younger than 1 year, with onset of the fatal episode apparently occurring during sleep, that remains unexplained after a thorough investigation, including performance of a complete autopsy and review of the circumstances of death and the clinical history.[100] Although SIDS is a heterogeneous entity with a largely unexplained multifactorial pathogenesis, an estimated 10% of SIDS cases stem from cardiac channelopathies, with approximately half involving a mutation in SCN5A.[101] In a large SIDS cohort, seven SCN5A missense mutations and one in-frame deletion were identified (N = 201; 4%).[102] All of these variants exhibited defects in the kinetics and voltage-dependence of inactivation, associated with gain-of-function.[102] In this study, the lack of clinical and family data on probands prevented demonstration of cosegregation of LQTS phenotypes in families with SIDS victims or demonstration of a de novo effect. Additionally, mutations in *SCN3B* and *SCN4B* identified in SIDS cases were associated with loss- and gain-of-function effects on the sodium current, respectively.[13] Mutations in genes encoding sodium channel–interacting proteins (ie, *CAV3, GPD1L,* and *SNTA1*) that have been associated with LQTS and Brugada syndrome have also recently been linked to SIDS (see **Table 1**).[16,18,20]

OVERLAP SYNDROMES

Several *SCN5A* mutations have been identified to segregate in families that express a more complex phenotype, displaying combinations of LQTS, Brugada syndrome, and conduction disease, a phenomenon commonly referred to as *cardiac sodium channel overlap syndromes.*[103] The first case of overlap syndrome was described in a large Dutch family segregating the *SCN5A*-1795insD mutation.[92] Right precordial ST-elevation, bradycardia-dependent QT prolongation, sinus node dysfunction, and conduction disease were present in isolation or some combination in mutation carriers from this family. Mice carrying the equivalent of the *SCN5A*-1795insD mutation recapitulated the multiple disease manifestations.[30] In vitro electrophysiologic studies on 1795insD-mutant channels have shown gating changes associated with both gain- and loss-of function effects of the mutation: a persistent inward sodium current (resulting in prolongation of the action potential, consistent with gain-of-function) and reduced current and enhanced slow inactivation (resulting in reduced channel availability, consistent with loss-of-function).

The biophysical complexity of *SCN5A* mutations associated with a mixed phenotype was also illustrated by the delK1500 mutation, segregating in a family with a heterogeneous clinical phenotype of LQTS, Brugada syndrome, and PCCD. This mutation exhibits sustained inward current in combination with a negative shift in voltage dependence of inactivation and a positive shift in voltage dependence of activation, resulting in reduced channel availability.[104] A considerable number of overlap syndromes with distinct combinations of clinical phenotypes have since been reported, including LQTS in combination with PCCD[105] and sinus node dysfunction in combination with Brugada syndrome and PCCD.[85] The most prevalent overlap syndrome is that of Brugada syndrome and PCCD,[106] which is expected because

mutations associated with both disorders exhibit loss-of-function characteristics.

The occurrence of multiple phenotypic manifestations is typically observed for mutations segregating in larger families, and one could argue that this could apply to a larger number of mutations if the respective families were sufficiently large to observe this effect. Factors thought to modulate the ultimate disease expression in the individual patient are believed to include genetic background effects (encompassing common genetic variants at the same or a different locus, and coinheritance of other rare variants), and physiologic (eg, age, gender, heart rate) and environmental factors (eg, exercise, infection).[103]

DILATED CARDIOMYOPATHY

Sodium channelopathies, including the Brugada syndrome, long QT syndrome, and sick sinus syndrome, were originally considered as primary and purely electrical disorders occurring in the absence of structural heart disease. However, current evidence has expanded the clinical spectrum of sodium channelopathies to include cardiac fibrosis, dilatation, and dysfunction.[82,107] Genome-wide linkage analysis in a family originally described in 1986 by Greenlee and colleagues[108] led to the discovery of an *SCN5A* missense mutation (D1275 N) that cosegregated with a variable phenotype, including dilated cardiomyopathy, sinus node dysfunction, conduction disease and atrial arrhythmias.[109,110] Various other *SCN5A* mutations associated with a similar clinical presentation have since been reported (**Table 3**). All mutations reported to date show an autosomal dominant pattern of inheritance, with the exception of *SCN5A*-R814Q occurring homozygously.[113] Most of the dilated cardiomyopathy–associated *SCN5A* mutations studied in heterologous expression systems has been predicted to cause loss-of-function effects through diverse kinetic effects altering both activation (D1275 N,[93] R814 W[112]) and inactivation (D1595H[112]). The A1180 V mutation has been associated with an increase in late sodium current, resulting in a gain-of-function effect.[114] The pathomechanism through which mutations lead to myocardial damage and structural abnormalities remains unknown. Proposed mechanisms include an abnormal calcium homeostasis and a disruption of the interaction between the sodium channel and cytoskeletal components such as the dystrophin complex.[112,116]

Atrial tachyarrhythmias seem to be a common clinical feature in *SCN5A* mutation carriers displaying dilated cardiomyopathy. Olson and

Table 3
SCN5A mutations associated with dilated cardiomyopathy

Mutation	Location	Phenotype	Effect on Na$^+$ Current	Comments	References
D1275 N	DIII S3	SND, CD, AF, VA	Decreased I_{NA}	Also associated with atrial standstill[93]	McNair et al[109] Olson et al[110]
T220I	DI S4	SND, CD, AF, VA	Decreased I_{NA}	Also associated with SSS[84]	Olson et al[110]
D1595H	DIV S3	SND, AF, VA	Decreased I_{NA}	D1595 N associated with atrioventricular block[111]	Olson et al[110] Nguyen et al[112]
2550–2551insTG	DII S5	SND, CD	NA		Olson et al[110]
R814 W	DII S4	AF	Decreased I_{NA}	De novo; decreased current rate-dependent (at faster rates)	Olson et al[110] Nguyen et al[112]
R814Q	DII S4	CD, VA	NA	Homozygous mutation	Frigo et al[113]
W156X and R225 W	D1 S1–S2 linker and D1 S4	CD, VA, fibrosis	Abolished I_{NA} (W156X) Decreased I_{NA} (R225 W)	Heterozygous single-mutation carriers clinically not affected	Bezzina et al[82]
A1180 V	DII–DIII linker	CD, AF	Decreased I_{NA}, late I_{NA}	Decreased current rate-dependent (at faster rates)	Ge et al[114]
R222Gln	D1 S4	IVCD, HF	NA	Associated with postpartum cardiomyopathy	Morales et al[115]

Abbreviations: AF, atrial fibrillation; CD, conduction disease; HF, heart failure; IVCD, intraventricular conduction delay; Na+, sodium; NA, not available; SND, sinus node dysfunction; SSS, sick sinus syndrome; VA, ventricular arrhythmias.

colleagues[110] reported documented atrial fibrillation in 43% of 37 individuals in five families that carried a dilated cardiomyopathy–related SCN5A mutation (mean age at diagnosis, 27.8 years). Although not completely excluded, cardiomyopathy did not seem to be secondary to atrial tachyarrhythmias. In line with this, Bezzina and colleagues[82] described a 1-year-old girl with compound heterozygosity for W156X/R225 W who exhibited overt dilated cardiomyopathy with replacement fibrosis and short episodes of arrhythmia, thereby rendering the possibility of tachyarrhythmia-induced cardiomyopathy unlikely.

ARRHYTHMOGENIC RIGHT VENTRICULAR CARDIOMYOPATHY

Arrhythmogenic right ventricular dysplasia/cardiomyopathy (ARVD/C) is a heritable disorder characterized by fibrosis and fibrofatty replacement affecting primarily the right ventricular myocardium. Progressive loss of myocardium can result in severe right ventricular dysfunction, ventricular tachyarrhythmias, and sudden death. Patients with ARVC typically present between the second and fifth decade of life with palpitations, syncope, or sudden death. Mutations in genes encoding components of the cardiac desmosome are associated with ARVC, and a genetic defect in one of these genes is identified in approximately 50% of patients.[117]

Among these patients, a subpopulation displays clinical and electrocardiographic features (right precordial ST-segment elevation in the absence or presence of sodium channel blockade) similar to patients with Brugada syndrome.[118] Conversely, several groups have identified (minor) structural and histologic abnormalities, consistent with ARVC in patients with Brugada syndrome.

In 1996, Corrado and colleagues[119] described a family with autosomal dominant inheritance with variable expressivity of distinct clinical features of Brugada syndrome, including right precordial ST-segment elevation, right bundle branch block, and sudden death. The index case (ie, the earliest documented case of the family) underwent ß-adrenergic blocking therapy but died suddenly at rest. Postmortem investigation revealed right ventricular dilatation, myocardial atrophy, and fibrofatty replacement of the right ventricular free wall.

In a study of 273 young (≤35 years of age) sudden death victims, the same group from Padua reported Brugada ECG patterns, including ST elevation in V1–V3 and polymorphic VT, in 13 of 96 subjects for whom ECGs were available. At autopsy, 12 of these 13 showed structural and histologic lesions characteristic of ARVC.[120] Compared with 19 young sudden death victims with ARVC but without right precordial ST-segment elevation from the same series, 83% (10/12) versus 26% (5/19) died suddenly at rest or during sleep. The presence and distribution of SCN5A mutations within these young sudden death series is unknown.

Frustaci and colleagues[121] found pathologic features in endomyocardial biopsies of 18 patients with Brugada syndrome with normal heart structure and function on noninvasive examinations, consistent with myocarditis (n = 14) and with right ventricular cardiomyopathy (n = 3) and fatty infiltration (n = 1). Remarkably, SCN5A mutations with loss-of-function effects when expressed heterologously were identified in the four subjects with cardiomyopathy and fatty infiltration. In addition, in the explanted heart of an SCN5A mutation–positive patient with Brugada syndrome without clinically detected structural abnormalities, right ventricular hypertrophy and fibrosis with epicardial fatty infiltration (but not myocyte replacement) were present.[107] However, (clinically detectable) structural abnormalities in patients with Brugada syndrome remain often either absent or subtle, as opposed to ARVC with right ventricular structural and histologic alterations as key features.[122]

A genetic link between ARVC and Brugada syndrome remains to be established. Peters and colleagues[118] showed that ajmaline could provoke the coved-type Brugada pattern ECG in 16% (9/55) of patients with ARVC according to the International Society and Federation of Cardiology Task Force/European Society of Cardiology criteria. In a follow-up study, repeated ajmaline testing after at least 3 years remained positive in only 50% (4/8); however, endomyocardial biopsies were not taken in the first study to exclude myocarditic changes of the myocardium. Additionally, the SCN5A-E746 K mutation was identified in one patient with ARVC with a positive ajmaline provocation test.[123] Thus, clinical and experimental studies show a convincing overlap, and a yet-undefined fine line, among the clinical, electrocardiographic, and histologic features of Brugada syndrome and ARVC.

DISTINGUISHING PATHOGENIC MUTATIONS FROM BENIGN SEQUENCE VARIANTS

The identification of a sequence variant in a gene that has been associated with arrhythmia is by itself not sufficient to claim that it is the cause of the disease. In fact, one of the most difficult aspects of genetic studies in the familial arrhythmia syndromes is the identification of large extended families necessary for rigorous segregation analysis. Assignment of a mutation as pathogenic often relies on the following criteria: (1) alteration of an evolutionarily conserved amino acid (in the case of nonsynonymous mutations), (2) alteration of protein structure (nonsense, frameshift, or splice site mutations), (3) absence of the variant in a sufficiently large (eg, >200) sample of unrelated, ethnically matched, unaffected individuals, and (4) alteration of protein function (eg, abnormal channel biophysical properties in vitro). However, the possibility of comprehensive functional assays is not widely available.

Rare, nonsynonymous (amino-acid substituting) SCN5A variants have been identified in 3.2% (42/1300) healthy controls.[87] A similar rate of genetic background noise has been reported in a large panel of healthy subjects from four ethnic groups (28 novel variants among 829 subjects; 3.4%).[124] This finding further supports the notion that genetic testing is not always straightforward and that a proper interpretation of the genetic test result is critical considering the implications of mutation identification. Distinguishing pathogenic mutations from innocuous and clinically silent gene variants remains a major challenge in many instances. For the sodium channel, mutation type (eg, nonsense vs missense), mutation location in channel subdomain (eg, pore vs transmembrane vs linker), and ethnic-specific background rates have been shown to be critical factors in predicting the pathogenicity of novel mutations.[125] For instance, in LQTS, a novel mutation (an unclassified variant) identified in the transmembrane regions of the SCN5A-encoded sodium channel is much more likely to be pathogenic than when located in an interdomain linker.[125] Thus, genetic tests should be viewed as probabilistic (taking into account factors such as location of mutation, ethnicity, lack of testing for other unknown susceptibility genes) and not as binary.

DISEASE VARIABILITY AND COMMON GENETIC VARIATION IN SODIUM CHANNELOPATHY

Individuals within a family who have the same pathogenic mutation as the proband may remain clinically unaffected (a phenomenon referred to as reduced penetrance), present with milder or more severe symptoms (referred to as variable expressivity), or even express different manifestations (pleiotropy). These genetic concepts are thought to stem from several factors, including (1) genetic background (the presence of modifying common or rare variants), (2) effects of physiologic factors (eg, age, gender), (3) environmental factors, and (4) complex gene-by-environment interactions.

Common genetic variants that modulate mutation-specific effects and influence the ultimate clinical presentation of a (monogenic) disease phenotype may reside within the same gene that carries the disease-causing mutation or at a distance, in another gene. The SCN5A-H558R polymorphism, located in the sodium channel DI—DII cytoplasmic linker, was shown through coexpression studies in vitro to (partly) rescue loss-of-function mutations, increasing sodium current.[126,127] The effect of a common modifying variant outside of the SCN5A gene itself is exemplified in a family segregating the SCN5A-D1275 N mutation and polymorphisms in the atrial-specific connexin40. Individuals who carried the SCN5A mutation and were homozygous for the Cx40 polymorphisms exhibited atrial standstill, whereas those who inherited the SCN5A mutations but were not homozygous for the Cx40 polymorphisms manifested with mild PR interval prolongation only.[93] Likewise, (compound) rare variants may also play a role in variable disease expressivity. This finding is exemplified by carriers of a stop codon in SCN5A (W156X), which is predicted to cause a 50% reduction in available sodium channels, who were phenotypically silent, whereas progressive conduction disease was diagnosed in W156X/R225 W compound mutation carriers.[82]

ECG parameters, including heart rate, PR, QRS, and QT interval, are known to be heritable traits and are therefore influenced by genetic variation.[128,129] Recent genome-wide association studies in large cohorts have tested for the association between common genetic variation in the form of single nucleotide polymorphisms, occurring at a frequency of approximately 5% or more in the general population and these parameters. Newton-Cheh and colleagues[130] (representing the QTGEN consortium) and Pfeufer and colleagues[131] (representing the QT Interval and Sudden Cardiac Death (QTSCD) consortium) each conducted a meta-analysis of genome-wide association studies performed in population-based cohorts for QT-interval duration, and independently observed (genome-wide significant) associations at multiple loci, including SCN5A. This finding implies that common genetic variation within this gene impacts on the extent of QT duration in the general population.

Similarly, a meta-analysis of genome-wide association studies for PR interval in the general population identified the chromosomal region harboring the neighboring SCN5A and SCN10A genes impacting on this parameter.[132] Some of these polymorphisms have been shown to modulate risk of atrial firbillation.[132] Future research will likely investigate whether these identified variants also impact on disease expression in the monogenic arrhythmia syndromes and in other common arrhythmias, such as ischemia-induced VF.

The frequency of common genetic variants in different populations may vary substantially and may underlie ethnic diversity in arrhythmia susceptibility. The SCN5A-S1103Y polymorphism, which occurs at a frequency of 8% to 13% among individuals of Africans descent and is absent in Caucasians, is associated with increased risk of ventricular arrhythmia and has been linked to sudden infant death syndrome and drug-induced LQTS.[2,133,134] In addition, certain common SCN5A promoter variants thought to be associated with decreased sodium channel levels, and impacting on PR interval and QRS duration, are specific for the Asian population.[135]

SUMMARY

The identification of the genetic defects underlying the inherited arrhythmia syndromes is crucial because it provides insight into important aspects of these disease entities, including prognosis and optimal treatment options for the specific molecular genetic subtypes, and enables presymptomatic identification and treatment of patients at risk. The observation of reduced penetrance and variable disease expressivity, in addition to the discovery that Brugada syndrome and LQTS are associated with mutations in the same gene, highlight the complexity of SCN5A-associated arrhythmia syndromes. Future research will provide more insight into aspects of the disease that are not understood, such as mutation-specific management and therapy, the nature of the mechanistic link between SCN5A mutations and cardiac remodeling, and the nature of genetic modifiers impacting on disease expression.

REFERENCES

1. Wilde AA, Bezzina CR. Genetics of cardiac arrhythmias. Heart 2005;91(10):1352–8.
2. Splawski I, Timothy KW, Tateyama M, et al. Variant of SCN5A sodium channel implicated in risk of cardiac arrhythmia. Science 2002;297(5585): 1333–6.
3. Makita N, Horie M, Nakamura T, et al. Drug-induced long-QT syndrome associated with a subclinical SCN5A mutation. Circulation 2002; 106(10):1269–74.
4. George AL Jr, Varkony TA, Drabkin HA, et al. Assignment of the human heart tetrodotoxin-resistant voltage-gated Na+ channel alpha-subunit gene (SCN5A) to band 3p21. Cytogenet Cell Genet 1995;68(1–2):67–70.
5. Wang Q, Li Z, Shen J, et al. Genomic organization of the human SCN5A gene encoding the cardiac sodium channel. Genomics 1996;34(1):9–16.
6. Guy HR, Seetharamulu P. Molecular model of the action potential sodium channel. Proc Natl Acad Sci U S A 1986;83(2):508–12.
7. Mantegazza M, Yu FH, Catterall WA, et al. Role of the C-terminal domain in inactivation of brain and cardiac sodium channels. Proc Natl Acad Sci U S A 2001;98(26):15348–53.
8. Hodgkin AL, Huxley AF. Currents carried by sodium and potassium ions through the membrane of the giant axon of Loligo. J Physiol 1952;116(4): 449–72.
9. Vilin YY, Ruben PC. Slow inactivation in voltage-gated sodium channels: molecular substrates and contributions to channelopathies. Cell Biochem Biophys 2001;35(2):171–90.
10. Horn R, Patlak J, Stevens CF. Sodium channels need not open before they inactivate. Nature 1981;291(5814):426–7.
11. Watanabe H, Koopmann TT, Le SS, et al. Sodium channel beta1 subunit mutations associated with Brugada syndrome and cardiac conduction disease in humans. J Clin Invest 2008;118(6): 2260–8.
12. Watanabe H, Darbar D, Kaiser DW, et al. Mutations in sodium channel beta1- and beta2-subunits associated with atrial fibrillation. Circ Arrhythm Electrophysiol 2009;2(3):268–75.
13. Tan BH, Pundi KN, Van Norstrand DW, et al. Sudden infant death syndrome-associated mutations in the sodium channel beta subunits. Heart Rhythm 2010;7(6):771–8.
14. Hu D, Barajas-Martinez H, Burashnikov E, et al. A mutation in the beta 3 subunit of the cardiac sodium channel associated with Brugada ECG phenotype. Circ Cardiovasc Genet 2009;2(3):270–8.
15. Medeiros-Domingo A, Kaku T, Tester DJ, et al. SCN4B-encoded sodium channel beta4 subunit in congenital long-QT syndrome. Circulation 2007; 116(2):134–42.
16. Cronk LB, Ye B, Kaku T, et al. Novel mechanism for sudden infant death syndrome: persistent late sodium current secondary to mutations in caveolin-3. Heart Rhythm 2007;4(2):161–6.
17. Vatta M, Ackerman MJ, Ye B, et al. Mutant caveolin-3 induces persistent late sodium current and is associated with long-QT syndrome. Circulation 2006;114(20):2104–12.
18. Cheng J, Van Norstrand DW, Medeiros-Domingo A, et al. Alpha1-syntrophin mutations identified in

sudden infant death syndrome cause an increase in late cardiac sodium current. Circ Arrhythm Electrophysiol 2009;2(6):667–76.

19. Ueda K, Valdivia C, Medeiros-Domingo A, et al. Syntrophin mutation associated with long QT syndrome through activation of the nNOS-SCN5A macromolecular complex. Proc Natl Acad Sci U S A 2008;105(27):9355–60.

20. Van Norstrand DW, Valdivia CR, Tester DJ, et al. Molecular and functional characterization of novel glycerol-3-phosphate dehydrogenase 1 like gene (GPD1-L) mutations in sudden infant death syndrome. Circulation 2007;116(20):2253–9.

21. London B, Michalec M, Mehdi H, et al. Mutation in glycerol-3-phosphate dehydrogenase 1 like gene (GPD1-L) decreases cardiac Na+ current and causes inherited arrhythmias. Circulation 2007; 116(20):2260–8.

22. Yang Y, Yang Y, Liang B, et al. Identification of a Kir3.4 mutation in congenital long QT syndrome. Am J Hum Genet 2010;86(6):872–80.

23. Schwartz PJ, Stramba-Badiale M, Crotti L, et al. Prevalence of the congenital long-QT syndrome. Circulation 2009;120(18):1761–7.

24. Karhunen P, Luomanmaki K, Heikkila J, et al. Syncope and Q-T prolongation without deafness: the Romano-Ward syndrome. Am Heart J 1970; 80(6):820–3.

25. Splawski I, Shen J, Timothy KW, et al. Spectrum of mutations in long-QT syndrome genes. KVLQT1, HERG, SCN5A, KCNE1, and KCNE2. Circulation 2000;102(10):1178–85.

26. Tester DJ, Will ML, Haglund CM, et al. Compendium of cardiac channel mutations in 541 consecutive unrelated patients referred for long QT syndrome genetic testing. Heart Rhythm 2005;2(5):507–17.

27. Hedley PL, Jorgensen P, Schlamowitz S, et al. The genetic basis of long QT and short QT syndromes: a mutation update. Hum Mutat 2009;30(11): 1486–511.

28. Bennett PB, Yazawa K, Makita N, et al. Molecular mechanism for an inherited cardiac arrhythmia. Nature 1995;376(6542):683–5.

29. Papadatos GA, Wallerstein PM, Head CE, et al. Slowed conduction and ventricular tachycardia after targeted disruption of the cardiac sodium channel gene Scn5a. Proc Natl Acad Sci U S A 2002;99(9):6210–5.

30. Remme CA, Verkerk AO, Nuyens D, et al. Overlap syndrome of cardiac sodium channel disease in mice carrying the equivalent mutation of human SCN5A-1795insD. Circulation 2006;114(24): 2584–94.

31. Nuyens D, Stengl M, Dugarmaa S, et al. Abrupt rate accelerations or premature beats cause life-threatening arrhythmias in mice with long-QT3 syndrome. Nat Med 2001;7(9):1021–7.

32. Tian XL, Yong SL, Wan X, et al. Mechanisms by which SCN5A mutation N1325S causes cardiac arrhythmias and sudden death in vivo. Cardiovasc Res 2004;61(2):256–67.

33. Ruan Y, Liu N, Bloise R, et al. Gating properties of SCN5A mutations and the response to mexiletine in long-QT syndrome type 3 patients. Circulation 2007;116(10):1137–44.

34. Veldkamp MW, Wilders R, Baartscheer A, et al. Contribution of sodium channel mutations to bradycardia and sinus node dysfunction in LQT3 families. Circ Res 2003;92(9):976–83.

35. Moss AJ, Zareba W, Benhorin J, et al. ECG T-wave patterns in genetically distinct forms of the hereditary long QT syndrome. Circulation 1995;92(10):2929–34.

36. Zhang L, Timothy KW, Vincent GM, et al. Spectrum of ST-T-wave patterns and repolarization parameters in congenital long-QT syndrome: ECG findings identify genotypes. Circulation 2000;102(23): 2849–55.

37. Schwartz PJ, Priori SG, Locati EH, et al. Long QT syndrome patients with mutations of the SCN5A and HERG genes have differential responses to Na+ channel blockade and to increases in heart rate. Implications for gene-specific therapy. Circulation 1995;92(12):3381–6.

38. Chang CC, Acharfi S, Wu MH, et al. A novel SCN5A mutation manifests as a malignant form of long QT syndrome with perinatal onset of tachycardia/bradycardia. Cardiovasc Res 2004;64(2):268–78.

39. Priori SG, Schwartz PJ, Napolitano C, et al. Risk stratification in the long-QT syndrome. N Engl J Med 2003;348(19):1866–74.

40. Jons C, Moss AJ, Goldenberg I, et al. Risk of fatal arrhythmic events in long QT syndrome patients after syncope. J Am Coll Cardiol 2010;55(8):783–8.

41. Zareba W, Moss AJ, Locati EH, et al. Modulating effects of age and gender on the clinical course of long QT syndrome by genotype. J Am Coll Cardiol 2003;42(1):103–9.

42. Zareba W, Moss AJ, Schwartz PJ, et al. Influence of genotype on the clinical course of the long-QT syndrome. International long-QT syndrome registry research group. N Engl J Med 1998;339(14): 960–5.

43. Liu JF, Moss AJ, Jons C, et al. Mutation-specific risk in two genetic forms of type 3 long QT syndrome. Am J Cardiol 2010;105(2):210–3.

44. Priori SG, Napolitano C, Schwartz PJ, et al. Association of long QT syndrome loci and cardiac events among patients treated with beta-blockers. JAMA 2004;292(11):1341–4.

45. Schwartz PJ, Spazzolini C, Crotti L. All LQT3 patients need an ICD: true or false? Heart Rhythm 2009;6(1):113–20.

46. Hofman N, Tan HL, Alders M, et al. Active cascade screening in primary inherited arrhythmia

syndromes: does it lead to prophylactic treatment? J Am Coll Cardiol 2010;55(23):2570–6.

47. Benhorin J, Taub R, Goldmit M, et al. Effects of flecainide in patients with new SCN5A mutation: mutation-specific therapy for long-QT syndrome? Circulation 2000;101(14):1698–706.

48. Moss AJ, Zareba W, Schwarz KQ, et al. Ranolazine shortens repolarization in patients with sustained inward sodium current due to type-3 long-QT syndrome. J Cardiovasc Electrophysiol 2008; 19(12):1289–93.

49. Priori SG, Napolitano C, Schwartz PJ, et al. The elusive link between LQT3 and Brugada syndrome: the role of flecainide challenge. Circulation 2000; 102(9):945–7.

50. Zipes DP, Camm AJ, Borggrefe M, et al. ACC/AHA/ ESC 2006 guidelines for management of patients with ventricular arrhythmias and the prevention of sudden cardiac death: a report of the American College of Cardiology/American Heart Association Task Force and the European Society of Cardiology Committee for Practice Guidelines (Writing Committee to Develop Guidelines for Management of Patients With Ventricular Arrhythmias and the Prevention of Sudden Cardiac Death). J Am Coll Cardiol 2006;48(5):e247–346.

51. Brugada P, Brugada J. Right bundle branch block, persistent ST segment elevation and sudden cardiac death: a distinct clinical and electrocardiographic syndrome. A multicenter report. J Am Coll Cardiol 1992;20(6):1391–6.

52. Priori SG, Napolitano C, Giordano U, et al. Brugada syndrome and sudden cardiac death in children. Lancet 2000;355(9206):808–9.

53. Antzelevitch C, Brugada P, Borggrefe M, et al. Brugada syndrome: report of the second consensus conference. Heart Rhythm 2005;2(4):429–40.

54. Fowler SJ, Priori SG. Clinical spectrum of patients with a Brugada ECG. Curr Opin Cardiol 2009; 24(1):74–81.

55. Tsuji H, Sato T, Morisaki K, et al. Prognosis of subjects with Brugada-type electrocardiogram in a population of middle-aged Japanese diagnosed during a health examination. Am J Cardiol 2008; 102(5):584–7.

56. Probst V, Veltmann C, Eckardt L, et al. Long-term prognosis of patients diagnosed with Brugada syndrome: results from the FINGER Brugada Syndrome Registry. Circulation 2010;121(5):635–43.

57. Wilde AA, Antzelevitch C, Borggrefe M, et al. Proposed diagnostic criteria for the Brugada syndrome: consensus report. Circulation 2002; 106(19):2514–9.

58. Eckardt L, Probst V, Smits JP, et al. Long-term prognosis of individuals with right precordial ST-segment-elevation Brugada syndrome. Circulation 2005;111(3):257–63.

59. Litovsky SH, Antzelevitch C. Differences in the electrophysiological response of canine ventricular subendocardium and subepicardium to acetylcholine and isoproterenol. A direct effect of acetylcholine in ventricular myocardium. Circ Res 1990; 67(3):615–27.

60. Miyazaki T, Mitamura H, Miyoshi S, et al. Autonomic and antiarrhythmic drug modulation of ST segment elevation in patients with Brugada syndrome. J Am Coll Cardiol 1996;27(5):1061–70.

61. Amin AS, Meregalli PG, Bardai A, et al. Fever increases the risk for cardiac arrest in the Brugada syndrome. Ann Intern Med 2008;149(3):216–8.

62. Postema PG, Wolpert C, Amin AS, et al. Drugs and Brugada syndrome patients: review of the literature, recommendations, and an up-to-date website. (http://www.brugadadrugs.org). Heart Rhythm 2009;6(9):1335–41.

63. Chen Q, Kirsch GE, Zhang D, et al. Genetic basis and molecular mechanism for idiopathic ventricular fibrillation. Nature 1998;392(6673):293–6.

64. Priori SG, Napolitano C, Gasparini M, et al. Natural history of Brugada syndrome: insights for risk stratification and management. Circulation 2002; 105(11):1342–7.

65. Kurita T, Shimizu W, Inagaki M, et al. The electrophysiologic mechanism of ST-segment elevation in Brugada syndrome. J Am Coll Cardiol 2002; 40(2):330–4.

66. Tukkie R, Sogaard P, Vleugels J, et al. Delay in right ventricular activation contributes to Brugada syndrome. Circulation 2004;109(10):1272–7.

67. Meregalli PG, Wilde AA, Tan HL. Pathophysiological mechanisms of Brugada syndrome: depolarization disorder, repolarization disorder, or more? Cardiovasc Res 2005;67(3):367–78.

68. Nabauer M, Beuckelmann DJ, Uberfuhr P, et al. Regional differences in current density and rate-dependent properties of the transient outward current in subepicardial and subendocardial myocytes of human left ventricle. Circulation 1996; 93(1):168–77.

69. Yan GX, Antzelevitch C. Cellular basis for the Brugada syndrome and other mechanisms of arrhythmogenesis associated with ST-segment elevation. Circulation 1999;100(15):1660–6.

70. Probst V, Wilde AA, Barc J, et al. SCN5A mutations and the role of genetic background in the pathophysiology of Brugada syndrome. Circ Cardiovasc Genet 2009;2(6):552–7.

71. Remme CA, Scicluna BP, Verkerk AO, et al. Genetically determined differences in sodium current characteristics modulate conduction disease severity in mice with cardiac sodium channelopathy. Circ Res 2009;104(11):1283–92.

72. Brugada J, Brugada R, Brugada P. Determinants of sudden cardiac death in individuals with the

electrocardiographic pattern of Brugada syndrome and no previous cardiac arrest. Circulation 2003; 108(25):3092–6.

73. Gehi AK, Duong TD, Metz LD, et al. Risk stratification of individuals with the Brugada electrocardiogram: a meta-analysis. J Cardiovasc Electrophysiol 2006;17(6):577–83.

74. Nademanee K, Veerakul G, Mower M, et al. Defibrillator Versus beta-Blockers for Unexplained Death in Thailand (DEBUT): a randomized clinical trial. Circulation 2003;107(17):2221–6.

75. Sacher F, Probst V, Iesaka Y, et al. Outcome after implantation of a cardioverter-defibrillator in patients with Brugada syndrome: a multicenter study. Circulation 2006;114(22):2317–24.

76. Belhassen B, Glick A, Viskin S. Efficacy of quinidine in high-risk patients with Brugada syndrome. Circulation 2004;110(13):1731–7.

77. Viskin S, Wilde AA, Tan HL, et al. Empiric quinidine therapy for asymptomatic Brugada syndrome: time for a prospective registry. Heart Rhythm 2009;6(3): 401–4.

78. Schott JJ, Alshinawi C, Kyndt F, et al. Cardiac conduction defects associate with mutations in SCN5A. Nat Genet 1999;23(1):20–1.

79. Kyndt F, Probst V, Potet F, et al. Novel SCN5A mutation leading either to isolated cardiac conduction defect or Brugada syndrome in a large French family. Circulation 2001;104(25):3081–6.

80. Royer A, van Veen TA, Le BS, et al. Mouse model of SCN5A-linked hereditary Lenegre's disease: age-related conduction slowing and myocardial fibrosis. Circulation 2005;111(14):1738–46.

81. Probst V, Kyndt F, Potet F, et al. Haploinsufficiency in combination with aging causes SCN5A-linked hereditary Lenegre disease. J Am Coll Cardiol 2003;41(4):643–52.

82. Bezzina CR, Rook MB, Groenewegen WA, et al. Compound heterozygosity for mutations (W156X and R225W) in SCN5A associated with severe cardiac conduction disturbances and degenerative changes in the conduction system. Circ Res 2003;92(2):159–68.

83. Short DS. The syndrome of alternating bradycardia and tachycardia. Br Heart J 1954;16(2): 208–14.

84. Benson DW, Wang DW, Dyment M, et al. Congenital sick sinus syndrome caused by recessive mutations in the cardiac sodium channel gene (SCN5A). J Clin Invest 2003;112(7):1019–28.

85. Smits JP, Koopmann TT, Wilders R, et al. A mutation in the human cardiac sodium channel (E161K) contributes to sick sinus syndrome, conduction disease and Brugada syndrome in two families. J Mol Cell Cardiol 2005;38(6):969–81.

86. Gui J, Wang T, Jones RP, et al. Multiple loss-of-function mechanisms contribute to SCN5A-related

familial sick sinus syndrome. PLoS One 2010; 5(6):e10985.

87. Kapplinger JD, Tester DJ, Alders M, et al. An international compendium of mutations in the SCN5A-encoded cardiac sodium channel in patients referred for Brugada syndrome genetic testing. Heart Rhythm 2010;7(1):33–46.

88. Maier SK, Westenbroek RE, Yamanushi TT, et al. An unexpected requirement for brain-type sodium channels for control of heart rate in the mouse sino-atrial node. Proc Natl Acad Sci U S A 2003;100(6): 3507–12.

89. Butters TD, Aslanidi OV, Inada S, et al. Mechanistic links between Na+ channel (SCN5A) mutations and impaired cardiac pacemaking in sick sinus syndrome. Circ Res 2010;107(1):126–37.

90. Lei M, Zhang H, Grace AA, et al. SCN5A and sinoatrial node pacemaker function. Cardiovasc Res 2007;74(3):356–65.

91. Abriel H, Wehrens XH, Benhorin J, et al. Molecular pharmacology of the sodium channel mutation D1790G linked to the long-QT syndrome. Circulation 2000;102(8):921–5.

92. Bezzina C, Veldkamp MW, van den Berg MP, et al. A single Na(+) channel mutation causing both long-QT and Brugada syndromes. Circ Res 1999; 85(12):1206–13.

93. Groenewegen WA, Firouzi M, Bezzina CR, et al. A cardiac sodium channel mutation cosegregates with a rare connexin40 genotype in familial atrial standstill. Circ Res 2003;92(1):14–22.

94. Roberts JD, Gollob MH. Impact of genetic discoveries on the classification of lone atrial fibrillation. J Am Coll Cardiol 2010;55(8):705–12.

95. Darbar D, Kannankeril PJ, Donahue BS, et al. Cardiac sodium channel (SCN5A) variants associated with atrial fibrillation. Circulation 2008;117(15): 1927–35.

96. Makiyama T, Akao M, Shizuta S, et al. A novel SCN5A gain-of-function mutation M1875T associated with familial atrial fibrillation. J Am Coll Cardiol 2008;52(16):1326–34.

97. Li Q, Huang H, Liu G, et al. Gain-of-function mutation of Nav1.5 in atrial fibrillation enhances cellular excitability and lowers the threshold for action potential firing. Biochem Biophys Res Commun 2009;380(1):132–7.

98. Ellinor PT, Nam EG, Shea MA, et al. Cardiac sodium channel mutation in atrial fibrillation. Heart Rhythm 2008;5(1):99–105.

99. Letsas KP, Sideris A, Efremidis M, et al. Prevalence of paroxysmal atrial fibrillation in Brugada syndrome: a case series and a review of the literature. J Cardiovasc Med (Hagerstown) 2007;8(10): 803–6.

100. Krous HF, Beckwith JB, Byard RW, et al. Sudden infant death syndrome and unclassified sudden

infant deaths: a definitional and diagnostic approach. Pediatrics 2004;114(1):234—8.

101. Arnestad M, Crotti L, Rognum TO, et al. Prevalence of long-QT syndrome gene variants in sudden infant death syndrome. Circulation 2007;115(3): 361—7.

102. Wang DW, Desai RR, Crotti L, et al. Cardiac sodium channel dysfunction in sudden infant death syndrome. Circulation 2007;115(3):368—76.

103. Remme CA, Wilde AA, Bezzina CR. Cardiac sodium channel overlap syndromes: different faces of SCN5A mutations. Trends Cardiovasc Med 2008;18(3):78—87.

104. Grant AO, Carboni MP, Neplioueva V, et al. Long QT syndrome, Brugada syndrome, and conduction system disease are linked to a single sodium channel mutation. J Clin Invest 2002;110(8): 1201—9.

105. Surber R, Hensellek S, Prochnau D, et al. Combination of cardiac conduction disease and long QT syndrome caused by mutation T1620K in the cardiac sodium channel. Cardiovasc Res 2008; 77(4):740—8.

106. Probst V, Allouis M, Sacher F, et al. Progressive cardiac conduction defect is the prevailing phenotype in carriers of a Brugada syndrome SCN5A mutation. J Cardiovasc Electrophysiol 2006;17(3): 270—5.

107. Coronel R, Casini S, Koopmann TT, et al. Right ventricular fibrosis and conduction delay in a patient with clinical signs of Brugada syndrome: a combined electrophysiological, genetic, histopathologic, and computational study. Circulation 2005;112(18):2769—77.

108. Greenlee PR, Anderson JL, Lutz JR, et al. Familial automaticity-conduction disorder with associated cardiomyopathy. West J Med 1986;144(1):33—41.

109. McNair WP, Ku L, Taylor MR, et al. SCN5A mutation associated with dilated cardiomyopathy, conduction disorder, and arrhythmia. Circulation 2004; 110(15):2163—7.

110. Olson TM, Michels VV, Ballew JD, et al. Sodium channel mutations and susceptibility to heart failure and atrial fibrillation. JAMA 2005;293(4): 447—54.

111. Wang DW, Viswanathan PC, Balser JR, et al. Clinical, genetic, and biophysical characterization of SCN5A mutations associated with atrioventricular conduction block. Circulation 2002;105(3):341—6.

112. Nguyen TP, Wang DW, Rhodes TH, et al. Divergent biophysical defects caused by mutant sodium channels in dilated cardiomyopathy with arrhythmia. Circ Res 2008;102(3):364—71.

113. Frigo G, Rampazzo A, Bauce B, et al. Homozygous SCN5A mutation in Brugada syndrome with monomorphic ventricular tachycardia and structural heart abnormalities. Europace 2007;9(6):391—7.

114. Ge J, Sun A, Paajanen V, et al. Molecular and clinical characterization of a novel SCN5A mutation associated with atrioventricular block and dilated cardiomyopathy. Circ Arrhythm Electrophysiol 2008;1(2):83—92.

115. Morales A, Painter T, Li R, et al. Rare variant mutations in pregnancy-associated or peripartum cardiomyopathy. Circulation 2010;121(20): 2176—82.

116. Bezzina CR, Remme CA. Dilated cardiomyopathy due to sodium channel dysfunction: what is the connection? Circ Arrhythm Electrophysiol 2008; 1(2):80—2.

117. Hamid MS, Norman M, Quraishi A, et al. Prospective evaluation of relatives for familial arrhythmogenic right ventricular cardiomyopathy/dysplasia reveals a need to broaden diagnostic criteria. J Am Coll Cardiol 2002;40(8): 1445—50.

118. Peters S, Trummel M, Denecke S, et al. Results of ajmaline testing in patients with arrhythmogenic right ventricular dysplasia-cardiomyopathy. Int J Cardiol 2004;95(2—3):207—10.

119. Corrado D, Nava A, Buja G, et al. Familial cardiomyopathy underlies syndrome of right bundle branch block, ST segment elevation and sudden death. J Am Coll Cardiol 1996;27(2):443—8.

120. Corrado D, Basso C, Buja G, et al. Right bundle branch block, right precordial ST-segment elevation, and sudden death in young people. Circulation 2001;103(5):710—7.

121. Frustaci A, Priori SG, Pieroni M, et al. Cardiac histological substrate in patients with clinical phenotype of Brugada syndrome. Circulation 2005;112(24): 3680—7.

122. Remme CA, Wever EF, Wilde AA, et al. Diagnosis and long-term follow-up of the Brugada syndrome in patients with idiopathic ventricular fibrillation. Eur Heart J 2001;22(5):400—9.

123. Peters S. Arrhythmogenic right ventricular dysplasia-cardiomyopathy and provocable coved-type ST-segment elevation in right precordial leads: clues from long-term follow-up. Europace 2008;10(7):816—20.

124. Ackerman MJ, Splawski I, Makielski JC, et al. Spectrum and prevalence of cardiac sodium channel variants among black, white, Asian, and Hispanic individuals: implications for arrhythmogenic susceptibility and Brugada/long QT syndrome genetic testing. Heart Rhythm 2004; 1(5):600—7.

125. Kapa S, Tester DJ, Salisbury BA, et al. Genetic testing for long-QT syndrome: distinguishing pathogenic mutations from benign variants. Circulation 2009;120(18):1752—60.

126. Poelzing S, Forleo C, Samodell M, et al. SCN5A polymorphism restores trafficking of a Brugada

syndrome mutation on a separate gene. Circulation 2006;114(5):368–76.

127. Viswanathan PC, Benson DW, Balser JR. A common SCN5A polymorphism modulates the biophysical effects of an SCN5A mutation. J Clin Invest 2003;111(3):341–6.

128. Newton-Cheh C, Larson MG, Corey DC, et al. QT interval is a heritable quantitative trait with evidence of linkage to chromosome 3 in a genome-wide linkage analysis: the Framingham Heart Study. Heart Rhythm 2005;2(3):277–84.

129. Busjahn A, Knoblauch H, Faulhaber HD, et al. QT interval is linked to 2 long-QT syndrome loci in normal subjects. Circulation 1999;99(24):3161–4.

130. Newton-Cheh C, Eijgelsheim M, Rice KM, et al. Common variants at ten loci influence QT interval duration in the QTGEN Study. Nat Genet 2009; 41(4):399–406.

131. Pfeufer A, Sanna S, Arking DE, et al. Common variants at ten loci modulate the QT interval duration in the QTSCD Study. Nat Genet 2009;41(4): 407–14.

132. Pfeufer A, van Noord C, Marciante KD, et al. Genome-wide association study of PR interval. Nat Genet 2010;42(2):153–9.

133. Burke A, Creighton W, Mont E, et al. Role of SCN5A Y1102 polymorphism in sudden cardiac death in blacks. Circulation 2005;112(6):798–802.

134. Plant LD, Bowers PN, Liu Q, et al. A common cardiac sodium channel variant associated with sudden infant death in African Americans, SCN5A S1103Y. J Clin Invest 2006;116(2):430–5.

135. Bezzina CR, Shimizu W, Yang P, et al. Common sodium channel promoter haplotype in Asian subjects underlies variability in cardiac conduction. Circulation 2006;113(3):338–44.

Inherited Cardiac Arrhythmia Syndrome: Role of Potassium Channels

Lia Crotti, MD, PhD[a,b], Roberto Insolia, PhD[a,b],
Peter J. Schwartz, MD, FESC[a,b,c,d,e,f,*]

KEYWORDS
- Potassium channels • Channelopathies
- Sudden cardiac death • Genetics • Arrhythmias

Potassium channels are the main contributors to repolarizing outward currents acting during cardiac action potential. Quantitative and qualitative variations in the expression and biophysical properties of voltage-gated potassium channels seem to be largely responsible for action potential differences observed among regions of the heart and between normal and diseased myocardium.

This review discusses the role of potassium-channel dysfunctions in inherited cardiac arrhythmia syndromes classified as channelopathies caused by either loss-of-function mutations (long QT syndrome [LQTS] and Andersen-Tawil syndrome [ATS]) or gain-of-function mutations in genes encoding potassium channels (short QT syndrome [SQTS] and familial atrial fibrillation [AF]). Early repolarization syndrome and Brugada syndrome are not included in the gain-of-function mutations although they can also be caused by a gain of function in the cardiac K_{ATP} Kir 6.1 channel (*KCNJ8*-S422L)[1]; they are discussed by Yan and Antzelevitch elsewhere in this issue.

CHANNELOPATHIES CAUSED BY LOSS-OF-FUNCTION OF POTASSIUM CHANNELS
LQTS

Congenital LQTS is an inherited disorder characterized by prolongation of the QT interval and an increased risk for life-threatening ventricular arrhythmias.[2] Under the unifying name of LQTS, 2 hereditary variants are included: the recessive Jervell and Lange-Nielsen syndrome (J-LNS), associated with deafness,[3] and the autosomal-dominant Romano-Ward syndrome (R-WS).[2] The disease is genetically heterogeneous and caused by mutations in one of several genes, including *KCNQ1*, *KCNH2*, *KCNE1*, and *KCNE2*, encoding potassium-channel subunits that are responsible for most of the genotype-positive cases.

There are several reasons for the current widespread interest in LQTS. One is represented by the dramatic manifestations of the disease, namely syncopal episodes that often result in cardiac arrest and sudden death. These events usually occur in conditions of either physical or emotional stress in otherwise healthy young

[a] Section of Cardiology, Department of Lung, Blood and Heart, University of Pavia, c/o Fondazione IRCCS Policlinico S. Matteo, V.le Golgi 19, 27100 Pavia, Italy
[b] Department of Cardiology, Fondazione IRCCS Policlinico San Matteo, V.le Golgi 19, 27100 Pavia, Italy
[c] Laboratory of Cardiovascular Genetics, IRCCS Istituto Auxologico Italiano, Milan, Italy
[d] Department of Medicine, University of Stellenbosch, PO Box 19063, Tygerberg 7505, Cape Town, South Africa
[e] Department of Medicine, Cardiovascular Genetics Laboratory, Hatter Institute for Cardiology Research, Cape Heart Centre, Faculty of Health Sciences, University of Cape Town, Observatory 7925, South Africa
[f] Department of Family and Community Medicine, College of Medicine, King Saud University, PO Box 2925, Riyadh 11461, Saudi Arabia
* Corresponding author. Department of Cardiology, Fondazione IRCCS Policlinico San Matteo, V. le Golgi 19, 27100 Pavia, Italy.
E-mail address: peter.schwartz@unipv.it

Card Electrophysiol Clin 3 (2011) 113–124
doi:10.1016/j.ccep.2010.10.008
1877-9182/11/$ — see front matter © 2011 Published by Elsevier Inc.

individuals, mostly children and teenagers. Another reason is that, although LQTS is a disease with high mortality among untreated patients, effective therapies are available; this makes the existence of symptomatic and undiagnosed or misdiagnosed patients unacceptable and inexcusable. The identification of genes associated with the congenital LQTS had a major effect on understanding the molecular basis for ventricular arrhythmias and sudden cardiac death.[2] The impressive correlation between specific mutations and critical alterations in the ionic control of ventricular repolarization makes this syndrome a unique paradigm that allows correlation of genotype and phenotype, thus providing a direct bridge between molecular biology and clinical cardiology in sudden cardiac death.

Molecular basis of LQTS

Many genes have been identified at the basis of the disease. Interestingly, most the genotype-positive patients with LQTS carry a disease-causing mutation in potassium-channel genes, the focus of this review.[2]

KCNQ1 (LQT1) and KCNE1 (LQT5) The delayed rectifier current (I_K) is a major determinant of phase 3 of the cardiac action potential. It comprises 2 independent components: one rapid (I_{Kr}) and one slow (I_{Ks}).

The KCNQ1 gene and the KCNE1 gene encode respectively the α (KvLQT1) and the β (MinK) subunit of the potassium channel conducting the I_{Ks} current. KCNQ1 mutations are found in the LQT1 variant of LQTS, which is also the most prevalent.

Homozygous or compound heterozygous mutations of KCNQ1 and of KCNE1 have been associated with the recessive J-LNS (JLN1). LQT5 is an uncommon (2%–3%) variant caused by mutations in the KCNE1 gene. These mutations cause both R-WS (LQT5) and J-LNS (JLN2).

Expression studies of mutated proteins have suggested multiple mechanisms of functional failure. Defective proteins may coassemble with the wild-type protein and exert a dominant-negative effect. Other mutations lead to defective proteins that do not assemble with wild-type peptides, resulting in a loss of function that reduces the I_{Ks} current by 50% or less (haploinsufficiency). Defective peptides may not even reach the membrane of the cardiac cell because the mutations interfere with intracellular protein trafficking.[2]

KCNH2 (LQT2) and KCNE2 (LQT6) The KCNH2 gene and the KCNE2 gene encode respectively the α (HERG) and the β (MiRP) subunit of the potassium channel conducting the I_{Kr} current. This is the second most common variant of LQTS, accounting for 35% to 40% of mutations in LQTS-genotyped patients. Mutations in KCNH2 cause a reduction of I_{Kr} current. Defective proteins may either cause a dominant-negative effect on the wild-type subunits or they may not interfere with the function of the normal subunits, thus causing haploinsufficiency. Trafficking abnormalities are another consequence of KCNH2 mutations.[2]

Mutations in the KCNE2 gene are found in the LQT6 variant of LQTS. This gene encodes MiRP1 (MinK Related Peptide 1), a small peptide that coassembles with the HERG protein to form the I_{Kr} channel. There are a few examples of KCNE2 mutations associated with LQTS.

Prevalence

The first data-driven indication of the prevalence of LQTS comes from the largest prospective study of neonatal electrocardiography ever performed[4] and involving 44,596 infants of 3 to 4 weeks of age. Among them, 0.5% had a corrected QT (QTc) between 450 and 469 ms and 0.7/1,000 had a QTc of 470 ms or greater, regarded as markedly prolonged by the European Task Force on Neonatal Electrocardiography.[5] In the latter group (n = 31) more than 90% of infants underwent molecular screening and mutations causing LQTS disease were found in 12 of 28 (43%), whereas among infants with a QTc of 461 to 470 ms, only 14 were screened and a disease-causing mutation was identified in 4 (29%).[4] When considering the subgroup of White infants, 17/43,080 were affected by LQTS, showing a prevalence of at least 1:2534 apparently healthy live-births (95% confidence interval 1:1583–1:4350). This is the first time that the prevalence of a cardiac disease of genetic origin has been quantified based on actual data.

Clinical presentation (R-WS)

The typical clinical presentation of LQTS has been regarded as the occurrence of syncope or cardiac arrest, precipitated by emotional or physical stress, in a young individual with a prolonged QT interval on the electrocardiogram (ECG).

The syncopal episodes are caused by torsades de pointes (TdP), often degenerating into ventricular fibrillation. In 670 patients with LQTS of known genotype and who had all suffered symptoms (syncope, cardiac arrest, or sudden death), Schwartz and colleagues[6] examined possible relations between genotype and the conditions (triggers) associated with the events. As predicted by their impairment on the I_{Ks} current (essential for

QT shortening during increases in heart rate), most of the events in patients with LQT1 occurred during exercise or stress. Conversely, most of the events (including the lethal ones) in patients with LQT2 occurred during emotional stress such as auditory stimuli (sudden noises and telephone ringing, especially occurring while at rest) and most of the events of patients with LQT3 (those with a mutation on *SCN5A*) occurred while they were asleep or at rest. Patients with LQT2 and LQT3 are at low risk during exercise because they have a well-preserved I_{Ks} current and are therefore able to shorten their QT interval whenever their heart rate increases (**Fig. 1**).

Even in the postpartum period, genotype is important because risk is higher for patients with LQT2 than patients with LQT1.[7] The higher risk for women with LQT2 is probably partly related to sleep disruption; accordingly, we recommend that fathers contribute to infants' night-time feeding, thus allowing uninterrupted sleep for their partners with LQTS.

Clinical presentation (J-LNS)
J-LNS,[3] characterized by congenital deafness, is caused by the presence of 2 homozygous or compound heterozygous mutations on either the *KCNQ1* or *KCNE1* genes.[3]

Data on 187 patients with J-LNS have shown clear differences versus the other types of LQTS including LQT1, the variant that shares with J-LNS an impairment in the I_{Ks} current. J-LNS is a severe variant of LQTS. Almost 90% of the patients have cardiac events, 50% become symptomatic by age 3 (earlier than any other major genetic subgroup of LQTS), and their average QTc is markedly prolonged (557 ± 65 ms). Within patients with J-LNS it has been possible to identify subgroups at lower risk, namely those with a QTc less than 550 ms, those without syncope in the first year of life, and the smaller group with *KCNE1* mutations.[3] The therapeutic approach to patients with J-LNS is made complex by the early age at which most of them become symptomatic and especially by the fact that β-blockers seem to have limited efficacy. Left cardiac sympathetic denervation (LCSD) may be less effective than in other patients with LQTS. Thus, for many patients with J-LNS an implantable cardioverter defibrillator (ICD) should be seriously considered, in addition to the traditional therapies. For the subgroups at lower risk it may be reasonable to postpone a decision about ICD implant until age 8 to 10 years.[3]

ECG features
QT interval duration The Bazett correction for heart rate remains useful despite unrelenting criticism and despite hyper- and undercorrection at slow and fast rates. QTc values greater than 440 ms are considered prolonged; however, values up to 460 ms may still be normal among women. Despite exceptions, the longer the QT the greater the risk for malignant arrhythmias; when QTc exceeds 500 ms, risk definitely increases.

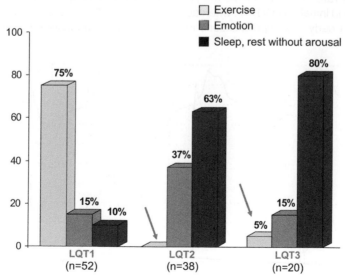

Fig. 1. Lethal cardiac events according to triggers and genotype. Numbers in parentheses are triggers, not patients. (*Modified from* Schwartz PJ, Priori SG, Spazzolini C, et al. Genotype-phenotype correlation in the long QT syndrome: gene-specific triggers for life-threatening arrhythmias. Circulation 2001;103:91; with permission.)

Given the incomplete penetrance of the disease, a normal QTc does not allow its exclusion, as proved by the existence of mutation carriers with a normal QT interval.[2] This concept has important practical and medicolegal implications because, for example, it no longer allows a cardiologist to state that a sibling of an affected patient with a normal QTc is definitely not affected by LQTS.

T-wave morphology The T wave is often biphasic or notched. These abnormalities are particularly evident in the precordial leads and contribute to the diagnosis of LQTS.

T-wave alternans T-wave alternans is a beat-to-beat alternation of the T wave, in polarity or amplitude, which may be present at rest but usually appears during emotional or physical stresses and may precede TdP. It is a marker of major electrical instability and it identifies patients at particularly high risk (**Fig. 2**).

Heart rate and its reflex control Recently, Brink and colleagues[8] and Schwartz and colleagues[9] in a large South African founder population with LQT1, in which all the affected members carry the *KCNQ1*-A341V mutation, reported that faster basal heart rates and brisk autonomic responses are associated with a greater probability of being symptomatic. This finding likely depends on the fact that patients with LQT1 have an impaired ability to shorten their QT interval during heart rate increases because of the mutation-dependent impairment in I_{Ks}, the current essential for QT adaptation. The lack of QT shortening during sudden heart rate increases favors the R-on-T phenomenon and initiation of VT/VF, whereas sudden pauses elicit early afterdepolarizations in patients with LQTS, which can trigger TdP. Blunted autonomic responses, revealed by relatively low values of baroreflex sensitivity, imply a reduced ability to change heart rate suddenly, which seems to be a protective mechanism for patients with LQT1.

Diagnosis

Given the characteristic features of LQTS, the typical cases present no diagnostic difficulty for physicians who are aware of the disease. However, borderline cases are more complex and require the evaluation of multiple variables besides clinical history and ECG. Diagnostic criteria were proposed in 1985[10] and subsequently updated in 1993 and in 2006.[2,11]

These diagnostic criteria were conceived in the premolecular era and should be used with common sense. They cannot be of value in identifying the so-called silent mutation carriers who have a normal QT interval. For these individuals, molecular screening is essential and when successful (70%–80% of cases in our laboratory), it allows the rapid screening of all the family members.[12] This situation has major clinical and medicolegal implications. Physicians who do not attempt to genotype their LQTS probands are willfully choosing to ignore the possibility that other family members might be mutation carriers at risk for sudden death, if their condition is not correctly recognized and treated.

Molecular genetics and risk stratification

Molecular genetics are important in risk stratification. In 1998,[13] based on 38 families, Zareba and colleagues suggested that patients with LQT1

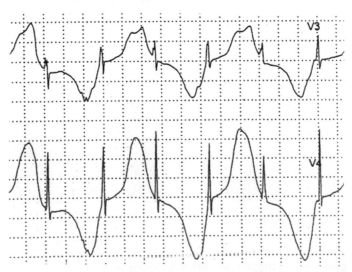

Fig. 2. T-wave alternans in a 23-month-old female patient with a first cardiac arrest at 7 months.

and LQT2 had more events, but that events in patients with LQT3 had greater lethality. In 2003[14] data on 647 patients of known genotype from 193 families indicated that the incidence of life-threatening events was lower among patients with LQT1, partly because of the high prevalence of silent mutation carriers (QTc <440 ms); the risk was higher among women with LQT2 versus men, and men with LQT3 versus women. Independently of genotype, the risk of becoming symptomatic was strongly correlated with QTc and was markedly greater with QTc greater than 500 ms.

After initial reports that mutations located in the C-terminal region were associated with a less severe clinical phenotype, in 2002 Moss and colleagues[15] indicated that patients with LQT2 with mutations in the pore region were at higher risk compared with patients with LQT2 with mutations in different regions of the same gene. In 2007 Moss and colleagues[16] reported in 600 patients with LQT1 that both the transmembrane location of the mutations and their dominant-negative effect are independent risk factors for cardiac events. Shortly afterwards, Crotti and colleagues[17] focused on the hot spot KCNQ1-A341V, a common mutation responsible for a founder effect in 25 South African families, and reported that the unusually high clinical severity already reported by Brink and colleagues[8] for the South African families is present also among patients with LQT1 from different ethnic backgrounds but carrying the same A341V mutation. Moreover, because KCNQ1-A341V has a mild dominant-negative effect (the current loss barely exceeds 50%) its striking clinically severe phenotype is explained neither by the location (transmembrane) nor by the functional consequence of the mutation (dominant-negative). This finding implies that the current biophysical assessments of the electrophysiologic effects of LQTS-causing mutations do not provide all the information necessary to make a complete genotype-phenotype correlation. In this regard, the study by Crotti and colleagues[17] paves the way toward a mutation-specific risk stratification.

The risk-stratification process is complicated by the presence of additional genetic variants that may modify clinical severity (genetic modifiers), as shown in an LQT2 family with the C-terminal A1116V mutation in whom the risk for life-threatening events was increased by the presence of the common KCNH2-K897T polymorphism. Electrophysiologic evidence did show that K897T produces an accentuation of the mutation-dependent I_{Kr} current loss, resulting in the unmasking of a clinically latent C-terminal LQT2 mutation.[18]

Recently, Crotti and colleagues[19] reported that common genetic variants of NOS1AP are significantly associated with clinical severity in the South African population with LQT1, with special reference to life-threatening arrhythmias, pointing to NOS1AP as a genetic modifier of LQTS. This knowledge should become clinically useful for risk stratification after validation in other populations with LQTS.

Therapy

The trigger for most of the episodes of life-threatening arrhythmias of LQTS is represented by a sudden increase in sympathetic activity, and antiadrenergic therapies provide the greatest degree of protection. Despite the passage of time, the most significant information on therapy still comes from a study from 1985.[10] That analysis included 233 symptomatic patients and reported a dramatic change in survival produced by pharmacologic or surgical antiadrenergic therapy when compared with any other therapy or no treatment. Such a large group of severely affected patients left without treatment is no longer available.

β-Adrenergic blocking agents represent the first-choice therapy in patients with LQTS, barring specific contraindications. In a large number of patients of unknown genotype, mortality on β-blocker therapy was 2%, and it was 1.6% when limited to patients with syncope (no cardiac arrest) and without events in the first year of life.[20] There is clear evidence that β-blockers are effective in patients with LQT1. Data from 2 large studies[21,22] indicate that mortality is around 0.5%, and sudden death combined with cardiac arrest reaches 1%. The impairment in the I_{Ks} current makes these patients particularly sensitive to catecholamines and responsive to β-blockade. These patients seldom need more than antiadrenergic therapy. Compared with patients with LQT1, patients with LQT2 have more life-threatening events despite β-blockers, but most of these have non fatal cardiac arrest (6%-7%).[6,21] There have been many doubts about the efficacy of β-blockers in patients with LQT3. Recently, albeit in a small population, it has been shown that antiadrenergic therapy (pharmacologic and/or surgical) is effective if the patients have not become symptomatic in the first year of life.[23] Approximately half of the patients with J-LNS are not adequately protected by β-blockers.[3]

Compliance is essential for patients with LQTS treated with β-blockers. Most of the so-called failures of β-blockers therapy are caused by incomplete compliance.[22]

LCSD After a small incision in the left subclavicular region, LCSD is performed by an extrapleural approach, which makes thoracotomy unnecessary. The average time for surgery is 35 to 40 minutes.[24,25] LCSD requires removal of the first 4 thoracic ganglia. The cephalic portion of the left stellate ganglion is left intact to avoid Horner syndrome.[24,25] The latest data published in 2004 include 147 patients with LQTS who had undergone LCSD during the preceding 35 years.[24] They represented a high-risk group, because 99% were symptomatic, their mean QTc was extremely long (563 ± 65 ms), 48% had a cardiac arrest, and 75% continued to have syncope despite full-dose β-blockers. The data most relevant to current clinical decisions are those regarding patients without cardiac arrest, who suffer syncope despite being treated with a full dose of β-blockers. During a mean follow-up of 8 years there was a 91% reduction in cardiac events. LCSD produced a mean QTc shortening of 39 ms, pointing to an action on the substrate as well as on the trigger. Mortality was 3% in this high-risk group. A postsurgery QTc of less than 500 ms predicted a favorable outcome. This series included 5 patients who underwent LCSD because of multiple ICD shocks and electrical storms: in this group, during a 4-year follow-up, there was a 95% decrease in the number of shocks (from an average of 29 shocks/y), with a dramatic improvement in the quality of life of the patients and of their families.

Whenever syncopal episodes recur despite a full-dose β-blocking therapy, LCSD should be considered and implemented whenever possible. Failure to discuss this option with the patients may carry medicolegal implications.[26]

ICDs There has been a major increase, largely unjustified, in the number of ICDs implanted in patients with LQTS. There is a consensus for immediately implanting an ICD in patients with documented cardiac arrest, either on or off therapy. In contrast, opinions differ regarding the use of ICDs in patients without cardiac arrest. ICDs do not prevent occurrence of malignant arrhythmias and TdP are frequently self-terminating in LQTS. The massive release of catecholamines, triggered by pain and fear, that follows an ICD discharge in a conscious patient (especially a young one) leads to further arrhythmias and to further discharges, which produce a vicious circle.

The US[27] and the European[28] ICD-LQTS Registries provide the disquieting information that most implanted patients had not suffered a cardiac arrest and, moreover, that many had not even

failed β-blocker therapy. In addition, in the European Registry 9% of the patients were asymptomatic before implantation and represented 45% of patients with LQT3.[28]

In the European LQTS ICD Registry 233 patients were enrolled and during follow-up (4.6 ± 3.2 years) at least one appropriate shock was received by 28% of patients, and adverse events occurred in 25%, excluding inappropriate shocks, and in 31% including inappropriate shocks.[28] Appropriate ICD therapies were predicted by age less than 20 years at implantation, a QTc more than 500 ms, and previous cardiac arrest and cardiac events despite therapy; within 7 years, appropriate shocks occurred in no patients with none of these factors and in 70% of those with all factors. From these data and in combination with our clinical experience in the management of patients with LQTS, the following groups of patients with LQTS seem logical candidates for an ICD implantation: (1) those who survived a cardiac arrest on therapy; (2) many of those who survived a cardiac arrest off therapy, except those with a preventable/reversible cause; (3) patients with syncope despite full-dose of β-blockers whenever LCSD either is not available or is discarded after discussion with the patients; (4) patients with 2 mutations who continue to have syncope despite β-blockade; (5) rare asymptomatic patients with QTc greater than 550 ms who also manifest signs of high electric instability (eg, T-wave alternans).

ATS

ATS is a multisystem disorder with a clinical spectrum characterized by ventricular arrhythmias, dysmorphic features, and periodic paralysis. The dysmorphic features are often subtle and the penetrance incomplete, thus complicating recognition of this disorder. ATS can occur either sporadically or as an autosomal-dominant trait. Clinical combination of periodic paralysis and ventricular arrhythmias was first published in the pediatric literature in 1963.[29]

Like the other features of ATS, the cardiac manifestations of the syndrome are also variable. Structural and functional heart disease has been described, and electrocardiographic and rhythm abnormalities are frequently observed. The most common arrhythmic episodes in ATS are polymorphic ventricular arrhythmias, although degeneration into lethal ventricular arrhythmias is uncommon. ATS, frequently and inappropriately classified as LQT7, is a complex clinical disorder in which the modest prolongation of the QT interval is only a secondary manifestation. Therefore, we believe that ATS should not be regarded as part of LQTS.[2]

Molecular basis of ATS

In 2001, mutations in the potassium-channel gene KCNJ2 were first identified as a cause of ATS[30] and as of today it remains the only genetic variants detected, accounting for nearly 60% of all clinical ATS cases. The KCNJ2 gene, also involved in SQTS type 3, encodes the strong inwardly rectifying channel protein Kir2.1. The generated inward-rectifier potassium current I_{K1} represents the major determinant of the resting membrane potential in the heart and contributes to the terminal phase of repolarization. I_{K1} is formed by coassembly of the Kir2.1.x subfamily of proteins (Kir 2.1, 2.2, and 2.3), with Kir2.1 being the most abundant subtype in ventricular tissue.

In 2001 study[30] the investigators mapped a potential disease-associated locus to chromosome 17q23, near the inward-rectifying potassium-channel gene KCNJ2. A missense mutation (D71V) in KCNJ2 was identified in the proband's family. Eight additional variants were detected in other unrelated patients. Expression of 2 of the identified mutations in Xenopus oocytes revealed loss of function and a dominant-negative effect in Kir2.1 current.[30]

Most ATS mutations so far described are located on the N-terminal and the C-terminal cytoplasmic domains of the channel. All KCNJ2 mutations cause a dominant-negative suppression of Kir2.1 channel function.[31] Most mutant subunits may coassemble with wild-type subunits and traffic appropriately to the cell surface, but they fail to function normally. Mutant channels show altered sensitivity to second-messenger phosphatidylinositol 4,5-biphosphate (PIP2), an essential activator of most inward-rectifier potassium channels. Nearly half of the identified KCNJ2 mutations occur at residues important for interaction between the potassium channel and PIP2.[32]

Management of ATS

Unlike catecholaminergic polymorphic ventricular tachycardia (CPVT), the arrhythmias in ATS, despite being frequently polymorphic, are not catecholamine sensitive and may even be suppressed at rapid heart rates. This finding explains the lack of efficacy of β-blocker therapy in patients with ATS. Recently, the efficacy of flecainide therapy in suppressing ventricular arrhythmias has been reported.[33] In the absence of confirmed therapeutic criteria, it may be reasonable to consider an ICD implant in the few patients with ATS with runs of rapid polymorphic ventricular tachycardia despite therapy.

Molecular diagnosis

Bidirectional ventricular tachycardia is an uncommon clinical problem uniquely associated with both ATS and CPVT.[34] Molecular screening on RYR2 and KCNJ2 should be performed in all these patients, as it is positive on RyR2 in most patients with CPVT and on KCNJ2 in nearly 60% of patients with ATS.

CHANNELOPATHIES CAUSED BY GAIN-OF-FUNCTION OF POTASSIUM CHANNELS
SQTS

SQTS is a recently described channelopathy, characterized by abnormally short QT interval, paroxysmal AF, and life-threatening ventricular arrhythmias. This autosomal-dominant syndrome can afflict infants, children, or young adults.[2]

Molecular basis of SQTS

Three main genetic variants have been described in SQTS, involving potassium-channel genes also associated with LQTS. However, whereas mutations on the potassium-channel genes causing LQTS are loss-of-function mutations, those observed in SQTS are gain-of-function mutations causing a shortening of the action potential duration.[2]

SQT1 is caused by mutations on KCNH2, the gene also responsible for LQTS type 2. Genetic screening in the first 2 reported families with SQTS and sudden cardiac death led to the identification of 2 different missense mutations on KCNH2 that resulted in the same amino acid change (KCNH2-N588K) of the cardiac I_{Kr} channel.[35] Whole-cell recordings showed that the mutation causes a significant increase of I_{Kr} during the action potential plateau.[36] Shortening of action potential is supposed to be linked to a shortening of the effective refractory period, thus causing an increased ventricular and atrial susceptibility to premature stimulation, leading to atrial and ventricular fibrillation.

Genetic heterogeneity in SQTS was made evident by the findings of Bellocq and colleagues,[37] who identified a mutation on KCNQ1 (V307L) in a 70-year-old patient with a QTc of 302 ms and aborted sudden cardiac death. The mutation, expressed in COS-7 cells, caused a gain of function of I_{Ks}.[37] The KCNQ1 gene is therefore not only responsible for LQTS type 1 but also for SQTS type 2 (SQT2). A second mutation (V141M) in the S1 segment of KCNQ1 was identified the following year by Hong and colleagues[38] in a baby girl born at 38 weeks after induction of delivery that was prompted by bradycardia and irregular rhythm.

The ECG revealed AF with slow ventricular response and short QT interval.

SQTS type 3 (SQT3) was described by Priori and colleagues[39] in 2005 and was associated with a gain-of-function mutation in the KCNJ2 gene, encoding for the strong inwardly rectifying channel protein Kir2.1, also involved in ATS.

Clinical presentation

SQTS has been described in few families worldwide; therefore, all the information available is based on fewer than 30 cases. Patients with this disease are likely to be at high risk for syncope and/or sudden cardiac death caused by ventricular tachyarrhythmias and episodes of AF are frequently documented at different ages even in adolescents and children. No information is available on whether specific triggers may precipitate cardiac events, because cardiac arrest has occurred both at rest and under stress.

The largest study published so far on SQTS[40] included 29 patients, 25 belonging to 8 families with SQTS and 4 sporadic cases, all with family and/or personal history of cardiac arrest/sudden cardiac death and documented short QT interval on the surface ECG. The first clinical presentation was sudden cardiac death in one-third of cases. The age of presentation varied from 4 months to 62 years. In 3 cases the first clinical manifestation occurred in the first year of life, 2 of which had aborted sudden death, suggesting a possible role for SQTS in some cases of sudden infant death syndrome (SIDS), the most frequent cause of mortality in the first year of life. The largest study to date, conducted on a cohort of SIDS victims,[41] identified a disease-causing mutation in LQTS genes in about 10% of cases, and one of those mutations, KCNQ1-I274V, causes a gain of function in I_{Ks}, predicting a short QT phenotype.[42] Therefore, SQTS can be considered, together with other channelopathies, as a contributing cause of SIDS.

Diagnosis

Diagnostic criteria for SQTS are not available and even the lower limit of the normal QT interval has not been fully established. In the reported cases of SQTS, the QTc interval using the Bazett formula was always less than 320 ms, except for the 3 cases, reported by Antzelevitch and colleagues,[43] in which the Brugada syndrome phenotype and a family history for sudden cardiac death were associated with QTc of 360 ms or less.

To better define the distribution and prognostic significance of short QT intervals, 2 different approaches have been used. Initially, a population of patients with idiopathic ventricular fibrillation

(IVF) was studied, and QTc values less than 360 ms were found more frequently among males with IVF than controls, but this was not true for females.[44] In addition, 2 normal populations were studied and no association between short QT and sudden cardiac death was observed.[45,46] These studies suggest that the presence of a short QT in the ECG is not sufficient to make a diagnosis of SQTS.

Apart from constantly short QTc intervals, affected patients have in common a short or even absent ST segment, with the T wave initiating immediately from the S wave. In patients with SQT1 the T waves often appear tall, narrow, and symmetric, with a prolonged Tpeak-Tend interval (**Fig. 3**).[2] In the 2 patients with SQT2 described (mutation on KCNQ1) the T waves appear to be symmetric, but not so tall and narrow.[2] By contrast, the 2 related patients with a mutation on the KCNJ2 gene (SQT3), showed an asymmetrical pattern with a less steep ascending section of the T wave, which is followed by a rapid descending and terminal phase of the T wave.[39] A further relevant feature in patients with SQTS is the lack of adaptation of the QT interval to heart rate.[2] When invasive electrophysiologic analysis is performed in patients with SQTS with a variety of ion-channel defects, a common finding is a short atrial and ventricular effective refractory period and, in some cases, inducible atrial and ventricular tachyarrhythmias. However, whether inducibility of ventricular arrhythmias is predictive of adverse clinical outcome remains unclear.

Therapy

Despite rapid advances in understanding the genetic basis of SQTS, the management of these patients is still poorly defined. In patients with mutations on the KCNH2 gene, it has been suggested that quinidine (and possibly disopyramide) may be effective in suppressing inducibility at programmed electrical stimulation, but whether this also confers long-term prevention of cardiac arrest is unknown. For the other genetic forms of SQTS, the efficacy of quinidine is less clear.

Fewer than 30 cases of SQTS have been reported and the present experience suggests that the disease may be lethal. For this reason the ICD is the therapy of choice in high-risk patients with SQTS. However, when only a limited cohort of patients is available, the severity of a disease tends to be overestimated, because symptomatic patients are identified because of their life-threatening arrhythmias, whereas asymptomatic patients remain underdiagnosed.

A common complication observed in patients with SQTS treated with an ICD implant is the

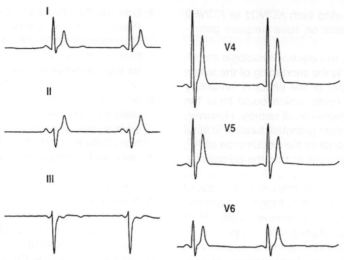

Fig. 3. Example of SQTS. Twelve-lead ECG (25 mm/s paper speed) of a patient in sinus rhythm, heart rate 52 beats per minute, left-axis deviation, QTc 280 ms. (*Modified from* Gaita F, Giustetto C, Bianchi F, et al. Short QT syndrome: a familial cause of sudden death. Circulation 2003;108:967; with permission.)

occurrence of inappropriate shocks, as a result of tall and narrow T-waves characteristic of this disorder[47] and to the prevalence of AF. The management of this disease is further complicated because sudden death events can occur in the first year of life, as well as in childhood, adolescence, and adulthood, and ICD implantation during childhood remains a problem for technical reasons and for its psychological effect in younger patients.[48]

Therefore, although there is a clear indication of ICD implant in previously symptomatic patients, this should be considered with caution in young asymptomatic patients, in whom oral quinidine may represent a bridge to ICD implant later in life when technical difficulties are decreased.

Familial AF

Even although most cases of AF are of acquired origin, a number yet to be defined (especially, but not only, the familial cases) seem to involve a genetic transmission. Historically, the first evidence of a genetic contribution in the development of AF was provided by Wolff in 1943,[49] documenting transmission of lone AF in a family with an autosomal-dominant pattern of inheritance. Since then, large epidemiologic studies have shown a heritability component in lone AF, showing that parental AF increased the risk of AF in the offspring to a relative risk up to 4.7, if parents were affected before age 60 years.[50,51] Although these results could be explained by common exposure to environmental factors, a genetic susceptibility to AF is likely. However, the genetic basis of acquired AF is not discussed in this

review, and the focus is on familial AF caused by potassium-channel dysfunctions.

Molecular basis of familial AF

Several potassium channels have been linked to familial AF. In most cases mutations in potassium-channel genes cause AF, reducing the atrial action potential duration, but some exceptions have been described.

In 2003 the identification of *KCNQ1* as responsible for the disease in a 4-generation family provided the first link of familial AF with channelopathy.[52] The mutation identified in this family was the substitution of a glycine in position 140 for a serine (S140G).[52] In vitro functional analysis revealed markedly increased current densities conducted by the mutant channel. Therefore, unlike the *KCNQ1* loss-of-function mutations observed in LQTS, the Ser140Gly substitution resulted in a gain of function. Nine of 16 affected patients showed QT prolongation, suggesting that the mutation may have opposing electrophysiologic effects in atrial and ventricular tissue. Subsequently, other *KCNQ1* gain-of-function mutations have been reported in association with familial and sporadic cases of AF.[53,54]

After the identification of *KCNQ1* as a causative gene for AF, other gain-of-function mutations within potassium-channel genes have been reported in association with AF, such as *KCNJ2*, encoding the strong inwardly rectifying channel protein Kir2.1,[55] and the potassium β subunits *KCNE2* and *KCNE5*, affecting the I_{Ks} current.[56,57]

The involvement of potassium channels in AF is supported by the evidence that as many as 30% of patients with SQTS, a condition that, as previously described, may develop from *KCNQ1* or *KCNH2* gain-of-function mutations, have frequent paroxysms of AF.[2]

In all these cases, the electrophysiologic mechanism leading to AF is the shortening of the action potential duration and of the effective refractory period in atrial myocytes, which could favor the occurrence of a multiple-circuit reentry. However, an increase of the action potential duration in atrial myocytes could also favor the occurrence of AF, as shown by the observation that the administration of cesium chloride, a potassium-channel blocker, into the sinus node artery of dogs induced early afterdepolarizations that triggered polymorphic atrial tachycardias, degenerating into AF.[58] These experimental studies are supported by scant evidence; even if AF is an uncommon finding in patients with LQTS, electrophysiologic studies on patients with LQTS revealed prolongation of both atrial action potential duration and effective refractory period along with short, spontaneous episodes of polymorphic atrial tachycardia.[59] In addition, in a family with hereditary lone AF, the disease-causing mutation identified was a loss-of-function mutation in the *KCNA5* gene,[60] encoding the Kv1.5 voltage-gated potassium channel. This potassium channel generates the ultrarapid component of the delayed-rectifier potassium current. The mutation identified in the family was an erroneous insertion of a stop codon at position 375 of the protein (E375X). This variant causes the expression of a truncated protein, unable to conduct any significant current[60] and therefore a delayed action potential repolarization and an increased effective refractory period.

ACKNOWLEDGMENTS

We are grateful to Pinuccia De Tomasi for expert editorial support.

REFERENCES

1. Medeiros-Domingo A, Tan BH, Crotti L, et al. Gain-of-function mutation, S422L, in the KCNJ8-encoded cardiac K ATP channel Kir6.1 as a pathogenic substrate for J wave syndromes. Heart Rhythm 2010;7:1466–71.
2. Schwartz PJ, Crotti L. Long and short QT syndrome. In: Zipes DP, Jalife J, editors. Cardiac electrophysiology: from cell to bedside. 5th edition. Philadelphia: Elsevier Saunders; 2009. p. 731–44.
3. Schwartz PJ, Spazzolini C, Crotti L, et al. The Jervell and Lange-Nielsen syndrome. Natural history, molecular basis, and clinical outcome. Circulation 2006;113:783–90.
4. Schwartz PJ, Stramba-Badiale M, Crotti L, et al. Prevalence of the congenital long-QT syndrome. Circulation 2009;120:1745–8.
5. Schwartz PJ, Garson A Jr, Paul T, et al. Guidelines for the interpretation of the neonatal electrocardiogram. Eur Heart J 2002;23:1329–44.
6. Schwartz PJ, Priori SG, Spazzolini C, et al. Genotype-phenotype correlation in the long-QT syndrome: gene-specific triggers for life-threatening arrhythmias. Circulation 2001;103:89–95.
7. Heradien MJ, Goosen A, Crotti L, et al. Does pregnancy increase cardiac risk for LQT1 patients? J Am Coll Cardiol 2006;48:1410–5.
8. Brink PA, Crotti L, Corfield V, et al. Phenotypic variability and unusual clinical severity of congenital long QT syndrome in a founder population. Circulation 2005;112:2602–10.
9. Schwartz PJ, Vanoli E, Crotti L, et al. Neural control of heart rate modifies arrhythmia risk in congenital long QT syndrome. J Am Coll Cardiol 2008;51:920–9.
10. Schwartz PJ. Idiopathic long QT syndrome: progress and questions. Am Heart J 1985;109:399–411.
11. Schwartz PJ. The congenital long QT syndromes from genotype to phenotype: clinical implications. J Intern Med 2006;259:39–47.
12. Schwartz PJ. Cascades or waterfalls, the cataracts of genetic screening are being opened on clinical cardiology. J Am Coll Cardiol 2010;55:2577–9.
13. Zareba W, Moss AJ, Schwartz PJ, et al; for the International Long-QT Syndrome Registry Research Group. Influence of genotype on the clinical course of the long-QT syndrome. N Engl J Med 1998;339:960–5.
14. Priori SG, Schwartz PJ, Napolitano C, et al. Risk stratification in the long-QT syndrome. N Engl J Med 2003;348:1866–74.
15. Moss AJ, Zareba W, Kaufman ES, et al. Increased risk of arrhythmic events in long-QT syndrome with mutations in the pore region of the human ether-a-go-go-related gene potassium channel. Circulation 2002;105:794–9.
16. Moss AJ, Shimizu W, Wilde AA, et al. Clinical aspects of type-1 long-QT syndrome by location, coding type, and biophysical function of mutations involving the KCNQ1 gene. Circulation 2007;115:2481–9.
17. Crotti L, Spazzolini C, Schwartz PJ, et al. The common long QT syndrome mutation KCNQ1/A341V causes unusually severe clinical manifestations in patients with different ethnic backgrounds: toward a mutation-specific risk stratification. Circulation 2007;116:2366–75.
18. Crotti L, Lundquist AL, Insolia R, et al. KCNH2-K897T is a genetic modifier of latent congenital long QT syndrome. Circulation 2005;112:1251–8. Corrections Circulation 2005;112:e295.

19. Crotti L, Monti MC, Insolia R, et al. NOS1AP is a genetic modifier of the long-QT syndrome. Circulation 2009;120:1657–63.

20. Moss AJ, Zareba W, Hall WJ, et al. Effectiveness and limitations of beta-blocker therapy in congenital long-QT syndrome. Circulation 2000;101:616–23.

21. Priori SG, Napolitano C, Schwartz PJ, et al. Association of long QT syndrome loci and cardiac events among patients treated with beta-blockers. JAMA 2004;292:1341–4.

22. Vincent GM, Schwartz PJ, Denjoy I, et al. High efficacy of beta-blockers in long QT syndrome type 1 and identification of the causes underlying events despite therapy. Circulation 2009;119:215–21.

23. Schwartz PJ, Spazzolini C, Crotti L. All LQT3 patients need an ICD: true or false? Heart Rhythm 2009;6:113–20.

24. Schwartz PJ, Priori SG, Cerrone M, et al. Left cardiac sympathetic denervation in the management of high-risk patients affected by the long QT syndrome. Circulation 2004;109:1826–33.

25. Odero A, Bozzani A, De Ferrari GM, et al. Left cardiac sympathetic denervation for the prevention of life-threatening arrhythmias. The surgical supraclavicular approach to cervico-thoracic sympathectomy. Heart Rhythm 2010;7:1161–5.

26. Schwartz PJ. Efficacy of left cardiac sympathetic denervation has an unforeseen side effect: medicolegal complications. Heart Rhythm 2010;7:1330–2.

27. Zareba W, Moss AJ, Daubert JP, et al. Implantable cardioverter defibrillator in high-risk long QT syndrome patients. J Cardiovasc Electrophysiol 2003;14:337–41.

28. Schwartz PJ, Spazzolini C, Priori SG, et al. Who are the long-QT syndrome patients who receive an implantable cardioverter-defibrillator and what happens to them? Data from the European Long-QT Syndrome Implantable Cardioverter-Defibrillator (LQTS ICD) Registry. Circulation 2010;122:1272–82.

29. Klein R, Ganelin R, Marks JF, et al. Periodic paralysis with cardiac arrhythmia. J Pediatr 1963;62:371–85.

30. Plaster NM, Tawil R, Tristani-Firouzi M, et al. Mutations in Kir2.1 cause the developmental and episodic electrical phenotypes of Andersen's syndrome. Cell 2001;105:511–9.

31. Tristani-Firouzi M, Jensen JL, Donaldson MR, et al. Functional and clinical characterization of KCNJ2 mutations associated with LQT7 (Andersen syndrome). J Clin Invest 2002;110:381–8.

32. Lopes CM, Zhang H, Rohacs T, et al. Alterations in conserved Kir channel-PIP2 interactions underlie channelopathies. Neuron 2002;34:933–44.

33. Pellizzon OA, Kalaizich L, Ptacek LJ, et al. Flecainide suppresses bidirectional ventricular tachycardia and reverses tachycardia-induced cardiomyopathy in Andersen-Tawil syndrome. J Cardiovasc Electrophysiol 2008;19:95–7.

34. Priori SG, Napolitano C, Tiso N, et al. Mutations in the cardiac ryanodine receptor gene (hRyR2) underlie catecholaminergic polymorphic ventricular tachycardia. Circulation 2001;103:196–200.

35. Brugada R, Hong K, Dumaine R, et al. Sudden death associated with short-QT syndrome linked to mutations in HERG. Circulation 2004;109:30–5.

36. Cordeiro JM, Brugada R, Wu YS, et al. Modulation of Ikr inactivation by mutation N588K in KCNH2: a link to arrhythmogenesis in short QT syndrome. Cardiovasc Res 2005;67:498–509.

37. Bellocq C, van Ginneken AC, Bezzina CR, et al. Mutation in the KCNQ1 gene leading to the short QT-interval syndrome. Circulation 2004;109:2394–7.

38. Hong K, Piper DR, Diaz-Valdecantos A, et al. De novo KCNQ1 mutation responsible for atrial fibrillation and short QT syndrome in utero. Cardiovasc Res 2005;68:433–40.

39. Priori SG, Pandit SV, Rivolta I, et al. A novel form of short QT syndrome (SQT3) is caused by a mutation in the KCNJ2 gene. Circ Res 2005;96:800–7.

40. Giustetto C, Di Monte F, Wolpert C, et al. Short QT syndrome: clinical findings and diagnostic-therapeutic implications. Eur Heart J 2006;27:2440–7.

41. Arnestad M, Crotti L, Rognum TO, et al. Prevalence of long-QT syndrome gene variants in sudden infant death syndrome. Circulation 2007;115:361–7.

42. Rhodes TE, Abraham RL, Welch RC, et al. Cardiac potassium channel dysfunction in sudden infant death syndrome. J Mol Cell Cardiol 2008;44:571–81.

43. Antzelevitch C, Pollevick GD, Cordeiro JM, et al. Loss-of-function mutations in the cardiac calcium channel underlie a new clinical entity characterized by ST-segment elevation, short QT intervals, and sudden cardiac death. Circulation 2007;115:442–9.

44. Viskin S, Zeltser D, Ish-Shalom M, et al. Is idiopathic ventricular fibrillation a short QT syndrome? Comparison of QT intervals of patients with idiopathic ventricular fibrillation and healthy controls. Heart Rhythm 2004;1:587–91.

45. Gallagher MM, Magliano G, Yap YG, et al. Distribution and prognostic significance of QT intervals in the lowest half centile in 12,012 apparently healthy persons. Am J Cardiol 2006;98:933–5.

46. Anttonen O, Junttila MJ, Rissanen H, et al. Prevalence and prognostic significance of short QT interval in a middle-aged Finnish population. Circulation 2002;116:714–20.

47. Schimpf R, Wolpert C, Bianchi F, et al. Congenital short QT syndrome and implantable cardioverter defibrillator treatment: inherent risk for inappropriate shock delivery. J Cardiovasc Electrophysiol 2003;14:1273–7.

48. Boriani G, Biffi M, Valzania C, et al. Short QT syndrome and arrhythmogenic cardiac diseases in

the young: the challenge of implantable cardioverter-defibrillator therapy for children. Eur Heart J 2006;27:2382—4.

49. Wolff L. Familial auricular fibrillation. N Engl J Med 1943;229:396—7.

50. Ellinor PT, Yoerger DM, Ruskin JN, et al. Familial aggregation in lone atrial fibrillation. Hum Genet 2005;118:179—84.

51. Christophersen IE, Ravn LS, Budtz-Joergensen E, et al. Familial aggregation of atrial fibrillation: a study in Danish twins. Circ Arrhythm Electrophysiol 2009; 2:378—83.

52. Chen YH, Xu WJ, Bendahhou S, et al. KCNQ1 gain-of-function mutation in familial atrial fibrillation. Science 2003;299:251—4.

53. Das S, Makino S, Melman YF, et al. Mutation in the S3 segment of KCNQ1 results in familial lone atrial fibrillation. Heart Rhythm 2009;6:1146—53.

54. Lundby A, Ravn LS, Svendsen JH, et al. KCNQ1 mutation Q147R is associated with atrial fibrillation and prolonged QT interval. Heart Rhythm 2007;4:1532—41.

55. Xia M, Jin Q, Bendahhaou S, et al. A Kir2.1 gain-of-function mutation underlies familial atrial fibrillation. Biochem Biophys Res Commun 2005; 332:1012—9.

56. Yang Y, Xia M, Jin Q, et al. Identification of a KCNE2 gain-of-function mutation in patients with familial atrial fibrillation. Am J Hum Genet 2004;75: 899—905.

57. Ravn LS, Aizawa Y, Pollevick GD, et al. Gain-of-function in IKs secondary to a mutation in KCNE5 associated with atrial fibrillation. Heart Rhythm 2008;5: 427—35.

58. Satoh T, Zipes DP. Cesium-induced atrial tachycardia degenerating into atrial fibrillation in dogs: atrial torsades de pointes? J Cardiovasc Electrophysiol 1998;9:970—5.

59. Kirchhof P, Eckardt L, Franz MR, et al. Prolonged atrial action potential durations and polymorphic atrial tachyarrhythmias in patients with long QT syndrome. J Cardiovasc Electrophysiol 2003;14: 1027—33.

60. Olson TM, Alekseev AE, Liu XK, et al. Kv1.5 channelopathy due to KCNA5 loss-of-function mutation causes human atrial fibrillation. Hum Mol Genet 2006;15:2185—91.

Role of Late Sodium Channel Current in Arrhythmogenesis

John C. Shryock, PhD

KEYWORDS

- Late I_{Na} • Angina • Heart failure • Arrhythmias • Ischemia
- Sodium channel • $Na_v1.5$

INTRODUCTION TO LATE SODIUM CHANNEL CURRENT

The property of cellular excitability in many tissues depends on the function of voltage-gated Na^+ channels. The relationship between membrane voltage and channel activation is steep; a small depolarization of the cell membrane leads to opening of Na^+ channels and a sudden regenerative depolarization that gives rise to the action potential (AP). The open conformation of the Na^+ channel is unstable, and opening is quickly followed by inactivation. During excitation of the heart, the voltage dependence and brevity of Na^+ channel openings restrict Na^+ entry in myocytes to a millisecond or so, which is sufficient to generate the AP upstroke. Inactivated Na^+ channels transition to a resting closed state in response to repolarization of the cell membrane.

Because repolarization of cardiac myocytes (unlike neurons) does not occur until hundreds of milliseconds after Na^+ channel opening, cardiac Na^+ channels spend a long time in inactivated states before closing. A failure of Na^+ channels to inactivate leads to continued depolarizing current (sodium channel late current [late I_{Na}]) and Na^+ entry that persists throughout the plateau of the cardiac AP. Many Na^+ channel mutations and pathologic conditions either delay or destabilize Na^+ channel inactivation and thereby enhance late I_{Na}. The detrimental effects of an enhanced late I_{Na} are depicted in **Fig. 1** and include 2 components: (1) the direct electric effect of an increased inward current during the AP plateau and (2) the indirect effects of increased cellular Na^+ loading. Both the components are arrhythmogenic. Because membrane resistance at the end of phase 2 (plateau) of the cardiac AP is high, a small inward current (ie, late I_{Na}) at this time can cause AP prolongation.[1–5] AP prolongation and slowing of repolarization, especially at low heart rates, may provide time for reactivation of L-type Ca^{2+} channels and formation of early afterdepolarizations (EADs).[6–9] EADs can trigger torsades de pointes (TdP) ventricular tachycardia.[10,11] Late I_{Na} is greater in some cells than in others,[3,12] and thus late I_{Na}–induced AP prolongation is not uniform and may create an increase of transmural dispersion of repolarization.[13,14]

The enhancement of late I_{Na} during the AP plateau may potentially lead to a doubling of cellular Na^+ influx.[15] An increased late I_{Na} is one explanation for the observed increase of the intracellular sodium concentration $[Na^+]_i$ in failing[15–20] and ischemic[21–23] hearts. The increase of $[Na^+]_i$ in turn causes the reversal potential of the sodium-calcium exchanger (NCX) to become more negative.[16] The result is a decreased driving force for Na^+ influx/Ca^{2+} efflux and an increased driving force for Na^+ efflux/Ca^{2+} influx from the cell via NCX (especially at depolarized potentials such as those during the AP plateau). Increased Ca^{2+} entry via NCX increases the intracellular calcium concentration $[Ca^{2+}]_i$ and Ca^{2+} uptake in the sarcoplasmic reticulum (SR). These events may lead to an increased leak of Ca^{2+} from the SR (ie, Ca^{2+} sparks) during diastole.[16] This leak leads to NCX-induced transient inward currents

Disclosure: Gilead Sciences markets ranolazine for treatment of chronic stable angina.
Biology, Cardiovascular Therapeutic Area, Gilead Sciences, Inc, 1651 Page Mill Road, Palo Alto, CA 94304, USA
E-mail address: John.Shryock@gilead.com

Card Electrophysiol Clin 3 (2011) 125–140
doi:10.1016/j.ccep.2010.10.005
1877-9182/11/$ – see front matter © 2011 Published by Elsevier Inc.

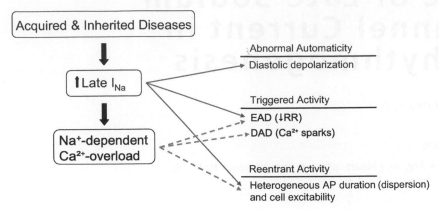

Fig. 1. Enhancement of late I_{Na} contributes to the genesis of atrial and ventricular tachyarrhythmias. AP, action potential; DAD, delayed afterdepolarization; EAD, early afterdepolarization; RR, repolarization reserve.

(I_{Ti}) and delayed afterdepolarizations (DADs),[24] as well as Ca^{2+} (and repolarization) alternans,[25,26] both of which are arrhythmogenic.

In normal cardiac cells and physiologic settings, Na^+ channel inactivation gating is stable throughout the cardiac AP plateau, and late I_{Na} is small (reported to be 0.2% of peak I_{Na} in the human left ventricle,[27] although higher values have been reported) and ranges from 21 to 24 pA in isolated cells.[5] Block of this small physiologic late I_{Na} has not been found to alter electric or contractile function of the heart. Block of late I_{Na} in the heart by tetrodotoxin (TTX) is reported to shorten AP duration (APD), especially of midmyocardial cells and Purkinje fibers, consistent with findings that the amplitude of late I_{Na} is large in these cells.[12,28] Block of late I_{Na} and reduction of APD in Purkinje fibers and midmyocardial cells has not been reported to be proarrhythmic; rather, it is associated with reduction of the dispersion of APD,[13] which is antiarrhythmic.

MECHANISMS OF ENHANCEMENT OF LATE I_{NA}

Many acute causes of an enhanced late I_{Na} have been identified: toxins,[29] angiotensin II,[30] hydrogen peroxide (H_2O_2),[4,31–33] nitric oxide,[34] peroxynitrite,[35] hypoxia,[36–39] the ischemic amphiphiles lysophosphatidylcholine[40,41] and palmitoyl-L-carnitine,[42] glycolytic pathway intermediates,[43] thrombin,[44] Ca^{2+} calmodulin,[45–47] and Na^+ channel phosphorylation.[48] The amplitude of late I_{Na} is also reported to be increased in myocytes from dogs and humans with heart failure[2,27,49–54]; in postinfarction remodeled myocardium[55]; in cells expressing mutant forms of scaffolding proteins such as ankyrin B,[56] syntrophin,[57] telethonin,[58] and caveolin 3[59]; and in cells expressing mutant forms of $Na_V1.5$.[60]

At a biophysical level, late I_{Na} has been shown to be the result of (1) rare bursts of openings and more abundant single late openings of channels[61–65] caused by destabilization of inactivation (which is normally considered to be an absorbing state), (2) a steady state window current caused by the overlap of voltages at which channels are both activated and inactivated (eg, −60 to −15 mV[66]), (3) a nonequilibrium resurgent current caused by unusually rapid recovery of channels from inactivation and subsequent reopening,[67,68] and (4) a slowing of the inactivation process. Mutations in the Na^+ channel gene SCN5A that are associated with the long QT (LQT) syndrome and an increase in late I_{Na}, are reported to increase late INa by one of these mechanisms.[69] At a molecular level, the modifications of channel structure responsible for late I_{Na} and failure of inactivation gating are little understood,[70] although the cytoplasmic III-IV linker and its IFM motif[71] as well as the channel cytoplasmic tail[72,73] are required for inactivation and both channel β subunits[74,75] and membrane structural proteins[49,57] can alter channel gating.[76] Many mutations in SCN5A are known to increase late I_{Na}.[69,77] The calmodulin-binding IQ motif and the EF handlike motif in the cytoplasmic tail of the pore-forming α subunit also modulate channel gating and excitability.[45,47] Evidence suggests that $Na_V1.5$ channel inactivation and thus the amplitude of late I_{Na} are altered by kinases, including Ca^{2+}/calmodulin-activated kinase II (CaMKII),[46,48] protein kinases A[78] and C,[79] AMP-activated protein kinase,[80] and the tyrosine kinase Fyn.[81,82] The specific $Na_V1.5$ amino acid phosphorylated by Fyn is reported to be Y1495, whereas phosphorylation of S1503 is reported to mediate the effect of PKC to decrease I_{Na}.[83] Both Y1495 and S1503 are in the III-IV linker. There are several consensus sites for protein kinase A–dependent phosphorylation, and both S36 and S525 have been implicated in destabilization of channel inactivation.[78] Although S-nitrosylation of the channel by nitric oxide has been proposed,[34] it has yet to be demonstrated.

PATHOLOGIC SETTINGS ASSOCIATED WITH AN INCREASE OF LATE I_{Na}

Ischemic environment, oxidative stress, and inflammation are settings in which late I_{Na} is increased.[4,7,15,31,33,35–38,40,42,44,48,80,83–89] In these settings, reactive oxygen species; intermediary lipid and glycolytic metabolites; acidosis; elevated intracellular Ca^{2+} levels; thrombin; activations of CaMKII, AMPK, PKC, and Fyn; and depolarization of myocyte membrane potential are present, and each alone is reported to enhance late I_{Na}, as noted earlier. The Na^+ window current contribution to late I_{Na} may also increase because of membrane depolarization of myocytes (ie, both excitable and inexcitable cells can have window current). Depolarization of cells by 20 to 30 mV or more would be expected to increase Na^+ window current and Na^+ loading of cells.

Late I_{Na} and Na^+ influx are reported to be enhanced by 58%,[49] 2-fold,[54] and up to 10-fold[27] in myocytes isolated from dogs that had heart failure. Late I_{Na} is enhanced by approximately 3-fold in myocytes treated with H_2O_2[31] and 10-fold in myocytes exposed to either of 2 lipid intermediates that accumulate rapidly during ischemia, namely, lysophosphatidylcholine[41] and palmitoyl-L-carnitine.[42]

Myocytes from failing hearts[2,27,49–54,90] or remodeled myocardium[55] have been shown to have an elevated late I_{Na}. For several reasons, the functional effect of an increased late I_{Na} may be greater in a diseased than in a normal myocardium. Both late INa and reverse mode NCX are increased in a failing heart, and late I_{Na} may therefore lead to a greater increase of Ca^{2+} loading via NCX in failing than in normal myocytes.[52] Second, K^+ outward currents such as background inward rectifier potassium current may be reduced in the failing heart, thus enabling a larger depolarization due to an inward current such as I_{Na} or forward mode sodium-calcium exchange current.[91] Third, depolarization of cells in an ischemic myocardium may lead to increased Na^+ window current and further Na^+ loading and depolarization. Depolarization reduces Na^+ influx during the AP upstroke, which may lead to conduction block. Lastly, electrotonic coupling of myocytes to other myocytes is decreased in a failing heart.[92] Loss of myocyte-myocyte electrotonic coupling in the failing heart may occur because of decreased expression or redistribution of connexin 43,[92,93] increased

fibrosis,[92,94] or myocyte Ca^{2+} overload.[16,90] Electrotonic coupling of adjacent myocytes dampens the variability of APD in the normal heart[95,96] and facilitates conduction of the AP. In the aged fibrotic heart in which electrotonic coupling is reduced, it is thus easier to induce fibrillation than in the normal heart.[94] Late I_{Na} is a cause of beat-to-beat variability of APD and arrhythmic activity in studies of myocytes isolated from failing hearts[2,49,52] or patients with atrial fibrillation.[97] Block of late I_{Na} was reported to decrease pacing- and H_2O_2-induced ventricular fibrillation in the aged heart, improve contractile function,[90,97] and reduce arrhythmogenesis in myocytes of failing hearts.[97] These findings suggest that late I_{Na} is more proarrhythmic in the setting of heart disease with structural and/or electric remodeling than in the normal heart.

A reduction of repolarization reserve because of a decrease of outward K^+ current may be associated with an increased proarrhythmic role of late I_{Na}. When repolarization reserve is reduced, the effect of an inward current (such as late I_{Na}) to increase APD is amplified.[13,98,99] Repolarization reserve is reduced in long QT syndromes and by drugs that reduce slow delayed rectifier potassium current (I_{Ks}) or rapid delayed rectifier potassium current (I_{Kr} (the hERG current). Reductions of I_{Ks} (LQT1) or I_{Kr} (LQT2) prolong APD and increase repolarization variability.[100,101] An enhancement of late I_{Na} has been shown to prolong APD and cause ventricular tachycardia in hearts wherein I_{Kr} and/or I_{Ks} is reduced.[99,102] Reduction of late I_{Na} by ranolazine, a drug known to inhibit late I_{Na}, decreases AP prolongation, arrhythmogenesis, and TdP caused by I_{Kr} blockers.[98,99,102,103] Thus, a reduction of late I_{Na} can reduce the proarrhythmic potential of I_{Kr} blockers and increase repolarization reserve. One may speculate that an increased coupling of myocytes to fibroblasts (via connexin 40) in the fibrotic heart has the potential to slow myocyte repolarization. The membrane capacitance of a fibroblast coupled to a myocyte needs to be charged or discharged each time the myocyte changes its membrane potential. When repolarization reserve is reduced because of either reduction of outward current or enhancement of late I_{Na}, myocyte coupling to fibroblasts further slows repolarization. In this case, reduction of late I_{Na} with an increase of repolarization reserve could be expected to speed repolarization. Because a reduction of late I_{Na} may also reduce $[Na^+]_i$ and thereby increase the transmembrane Na^+ gradient, it may also increase the safety factor for electrical conduction in the heart.

Atrial fibrillation is a condition associated with an increase of oxidative stress,[104] a reduction of atrial peak I_{Na}, and an increase of late I_{Na}.[97] Late I_{Na} is also reported to be increased in left atrial myocytes from rabbits with left ventricular hypertrophy.[105] Late I_{Na} has been shown to be a cause of EADs, DADs, diastolic depolarization, and triggered activity of atrial myocytes.[105–108]

WHY IS LATE I_{Na} PATHOLOGIC?

The paradigm for Na^+ and Ca^{2+} overload after enhancement of late I_{Na} is shown in **Figs. 2** and **3**. An elevation of late I_{Na} by 2- to 10-fold leads to acute electrical and contractile dysfunction within minutes in isolated myocytes.[4,33,40,42,90,108,109] Dysfunction observed in myocytes from dogs that had heart failure was associated with an elevation of late I_{Na} by as little as 30% to 50%.[49,52] Late I_{Na} leads to EADs, DADs, and triggered activity,[33,108,109] and late I_{Na}–induced phase 4 depolarization leads to spontaneous activity.[107] The increased variability of APD due to EADs, and occurrences of AP alternans due to Ca^{2+} loading, and DADs, may lead to both conduction block and reentrant activity (see **Fig. 1**). Results of in silico modeling studies suggest that a small increase of late I_{Na} (to 0.2% of peak I_{Na}) is sufficient to alter the transmural pattern of APD heterogeneity.[14] Because a failure of Na^+ channel inactivation leads to increased Na^+ influx and $[Na^+]_i$, and therefore to Ca^{2+} influx, enhancement of late I_{Na} increases $[Ca^{2+}]_i$ and alters cellular Ca^{2+} handling. The effect of these increases of late I_{Na}, $[Na^+]_i$, and $[Ca^{2+}]_i$ is to prolong the cellular Ca^{2+} transient, increase the diastolic level of intracellular Ca^{2+}, and slow the relaxation of ventricular contraction.[49] Ventricular relaxation at the onset of diastole enables the rapid increase of coronary blood flow during the diastolic interval. Thus, slowing of relaxation may lead to reduction of coronary

microvascular blood flow and exacerbation of ischemia. Inhibition of this pathologic "ischemia begets ischemia" feedback loop by the late I_{Na} inhibitor ranolazine seems to be the basis of its clinical antianginal and anti-ischemic effect.[110,111]

THE RELATIONSHIP OF LATE I_{Na} TO ARRHYTHMOGENESIS

Late I_{Na} generates both triggers and substrates for arrhythmic activity.[7] The arrhythmia triggers are spontaneous diastolic depolarizations, EADs, and DADs. H_2O_2[4,31,33] and anemone toxin II (ATX-II)[108,109] are late I_{Na} enhancers that increase late I_{Na}, prolong APD, and cause EADs and Ca^{2+} loading. ATX-II, a selective enhancer of late I_{Na}, is also reported to increase the rate of diastolic depolarization and AP firing of atrial myocytes.[108] Consistent with the proarrhythmic role of late I_{Na}, in the anesthetized dog, an increase of late I_{Na} was shown to prolong the QTc interval and sensitize the heart to adrenaline-induced arrhythmias.[1] The electrical and mechanical dysfunction induced by H_2O_2 and ATX-II is inhibited by ranolazine, TTX, and other Na^+ channel blockers, suggesting that it is attributable to the increase of late I_{Na}.[33,108,112,113] In the ischemic heart, drugs that reduce late I_{Na} also reduce ventricular arrhythmic activity[114–118] and infarct size (**Table 1**).[88,89,115,119]

Late I_{Na} and EADs

A prolonged APD and EADs are prominent features of myocytes isolated from failing hearts, and block of late I_{Na} in these cells reduces both APD and occurrences of EADs.[53,54] Low heart rates and prolongation of APD (ie, reduction of repolarization reserve) are the basis for the formation of EADs.[10] Reduction of I_{Kr} (hERG current) and

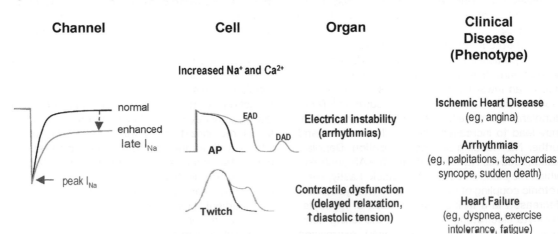

Fig. 2. Pathology of enhanced late I_{Na} from channel to clinical phenotype.

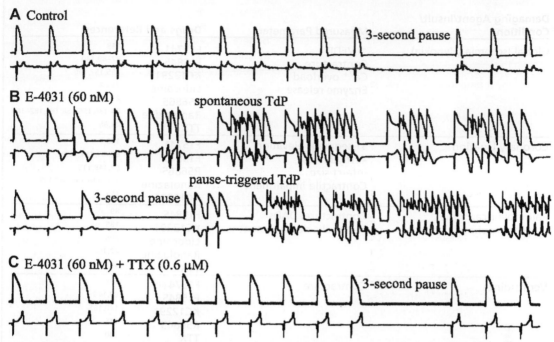

A Control

3-second pause

B E-4031 (60 nM) spontaneous TdP

pause-triggered TdP

3-second pause

C E-4031 (60 nM) + TTX (0.6 μM)

3-second pause

Fig. 3. TTX terminates I_{Kr} block–induced TdP. Representative recording of the effect of TTX (0.6 μM) to attenuate occurrences of TdP induced by the I_{Kr} blocker E-4031 (60 μM) in the female rabbit isolated heart. The heart was paced at 1 Hz and sequentially exposed to no drug, E-4031 alone, and E-4031 plus TTX. Spontaneous or 3-second pause-triggered episodes of TdP were induced by E-4031 (Panel *B*) but were not observed in the absence of drug (Panel *A*, control) or in the presence of E-4031 plus TTX (Panel *C*). The top and bottom traces in each panel are the monophasic AP and the electrocardiogram, respectively. (*From* Wu L, Rajamani S, Li H, et al. Reduction of repolarization reserve unmasks the proarrhythmic role of endogenous late Na+ current in the heart. Am J Physiol Heart Circ Physiol 2009;297:H1048–57; with permission.)

enhancement of late I_{Na} individually reduce repolarization reserve and increase APD (**Fig. 3**). Prolongation of APD, especially with AP triangulation, allows time for both Ca^{2+} and Na^+ channels to recover from inactivation and reactivate to generate further depolarization (an EAD).[112] Purkinje fibers seem to be susceptible to EAD formation due to I_{Kr} blockade.[28] Blockers of either Ca^{2+} or Na^+ channels can prevent occurrences of EADs.[2,6,11,33,50,53,54,102,105,109,112,113,120,121]

Late I_{Na} and DADs

High heart rates and cellular Na^+ and Ca^{2+} overload are the basis for the formation of DADs. I_{TI} is the cause of the DAD.[24,122] I_{TI} is a cell membrane Na^+-Ca^{2+} exchange current activated by spontaneous diastolic releases of Ca^{2+} (sparks) from the SR.[123] Phosphorylations of cardiac ryanodine receptors (RyR2; SR Ca^{2+} release channels) by CaMKII and of SERCA by β-adrenergic receptor–activated protein kinase A are associated with increased spontaneous Ca^{2+} sparks and waves in ventricular myocytes.[124] Overexpression of CaMKIIδc in the heart leads to increased

phosphorylation of ryanodine receptors and increased Ca^{2+} spark frequency.[125,126] Conditions associated with excessive Ca^{2+} loading, such as high heart rates; inhibition of Na^+,K^+-ATPase activity by cardiac glycosides; or enhancement of late I_{Na} (eg, by ischemia, oxidative stress) result in increased spark frequency and in I_{TI} and DADs.[16,24,108] In the failing heart, both diastolic leak of Ca^{2+} from the SR and NCX are increased and SR Ca^{2+} content and contractility are secondarily decreased,[124] thus potentially ameliorating a pathologic Ca^{2+} overload caused by excessive adrenergic stimulation and/or ischemia. An increase of late I_{Na} upsets this adaptive mechanism that is meant to reduce Ca^{2+} overload. The increased influx and concentration of intracellular Na^+ caused by late I_{Na} reduce Ca^{2+} extrusion via NCX. The resultant Ca^{2+} overload can lead to not only increased diastolic tension but also DADs. Reduction by ranolazine or TTX of an enhanced late I_{Na} has been shown to decrease the occurrence of DADs.[108,127] In summary, an enhanced late I_{Na} is a risk factor for EADs when combined with low heart rates and drug-induced or inherited reductions of I_{Kr} and is a risk factor

Table 1
Cardioprotective effects of late I_{Na} inhibitors

Damaging Agent/Insult/ Condition	Measured Parameters	Drugs and References	
Global Ischemia (Hypoxia)	↑LVEDP Contracture Ca^{2+} overload Enzyme release	F15741 F15845 KC12291 Lidocaine R56865 Ranolazine TTX	119 87–89,140 155,157,140 21,22 21,85 84,136,156,158,160,182–184 21,85
Coronary Ligation	ST-segment elevation Arrhythmias Infarct size Contractile impairment	F15741 F15845 R56865 Ranolazine KC12291	119 87–89,114,119 87,148,115 116–118,136,147,159 157
Palmitoyl-L-carnitine, Lysophosphatidylcholine	Contracture, DADs Metabolic derangement	F15845 KC12291 Lidocaine Ranolazine TTX	89 185 206 42,187 40,42
Veratridine	Contracture	F15741 F15845 KC12291 R56865 TTX	119 89,140 140,185 115 140
Aconitine	VT	F15845 R56865 TTX	114 188 188–190
Cardiac Glycoside	Arrhythmias, contracture	Lidocaine R56865	192 115,191,193,207
Heart Failure	Myocyte APD Remodeling Contraction, $[Ca^{2+}]_i$	Ranolazine TTX Lidocaine	50,52,90,194,195 2,52,53 54
Nonischemic Cardiomyopathy	VT suppression	Ranolazine	180
ROS (H_2O_2)	Contraction, metabolism, EADs	Ranolazine TTX	32,33,84,107 4,33,107
ATX-II	APD Arrhythmia, EAD, DAD, TdP Contracture/Ca^{2+} load Ca^{2+} cycling	Mexiletine Ranolazine TTX Lidocaine	113,196 13,25,102,106–109,196 107,108 197
I_{Kr} Blockers	APD, arrhythmias AP dispersion	Mexiletine Lidocaine Ranolazine TTX	197 198 98,103,120,199 98
ACh or Vagal Stimulation	AF Atrial rate (ERP)	Lidocaine Ranolazine	154 121,186,200
Electrically Induced Arrhythmia	Incidence of AF, VF ERP, VF threshold	Ranolazine	200–202
Isoproterenol	AF	Ranolazine	97,121,200
Previous MI	Diastolic function	Ranolazine	165
AF	Sinus rhythm Late I_{Na}, contraction	Ranolazine	97,178,202,203
Atrioventricular Block	Arrhythmias	Ranolazine	199
LQT3	QTc	Mexiletine Ranolazine	204 205
Left Ventricular Hypertrophy	EADs, spontaneous activity	TTX	105

Abbreviations: ACh, acetylcholine; AF, atrial fibrillation; APD, AP duration; DAD, delayed afterdepolarization; EAD, early afterdepolarization; ERP, effective refractory period; LVEDP, left ventricular end-diastolic pressure; MI, myocardial infarction; TdP, torsades de pointes; TTX, tetrodotoxin; ROS, reactive oxygen species; VF, ventricular fibrillation; VT, ventricular tachycardia (upword arrow), increase.

for DADs when combined with high heart rates, Ca^{2+} loading, adrenergic activity, and CaMKII activation.

Late I_{Na} and Dispersion of Repolarization

Dispersion of APD and therefore of electrical excitability among adjacent myocardial cells increases the potential for reentrant conduction of electric impulses in the heart and is temporally related to arrhythmic events.[128] The presence of greater late I_{Na} in some regions of the heart relative to others contributes to the dispersion of APD[3,9,12,113,129–131] and is increased in patients with either the LQT3[130,131] syndrome or heart failure[2] ranolazine and TTX have been found to reduce AP dispersion.[2,13,33,50,95,98,102,109,120,132] Na^+-induced Ca^{2+} overloading of myocytes also leads to increased dispersion of APD and Ca^{2+} alternans among adjacent cells in the heart.[25] The late I_{Na} inhibitor ranolazine has been shown to attenuate Ca^{2+} alternans–induced dysfunction.[25] In the failing human heart, APD is prolonged but the transmural dispersion of APD was reported to be decreased, although it was not clear whether local heterogeneity of repolarization or base to apical dispersion was decreased.[93] Regardless, inhibition of late I_{Na} decreases APD in myocytes isolated from failing human hearts and improves Ca^{2+} handling.

THE ANTIARRHYTHMIC BENEFITS OF INHIBITING LATE I_{NA} IN THE HEART

Many drugs, including amiodarone; propranolol; verapamil; the Na^+ channel blockers quinidine, mexiletine, lidocaine, and flecainide; and antiepileptic drugs including phenytoin, are known to reduce late I_{Na} but are rarely used for this purpose because of a lack of selectivity for inhibition of late I_{Na} relative to peak I_{Na} or other currents. TTX is a selective Na^+ channel blocker that inhibits late I_{Na} in the heart at concentrations 5- to 10-fold lower than it inhibits cardiac peak I_{Na}.[5,31,53,55,85,133–135] It is commonly used in myocyte preparations to validate effects of other late I_{Na} blockers. The antianginal drug ranolazine[132,136–139] and the Pierre Fabre compound F15845[87–89,114,119,140] are currently the most selective inhibitors of cardiac late I_{Na}.

A summary of the antiarrhythmic and cardioprotective effects reported in preclinical studies of ranolazine, F15845, and other late I_{Na} inhibitors is presented in **Table 1**. In animal models and isolated heart preparations, ranolazine and F15845 have been shown to attenuate ischemia-induced increases of intracellular Na^+ and Ca^{2+} concentrations, diastolic tension, arrhythmias,

and ST-segment elevation. Ranolazine not only decreased late I_{Na} and the duration and variability of the AP and the Ca^{2+} transient but also attenuated the increase of $[Ca^{2+}]_i$ caused by increased frequency of pacing, the frequency of occurrences of spontaneous Ca^{2+} release from the SR, and Ca^{2+} alternans observed in myocytes isolated from dogs that had heart failure. In the isolated rodent heart exposed to H_2O_2, which causes increases in APD, intracellular concentrations of Na^+ and Ca^{2+}, and EADs, ranolazine delays and reduces the H_2O_2-induced changes. Thus, when cardiac late I_{Na} is enhanced by ischemia, oxidative stress and inflammation, or heart failure, inhibition of late I_{Na} reduces arrhythmic activity associated with these pathologic states. No cardiovascular risks associated with the block of cardiac late I_{Na} have been identified to date.

Drug-induced proarrhythmia related to the use of I_{Kr} blocking drugs is associated with triangulation of the ventricular AP,[141] reverse use dependence of AP prolongation,[142] increased time and spatial variability (dispersion) of APD,[100,101,130,131,143] and the occurrence of EADs, DADs, Ca^{2+} overload, and triggered activity.[143,144] These effects are believed to be the result of a reduction of repolarization reserve (especially at low heart rates) that causes AP prolongation with Na^+ and Ca^{2+} loading. Reduction of late I_{Na} increases repolarization reserve and shortens APD in the presence of I_{Kr} blockers. Reduction of late I_{Na} by ranolazine, lidocaine, or TTX has been shown to prevent or reverse the proarrhythmic effects (eg, EADs) of I_{Kr} blocking drugs.[98,103,109,120,132,137] Increases of APD and occurrences of EADs caused by E-4031 and the selective I_{Ks} blocker chromanol 293B are reversed and suppressed by ranolazine, 10 μM.[109] Furthermore, EADs induced by the I_{Kr} blocker and the class III antiarrhythmic agent sotalol (100 μM) in canine Purkinje fibers and M cells,[120,132] and EADs and ventricular tachycardia induced by E-4031 (60 nM) in the rabbit isolated heart, are suppressed by ranolazine (5–10 μM).[98,102,132] Spontaneous and pause-triggered arrhythmic activity (ie, TdP) induced by amiodarone, quinidine, moxifloxacin, cisapride, and ziprasidone in the female rabbit isolated heart is reduced by ranolazine.[99,132,145,146] In ventricular tissue from the dog heart, ranolazine reduces APD more in cells with long APDs (Purkinje fibers and M cells) than in cells with short APD (epicardial cells) and thus decreases dispersion of repolarization.[132] Data suggest that reduction of late I_{Na} in the heart increases repolarization reserve and reduces repolarization variability and its proarrhythmic effects.

Inhibitors of late I_{Na} reduce ST-segment elevation during regional ischemia.[88,140,147,148] This is surprising, considering the many detrimental changes that occur during ischemia. Ischemic myocardium is without oxygen or metabolic substrate for ATP formation. Intracellular concentrations of ischemic metabolites (some of which act to increase late I_{Na}), H^+, Na^+, and Ca^{2+} increase, and K^+ exits cells and accumulates extracellularly. ATP-sensitive potassium current is activated, APD shortens, and rhythmic contractions cease. Cellular depolarization (caused by reduction of the transmembrane K^+ gradient) and reduction of AP amplitude lead to ST-segment elevation in the electrocardiogram.[149] Late I_{Na} inhibitors reduce the increase of Na^+_i in the ischemic myocardium.[21,22,84] Inhibition of late I_{Na} may play a major role in the reduction of Na^+ uptake, but reduction of peak I_{Na} may also be important. Inhibitors of late I_{Na} reduce peak I_{Na} in a use- and/or voltage-dependent manner.[114,150-152] Use-dependent block of Na^+ channels by lidocaine leads to activation failure and slows AP propagation with arrhythmia suppression.[153,154] Thus, high rates of channel activation (as during tachycardia) and even relatively small depolarizations of cells (as in ischemic tissue) facilitate use- and voltage-dependent block, respectively, of Na^+ channels by late I_{Na} inhibitors such as ranolazine,[150,151] presumably by increasing the fraction of channels in inactivated states that are stabilized by the drugs.[50,150,151] Studies of isolated cells have demonstrated that prolonged depolarization in the range of -70 to -40 mV inactivates most Na^+ channels, but some channels exhibit inactivation failure that is manifested as long bursts of rapid channel openings and closings.[5,31,53,63-66,133] This bursting activity is blocked by ranolazine and other late I_{Na} inhibitors[31,36]; ranolazine seems to decrease the rate at which inactivated Na^+ channels transition back to the open state. Late I_{Na} blockers such as ranolazine therefore reduce Na^+ influx during ischemia by reducing the enhanced late I_{Na}, by use- and voltage-dependent reduction of peak I_{Na}, and by block of Na^+ channel openings due to inactivation failure in depolarized cells. Prevention of the ischemia-induced increase of the intracellular Na^+ concentration maintains the Na^+ gradient that drives Ca^{2+} extrusion via NCX. In summary, a reduction of cellular Na^+ uptake in the ischemic myocardium could lead to reductions of cellular K^+ loss and depolarization of cells, as well as to reductions of metabolic,[155,156] electrical,[114,116,148] and contractile[42,89,157-159] derangements caused by NCX-mediated Ca^{2+} overload.

Drugs that selectively reduce late I_{Na} may be effective in the treatment of ischemic heart diseases, including chronic angina, heart failure, and atrial and ventricular arrhythmias, and acute ischemia without causing direct effects on heart rate or blood pressure. The underlying mechanism of therapeutic benefit is a reduction of the pathologic condition caused by late I_{Na}–induced Na^+ and Ca^{2+} overload in the myocardium[15,18,20-22,38,49,52,89-91,115,136,137,153,156,158-164] including contractile (increased diastolic tension and reduced myocardial compliance[90,97,165]) and electrical dysfunction. Ranolazine has been demonstrated to reduce anginal symptoms and increase exercise tolerance in clinical trials[138,139,166-176,181] and it is associated with reductions in recurrent ischemia[176,177] and both supraventricular[178,179] and ventricular[179,180] arrhythmic activity.

SUMMARY

Late I_{Na} is normally a small current in the heart. It is most prominent in Purkinje fibers and M cells and thus contributes to dispersion of repolarization in the normal myocardium. Inhibition of the normal small late I_{Na} has yet to be associated with any electric (or mechanical) consequence for cardiac function. An enhancement of late I_{Na} occurs as a result of congenital or acquired Na^+ channelopathies, including the commonly acquired conditions of myocardial ischemia, heart failure, oxidative stress, and cardiac remodeling (eg, atrial fibrillation or postmyocardial infarction). Enhancement of late I_{Na}, especially in association with reduction of repolarizing K^+ current, is proarrhythmic in both atrial and ventricular myocardium and may provide both the triggers and the substrate for arrhythmic activity. Enhancement of late I_{Na} may cause diastolic depolarization, reduction of repolarization reserve, APD prolongation and afterdepolarizations, triggered activity, increased dispersion of repolarization, reentrant arrhythmic activity, Na^+-induced Ca^{2+} overload associated with AP alternans, and diastolic contractile dysfunction. Reduction of an enhanced late I_{Na} has been shown to be protective during ischemia and to reduce arrhythmic activity in many preclinical models. Notwithstanding the lack of selectivity of ranolazine to block late I_{Na}, results of clinical studies with the drug can be viewed as supportive evidence for a pathologic role of late I_{Na} in the ischemic heart.

ACKNOWLEDGMENTS

The author thanks Luiz Belardinelli, Charles Antzelevitch, Lin Wu, Yejia Song, Sridharan

Rajamani, Cathy Smith-Maxwell, Lina Yao, Kirsten Hoyer, Yuzhi Wu, and many academic colleagues for their intellectual contributions to the understanding of the roles of late I_{Na} in the heart.

REFERENCES

1. Miyamoto S, Zhu BM, Aye NN, et al. Slowing Na+ channel inactivation prolongs QT interval and aggravates adrenaline-induced arrhythmias. Jpn J Pharmacol 2001;86:114–9.

2. Maltsev VA, Silverman N, Sabbah HN, et al. Chronic heart failure slows late sodium current in human and canine ventricular myocytes: implications for repolarization variability. Eur J Heart Fail 2007;9:219–27.

3. Sakmann BF, Spindler AJ, Bryant SM, et al. Distribution of a persistent sodium current across the ventricular wall in guinea pigs. Circ Res 2000;87:910–4.

4. Ward CA, Giles WR. Ionic mechanism of the effects of hydrogen peroxide in rat ventricular myocytes. J Physiol 1997;500(Pt 3):631–42.

5. Kiyosue T, Arita M. Late sodium current and its contribution to action potential configuration in guinea pig ventricular myocytes. Circ Res 1989;64:389–97.

6. January CT, Riddle JM. Early afterdepolarizations: mechanism of induction and block. A role for L-type Ca2+ current. Circ Res 1989;64:977–90.

7. Zaza A, Belardinelli L, Shryock JC, et al. Pathophysiology and pharmacology of the cardiac "late sodium current". Pharmacol Ther 2008;119:326–39.

8. Guo D, Zhou J, Zhao X, et al. L-type calcium current recovery versus ventricular repolarization: preserved membrane-stabilizing mechanism for different QT intervals across species. Heart Rhythm 2008;5:271–9.

9. Viswanathan PC, Rudy Y. Pause induced early afterdepolarizations in the long QT syndrome: a simulation study. Cardiovasc Res 1999;42:530–42.

10. Zabel M, Hohnloser SH, Behrens S, et al. Electrophysiologic features of torsades de pointes: insights from a new isolated rabbit heart model. J Cardiovasc Electrophysiol 1997;8:1148–58.

11. Volders PG, Vos MA, Szabo B, et al. Progress in the understanding of cardiac early afterdepolarizations and torsades de pointes: time to revise current concepts. Cardiovasc Res 2000;46:376–92.

12. Zygmunt AC, Eddlestone GT, Thomas GP, et al. Larger late sodium conductance in M cells contributes to electrical heterogeneity in canine ventricle. Am J Physiol Heart Circ Physiol 2001;281:H689–97.

13. Antzelevitch C, Belardinelli L. The role of sodium channel current in modulating transmural dispersion of repolarization and arrhythmogenesis.

J Cardiovasc Electrophysiol 2006;17(Suppl 1):S79–85.

14. Dos Santos RW, Otaviano CF, Neumann CL, et al. ATX-II effects on the apparent location of M cells in a computational model of a human left ventricular wedge. J Cardiovasc Electrophysiol 2006;17(Suppl 1):S86–95.

15. Makielski JC, Farley AL. Na(+) current in human ventricle: implications for sodium loading and homeostasis. J Cardiovasc Electrophysiol 2006;17(Suppl 1):S15–20.

16. Bers DM. Excitation-contraction coupling and cardiac contractile force. Dordrecht (The Netherlands): Kluwer Academic Publishers; 2001.

17. Despa S, Islam MA, Weber CR, et al. Intracellular Na(+) concentration is elevated in heart failure but Na/K pump function is unchanged. Circulation 2002;105:2543–8.

18. Maier LS, Hasenfuss G. Role of [Na+]i and the emerging involvement of the late sodium current in the pathophysiology of cardiovascular disease. Eur Heart J Suppl 2006;8:A6–9.

19. Pieske B, Maier LS, Piacentino V III, et al. Rate dependence of [Na+]i and contractility in nonfailing and failing human myocardium. Circulation 2002;106:447–53.

20. Pieske B, Houser SR. [Na+]i handling in the failing human heart. Cardiovasc Res 2003;57:874–86.

21. Haigney MC, Lakatta EG, Stern MD, et al. Sodium channel blockade reduces hypoxic sodium loading and sodium-dependent calcium loading. Circulation 1994;90:391–9.

22. Van Emous JG, Nederhoff MG, Ruigrok TJ, et al. The role of the Na+ channel in the accumulation of intracellular Na+ during myocardial ischemia: consequences for post-ischemic recovery. J Mol Cell Cardiol 1997;29:85–96.

23. Baetz D, Bernard M, Pinet C, et al. Different pathways for sodium entry in cardiac cells during ischemia and early reperfusion. Mol Cell Biochem 2003;242:115–20.

24. Lederer WJ, Tsien RW. Transient inward current underlying arrhythmogenic effects of cardiotonic steroids in Purkinje fibres. J Physiol 1976;263:73–100.

25. Wasserstrom JA, Sharma R, O'Toole MJ, et al. Ranolazine antagonizes the effects of increased late sodium current on intracellular calcium cycling in rat isolated intact heart. J Pharmacol Exp Ther 2009;331:382–91.

26. Pruvot EJ, Katra RP, Rosenbaum DS, et al. Role of calcium cycling versus restitution in the mechanism of repolarization alternans. Circ Res 2004;94:1083–90.

27. Valdivia CR, Chu WW, Pu J, et al. Increased late sodium current in myocytes from a canine heart failure model and from failing human heart. J Mol Cell Cardiol 2005;38:475–83.

28. Antzelevitch C, Shimizu W, Yan GX, et al. The M cell: its contribution to the ECG and to normal and abnormal electrical function of the heart. J Cardiovasc Electrophysiol 1999;10:1124–52.

29. Honerjager P. Cardioactive substances that prolong the open state of sodium channels. Rev Physiol Biochem Pharmacol 1982;92:1–74.

30. Shang LL, Sanyal S, Pfahnl AE, et al. NF-kappaB-dependent transcriptional regulation of the cardiac scn5a sodium channel by angiotensin II. Am J Physiol Cell Physiol 2008;294:C372–9.

31. Ma JH, Luo AT, Zhang PH. Effect of hydrogen peroxide on persistent sodium current in guinea pig ventricular myocytes. Acta Pharmacol Sin 2005;26:828–34.

32. Matsumura H, Hara A, Hashizume H, et al. Protective effects of ranolazine, a novel anti-ischemic drug, on the hydrogen peroxide-induced derangements in isolated, perfused rat heart: comparison with dichloroacetate. Jpn J Pharmacol 1998;77:31–9.

33. Song Y, Shryock JC, Wagner S, et al. Blocking late sodium current reduces hydrogen peroxide-induced arrhythmogenic activity and contractile dysfunction. J Pharmacol Exp Ther 2006;318: 214–22.

34. Ahern GP, Hsu SF, Klyachko VA, et al. Induction of persistent sodium current by exogenous and endogenous nitric oxide. J Biol Chem 2000;275: 28810–5.

35. Gautier M, Zhang H, Fearon IM. Peroxynitrite formation mediates LPC-induced augmentation of cardiac late sodium currents. J Mol Cell Cardiol 2008;44:241–51.

36. Ju YK, Saint DA, Gage PW. Hypoxia increases persistent sodium current in rat ventricular myocytes. J Physiol 1996;497(Pt 2):337–47.

37. Fearon IM, Brown ST. Acute and chronic hypoxic regulation of recombinant hNa(v)1.5 alpha subunits. Biochem Biophys Res Commun 2004; 324:1289–95.

38. Saint DA. The role of the persistent Na(+) current during cardiac ischemia and hypoxia. J Cardiovasc Electrophysiol 2006;17(Suppl 1): S96–103.

39. Ma JH, Wang XP, Zhang PH. Mechanisms on nitric oxide increasing persistent sodium current of ventricular myocytes in guinea pig during normoxia and hypoxia. Acta Pharmacol Sin 2004;56:603–8.

40. Wu J, Corr PB. Palmitoylcarnitine increases [Na+]i and initiates transient inward current in adult ventricular myocytes. Am J Physiol 1995;268: H2405–17.

41. Undrovinas AI, Fleidervish IA, Makielski JC. Inward sodium current at resting potentials in single cardiac myocytes induced by the ischemic metabolite lysophosphatidylcholine. Circ Res 1992;71: 1231–41.

42. Wu Y, Song Y, Belardinelli L, et al. The late INa inhibitor ranolazine attentuates effects of palmitoyl-L-carnitine to increase late INa and cause ventricular diastolic dysfunction. J Pharmacol Exp Ther 2009;330(2):550–7.

43. Kohlhardt M, Fichtner H, Frobe U. Metabolites of the glycolytic pathway modulate the activity of single cardiac Na+ channels. FASEB J 1989;3:1963–7.

44. Pinet C, Algalarrondo V, Sablayrolles S, et al. Protease-activated receptor-1 mediates thrombin-induced persistent sodium current in human cardiomyocytes. Mol Pharmacol 2008;73:1622–31.

45. Biswas S, DiSilvestre D, Tian Y, et al. Calcium-mediated dual-mode regulation of cardiac sodium channel gating. Circ Res 2009;104:870–8.

46. Aiba T, Hesketh GG, Liu T, et al. Na+ channel regulation by Ca2+/calmodulin and Ca2+/calmodulin-dependent protein kinase II in guinea-pig ventricular myocytes. Cardiovasc Res 2010;85:454–63.

47. Tan HL, Kupershmidt S, Zhang R, et al. A calcium sensor in the sodium channel modulates cardiac excitability. Nature 2002;415:442–7.

48. Wagner S, Dybkova N, Rasenack EC, et al. Ca2+/calmodulin-dependent protein kinase II regulates cardiac Na+ channels. J Clin Invest 2006;116: 3127–38.

49. Undrovinas A, Maltsev VA. Late sodium current is a new therapeutic target to improve contractility and rhythm in failing heart. Cardiovasc Hematol Agents Med Chem 2008;6:348–59.

50. Undrovinas AI, Belardinelli L, Undrovinas NA, et al. Ranolazine improves abnormal repolarization and contraction in left ventricular myocytes of dogs with heart failure by inhibiting late sodium current. J Cardiovasc Electrophysiol 2006;17(Suppl 1): S169–77.

51. Maltsev VA, Reznikov V, Undrovinas NA, et al. Modulation of late sodium current by Ca2+, calmodulin, and CaMKII in normal and failing dog cardiomyocytes: similarities and differences. Am J Physiol Heart Circ Physiol 2008;294:H1597–608.

52. Undrovinas NA, Maltsev VA, Belardinelli L, et al. Late sodium current contributes to diastolic cell Ca2+ accumulation in chronic heart failure. J Physiol Sci 2010;60:245–57.

53. Maltsev VA, Sabbah HN, Higgins RS, et al. Novel, ultraslow inactivating sodium current in human ventricular cardiomyocytes. Circulation 1998;98: 2545–52.

54. Undrovinas AI, Maltsev VA, Sabbah HN. Repolarization abnormalities in cardiomyocytes of dogs with chronic heart failure: role of sustained inward current. Cell Mol Life Sci 1999;55:494–505.

55. Huang B, El Sherif T, Gidh-Jain M, et al. Alterations of sodium channel kinetics and gene expression in the postinfarction remodeled myocardium. J Cardiovasc Electrophysiol 2001;12:218–25.

56. Chauhan VS, Tuvia S, Buhusi M, et al. Abnormal cardiac Na(+) channel properties and QT heart rate adaptation in neonatal ankyrin(B) knockout mice. Circ Res 2000;86:441–7.

57. Ueda K, Valdivia C, Medeiros-Domingo A, et al. Syntrophin mutation associated with long QT syndrome through activation of the nNOS-SCN5A macromolecular complex. Proc Natl Acad Sci U S A 2008; 105:9355–60.

58. Mazzone A, Strege PR, Tester DJ, et al. A mutation in telethonin alters Nav1.5 function. J Biol Chem 2008;283:16537–44.

59. Vatta M, Ackerman MJ, Ye B, et al. Mutant caveolin-3 induces persistent late sodium current and is associated with long-QT syndrome. Circulation 2006; 114:2104–12.

60. George AL Jr. Inherited disorders of voltage-gated sodium channels. J Clin Invest 2005;115:1990–9.

61. Li CZ, Wang XD, Wang HW, et al. Four types of late Na channel current in isolated ventricular myocytes with reference to their contribution to the lastingness of action potential plateau. Sheng Li Xue Bao 1997;49:241–8.

62. Maltsev VA, Undrovinas AI. A multi-modal composition of the late Na+ current in human ventricular cardiomyocytes. Cardiovasc Res 2006;69:116–27.

63. Liu YM, DeFelice LJ, Mazzanti M. Na channels that remain open throughout the cardiac action potential plateau. Biophys J 1992;63:654–62.

64. Patlak JB, Ortiz M. Slow currents through single sodium channels of the adult rat heart. J Gen Physiol 1985;86:89–104.

65. Zilberter Y, Starmer CF, Starobin J, et al. Late Na channels in cardiac cells: the physiological role of background Na channels. Biophys J 1994;67: 153–60.

66. Attwell D, Cohen I, Eisner D, et al. The steady state TTX-sensitive ("window") sodium current in cardiac Purkinje fibres. Pflugers Arch 1979;379:137–42.

67. Bean BP. The molecular machinery of resurgent sodium current revealed. Neuron 2005;45:185–7.

68. Clancy CE, Tateyama M, Liu H, et al. Non-equilibrium gating in cardiac Na+ channels: an original mechanism of arrhythmia. Circulation 2003;107: 2233–7.

69. Zimmer T, Surber R. SCN5A channelopathies–an update on mutations and mechanisms. Prog Biophys Mol Biol 2008;98:120–36.

70. Ulbricht W. Sodium channel inactivation: molecular determinants and modulation. Physiol Rev 2005; 85:1271–301.

71. West JW, Patton DE, Scheuer T, et al. A cluster of hydrophobic amino acid residues required for fast Na(+)-channel inactivation. Proc Natl Acad Sci U S A 1992;89:10910–4.

72. Deschenes I, Trottier E, Chahine M. Implication of the C-terminal region of the alpha-subunit of voltage-gated sodium channels in fast inactivation. J Membr Biol 2001;183:103–14.

73. Kass RS. Sodium channel inactivation in heart: a novel role of the carboxy-terminal domain. J Cardiovasc Electrophysiol 2006;17(Suppl 1):S21–5.

74. Johnson D, Bennett ES. Isoform-specific effects of the beta2 subunit on voltage-gated sodium channel gating. J Biol Chem 2006;281:25875–81.

75. Maltsev VA, Kyle JW, Undrovinas A. Late Na+ current produced by human cardiac Na+ channel isoform Nav1.5 is modulated by its beta1 subunit. J Physiol Sci 2009;59:217–25.

76. Abriel H. Cardiac sodium channel Nav1.5 and interacting proteins: physiology and pathophysiology. J Mol Cell Cardiol 2010;48:2–11.

77. Ruan Y, Liu N, Priori SG. Sodium channel mutations and arrhythmias. Nat Rev Cardiol 2009;6:337–48.

78. Tateyama M, Rivolta I, Clancy CE, et al. Modulation of cardiac sodium channel gating by protein kinase A can be altered by disease-linked mutation. J Biol Chem 2003;278:46718–26.

79. Murray KT, Hu NN, Daw JR, et al. Functional effects of protein kinase C activation on the human cardiac Na+ channel. Circ Res 1997;80:370–6.

80. Light PE, Wallace CH, Dyck JR. Constitutively active adenosine monophosphate-activated protein kinase regulates voltage-gated sodium channels in ventricular myocytes. Circulation 2003;107: 1962–5.

81. Ahern CA, Zhang JF, Wookalis MJ, et al. Modulation of the cardiac sodium channel NaV1.5 by Fyn, a Src family tyrosine kinase. Circ Res 2005; 96:991–8.

82. Jespersen T, Gavillet B, van Bemmelen MX, et al. Cardiac sodium channel Na(v)1.5 interacts with and is regulated by the protein tyrosine phosphatase PTPH1. Biochem Biophys Res Commun 2006;348:1455–62.

83. Valdivia CR, Ueda K, Ackerman MJ, et al. GPD1L links redox state to cardiac excitability by PKC-dependent phosphorylation of the sodium channel SCN5A. Am J Physiol Heart Circ Physiol 2009;297: H1446–52.

84. Zhang XQ, Yamada S, Barry WH. Ranolazine inhibits an oxidative stress-induced increase in myocyte sodium and calcium loading during simulated-demand ischemia. J Cardiovasc Pharmacol 2008;51(5):443–9.

85. Le Grand B, Vie B, Talmant JM, et al. Alleviation of contractile dysfunction in ischemic hearts by slowly inactivating Na+ current blockers. Am J Physiol 1995;269:H533–40.

86. Saint DA. The cardiac persistent sodium current: an appealing therapeutic target? Br J Pharmacol 2008;153:1133–42.

87. Letienne R, Bel L, Bessac AM, et al. Myocardial protection by F 15845, a persistent sodium current

blocker, in an ischemia-reperfusion model in the pig. Eur J Pharmacol 2009;624:16–22.

88. Vacher B, Pignier C, Letienne R, et al. F 15845 inhibits persistent sodium current in the heart and prevents angina in animal models. Br J Pharmacol 2009;156:214–25.

89. Vie B, Sablayrolles S, Letienne R, et al. 3-(R)-[3-(2-methoxyphenylthio-2-(S)-methylpropyl]amino-3,4-dihydro-2H-1,5- benzoxathiepine bromhydrate (F 15845) prevents ischemia-induced heart remodeling by reduction of the intracellular Na+ overload. J Pharmacol Exp Ther 2009;330:696–703.

90. Sossalla S, Wagner S, Rasenack E, et al. Ranolazine improves diastolic dysfunction in isolated myocardium from failing human hearts - role of late sodium current and intracellular ion accumulation. J Mol Cell Cardiol 2008;45:32–43.

91. Pogwizd SM, Schlotthauer K, Li L, et al. Arrhythmogenesis and contractile dysfunction in heart failure: roles of sodium-calcium exchange, inward rectifier potassium current, and residual beta-adrenergic responsiveness. Circ Res 2001;88:1159–67.

92. Burstein B, Comtois P, Michael G, et al. Changes in connexin expression and the atrial fibrillation substrate in congestive heart failure. Circ Res 2009;105:1213–22.

93. Glukhov AV, Fedorov VV, Lou Q, et al. Transmural dispersion of repolarization in failing and nonfailing human ventricle. Circ Res 2010;106:981–91.

94. Morita N, Sovari AA, Xie Y, et al. Increased susceptibility of aged hearts to ventricular fibrillation during oxidative stress. Am J Physiol Heart Circ Physiol 2009;297:H1594–605.

95. Zaniboni M, Pollard AE, Yang L, et al. Beat-to-beat repolarization variability in ventricular myocytes and its suppression by electrical coupling. Am J Physiol Heart Circ Physiol 2000;278:H677–87.

96. Spitzer KW, Pollard AE, Yang L, et al. Cell-to-cell electrical interactions during early and late repolarization. J Cardiovasc Electrophysiol 2006;17 (Suppl 1):S8–14.

97. Sossalla S, Kallmeyer B, Wagner S, et al. Altered Na(+) currents in atrial fibrillation. Effects of ranolazine on arrhythmias and contractility in human atrial myocardium. J Am Coll Cardiol 2010;55:2330–42.

98. Wu L, Rajamani S, Li H, et al. Reduction of repolarization reserve unmasks the proarrhythmic role of endogenous late Na(+) current in the heart. Am J Physiol Heart Circ Physiol 2009;297:H1048–57.

99. Wu L, Shryock JC, Song Y, et al. An increase in late sodium current potentiates the proarrhythmic activities of low-risk QT-prolonging drugs in female rabbit hearts. J Pharmacol Exp Ther 2006;316:718–26.

100. Di Diego JM, Belardinelli L, Antzelevitch C. Cisapride-induced transmural dispersion of repolarization and torsade de pointes in the canine left ventricular wedge preparation during epicardial stimulation. Circulation 2003;108:1027–33.

101. Thomsen MB, Verduyn SC, Stengl M, et al. Increased short-term variability of repolarization predicts d-sotalol-induced torsades de pointes in dogs. Circulation 2004;110:2453–9.

102. Wu L, Shryock JC, Song Y, et al. Antiarrhythmic effects of ranolazine in a guinea pig in vitro model of long-QT syndrome. J Pharmacol Exp Ther 2004;310:599–605.

103. Wang W, Robertson C, Dhalla AK, et al. Antitorsadogenic effects of ({+/-})-N-(2,6-dimethyl-phenyl)-(4 [2-hydroxy-3-(2-methoxyphenoxy)propyl]-1-piperazine (ranolazine) in anesthetized rabbits. J Pharmacol Exp Ther 2008;325:875–81.

104. Van Wagoner DR. Oxidative stress and inflammation in atrial fibrillation: role in pathogenesis and potential as a therapeutic target. J Cardiovasc Pharmacol 2008;52:306–13.

105. Guo D, Young L, Wu Y, et al. Increased late sodium current in left atrial myocytes of rabbits with left ventricular hypertrophy: its role in the genesis of atrial arrhythmias. Am J Physiol Heart Circ Physiol 2010;298:H1375–81.

106. Wu J, Cheng L, Lammers WJ, et al. Sinus node dysfunction in ATX-II-induced in-vitro murine model of long QT3 syndrome and rescue effect of ranolazine. Prog Biophys Mol Biol 2008;98:198–207.

107. Song Y, Shryock JC, Belardinelli L. A slowly-inactivating sodium current contributes to spontaneous diastolic depolarization of atrial myocytes. Am J Physiol Heart Circ Physiol 2009;297:H1254–62.

108. Song Y, Shryock JC, Belardinelli L. An increase of late sodium current induces delayed afterdepolarizations and sustained triggered activity in atrial myocytes. Am J Physiol Heart Circ Physiol 2008;294:H2031–9.

109. Song Y, Shryock JC, Wu L, et al. Antagonism by ranolazine of the pro-arrhythmic effects of increasing late INa in guinea pig ventricular myocytes. J Cardiovasc Pharmacol 2004;44:192–9.

110. Shryock JC, Belardinelli L. Inhibition of late sodium current to reduce electrical and mechanical dysfunction of ischaemic myocardium. Br J Pharmacol 2008;153:1128–32.

111. Boden WE. Ranolazine and its anti-ischemic effects: revisiting an old mechanistic paradigm anew? J Am Coll Cardiol 2010;56:943–5.

112. Fedida D, Orth PM, Hesketh JC, et al. The role of late I and antiarrhythmic drugs in EAD formation and termination in Purkinje fibers. J Cardiovasc Electrophysiol 2006;17(Suppl 1):S71–8.

113. Sicouri S, Antzelevitch D, Heilmann C, et al. Effects of sodium channel block with mexiletine to reverse action potential prolongation in in vitro models of the long term QT syndrome. J Cardiovasc Electrophysiol 1997;8:1280–90.

114. Pignier C, Rougier JS, Vie B, et al. Selective inhibition of persistent sodium current by F 15845 prevents ischaemia-induced arrhythmias. Br J Pharmacol 2010;161:79–91.

115. VerDonck L, Borgers M, Verdonck F. Inhibition of sodium and calcium overload pathology in the myocardium: a new cytoprotective principle. Cardiovasc Res 1993;27:349–57.

116. Dhalla AK, Wang WQ, Dow J, et al. Ranolazine, an antianginal agent, markedly reduces ventricular arrhythmias induced by ischemia and ischemia-reperfusion. Am J Physiol Heart Circ Physiol 2009;297:H1923–9.

117. Gralinski MR, Chi L, Park JL, et al. Protective effects of ranolazine on ventricular fibrillation induced by activation of the ATP-dependent potassium channel in the rabbit heart. J Cardiovasc Pharmacol Ther 1996;1:141–8.

118. Kloner RA, Dow JS, Bhandari A. The antianginal agent ranolazine is a potent antiarrhythmic agent that reduces ventricular arrhythmias: through a mechanism favoring inhibition of late sodium channel. Cardiovasc Ther 2010. [Epub ahead of print].

119. Le Grand B, Pignier C, Letienne R, et al. Na+ currents in cardioprotection: better to be late. J Med Chem 2009;52:4149–60.

120. Antzelevitch C, Belardinelli L, Wu L, et al. Electrophysiologic properties and antiarrhythmic actions of a novel antianginal agent. J Cardiovasc Pharmacol Ther 2004;9(Suppl 1):S65–83.

121. Sicouri S, Glass A, Belardinelli L, et al. Antiarrhythmic effects of ranolazine in canine pulmonary vein sleeve preparations. Heart Rhythm 2008;5:1019–26.

122. Wu Y, Roden DM, Anderson ME. Calmodulin kinase inhibition prevents development of the arrhythmogenic transient inward current. Circ Res 1999;84:906–12.

123. Katra RP, Laurita KR. Cellular mechanism of calcium-mediated triggered activity in the heart. Circ Res 2005;96:535–42.

124. Curran J, Brown KH, Santiago DJ, et al. Spontaneous Ca waves in ventricular myocytes from failing hearts depend on Ca(2+)-calmodulin-dependent protein kinase II. J Mol Cell Cardiol 2010;49:25–32.

125. Maier LS, Zhang T, Chen L, et al. Transgenic CaMKIIdeltaC overexpression uniquely alters cardiac myocyte Ca2+ handling: reduced SR Ca2+ load and activated SR Ca2+ release. Circ Res 2003;92:904–11.

126. Maier LS. Role of CaMKII for signaling and regulation in the heart. Front Biosci 2009;14:486–96.

127. Fredj S, Lindegger N, Sampson KJ, et al. Altered Na+ channels promote pause-induced spontaneous diastolic activity in long QT syndrome type 3 myocytes. Circ Res 2006;99:1225–32.

128. Antzelevitch C. Ionic, molecular, and cellular bases of QT-interval prolongation and torsade de pointes. Europace 2007;9(Suppl 4):4–15.

129. Flaim SN, Giles WR, McCulloch AD. Contributions of sustained INa and IKv43 to transmural heterogeneity of early repolarization and arrhythmogenesis in canine left ventricular myocytes. Am J Physiol Heart Circ Physiol 2006;291:H2617–29.

130. Restivo M, Caref EB, Kozhevnikov DO, et al. Spatial dispersion of repolarization is a key factor in the arrhythmogenicity of long QT syndrome. J Cardiovasc Electrophysiol 2004;15:323–31.

131. Milberg P, Reinsch N, Wasmer K, et al. Transmural dispersion of repolarization as a key factor of arrhythmogenicity in a novel intact heart model of LQT3. Cardiovasc Res 2005;65:397–404.

132. Antzelevitch C, Belardinelli L, Zygmunt AC, et al. Electrophysiological effects of ranolazine, a novel antianginal agent with antiarrhythmic properties. Circulation 2004;110:904–10.

133. Josephson IR, Sperelakis N. Tetrodotoxin differentially blocks peak and steady-state sodium channel currents in early embryonic chick ventricular myocytes. Pflugers Arch 1989;414:354–9.

134. Carmeliet E. Slow inactivation of the sodium current in rabbit cardiac Purkinje fibres. Pflugers Arch 1987;408:18–26.

135. Carmeliet E. Voltage-dependent block by tetrodotoxin of the sodium channel in rabbit cardiac Purkinje fibers. Biophys J 1987;51:109–14.

136. Hale SL, Shryock JC, Belardinelli L, et al. Late sodium current inhibition as a new cardioprotective approach. J Mol Cell Cardiol 2008;44:954–67.

137. Belardinelli L, Shryock JC, Fraser H. Inhibition of the late sodium current as a potential cardioprotective principle: effects of the late sodium current inhibitor ranolazine. Heart 2006;92(Suppl 4):iv6–14.

138. Keating GM. Ranolazine a review of its use in chronic stable angina pectoris. Drugs 2008;68(17):2483–503.

139. Nash DT, Nash SD. Ranolazine for chronic stable angina. Lancet 2008;372:1335–41.

140. Le Grand B, Pignier C, Letienne R, et al. Sodium late current blockers in ischemia reperfusion: is the bullet magic? J Med Chem 2008;51:3856–66.

141. Hondeghem LM, Carlsson L, Duker G. Instability and triangulation of the action potential predict serious proarrhythmia, but action potential duration prolongation is antiarrhythmic. Circulation 2001;103:2004–13.

142. Okada Y, Ogawa S, Sadanaga T, et al. Assessment of reverse use-dependent blocking actions of class III antiarrhythmic drugs by 24-hour Holter electrocardiography. J Am Coll Cardiol 1996;27:84–9.

143. Belardinelli L, Antzelevitch C, Vos MA. Assessing predictors of drug-induced torsade de pointes. Trends Pharmacol Sci 2003;24:619–25.

144. Belardinelli L, Shryock JC, Wu L, et al. Use of preclinical assays to predict risk of drug-induced torsades de pointes. Heart Rhythm 2005;2:S16–22.

145. Wu L, Guo D, Li H, et al. Role of late sodium current in modulating the proarrhythmic and anti-arrhythmic effects of quinidine. Heart Rhythm 2008;5:1726–34.

146. Wu L, Rajamani S, Shryock JC, et al. Augmentation of late sodium current unmasks the proarrhythmic effects of amiodarone. Cardiovasc Res 2008;77:481–8.

147. Wang JX, Maruyama K, Murakami M, et al. Antianginal effects of ranolazine in various experimental models of angina. Arzneimittelforschung 1999;49:193–9.

148. Verscheure Y, Pouget G, De Court, et al. Attenuation by R 56865, a novel cytoprotective drug, of regional myocardial ischemia- and reperfusion-induced electrocardiographic disturbances in anesthetized rabbits. J Cardiovasc Pharmacol 1995;25:126–33.

149. Janse MJ. Electrophysiology and electrocardiology of acute myocardial ischemia. Can J Cardiol 1986;(Suppl A):46A–52A.

150. Rajamani S, El Bizri N, Shryock JC, et al. Use-dependent block of cardiac late Na(+) current by ranolazine. Heart Rhythm 2009;6:1625–31.

151. Rajamani S, Shryock JC, Belardinelli L. Block of tetrodotoxin-sensitive, Na(V)1.7 and tetrodotoxin-resistant, Na(V)1.8, Na+ channels by ranolazine. Channels (Austin) 2008;2:449–60.

152. Carmeliet E, Tytgat J. Agonistic and antagonistic effect of R56865 on the Na+ channel in cardiac cells. Eur J Pharmacol 1991;196:53–60.

153. Noble D, Varghese A. Modelling of sodium-overload arrhythmias and their suppression. Can J Cardiol 1998;14:97–100.

154. Comtois P, Sakabe M, Vigmond EJ, et al. Mechanisms of atrial fibrillation termination by rapidly unbinding Na+ channel blockers: insights from mathematical models and experimental correlates. Am J Physiol Heart Circ Physiol 2008;295:H1489–504.

155. Hartmann M, Decking UK, Schrader J. Cardioprotective actions of KC 12291. II. Delaying Na+ overload in ischemia improves cardiac function and energy status in reperfusion. Naunyn Schmiedebergs Arch Pharmacol 1998;358:554–60.

156. Gralinski MR, Black SC, Kilgore KS, et al. Cardioprotective effects of ranolazine (RS-43285) in the isolated perfused rabbit heart. Cardiovasc Res 1994;28:1231–7.

157. John GW, Letienne R, Le Grand B, et al. KC 12291: an atypical sodium channel blocker with myocardial antiischemic properties. Cardiovasc Drug Rev 2004;22:17–26.

158. Fraser H, Belardinelli L, Wang L, et al. Ranolazine decreases diastolic calcium accumulation caused by ATX-II or ischemia in rat hearts. J Mol Cell Cardiol 2006;41:1031–8.

159. Hale SL, Kloner RA. Ranolazine, an inhibitor of the late sodium channel current, reduces postischemic myocardial dysfunction in the rabbit. J Cardiovasc Pharmacol Ther 2006;11:249–55.

160. Belardinelli L, Antzelevitch C, Fraser H. Inhibition of late (sustained/persistent) sodium current: a potential drug target to reduce intracellular sodium-dependent effects on cardiomyocyte function. Eur Heart J 2004;6(Suppl 1):13–7.

161. Belardinelli L, Shryock JC, Fraser H. The mechanism of ranolazine action to reduce ischemia-induced diastolic dysfunction. Eur Heart J 2006;8(Suppl A):A10–3.

162. Hasenfuss G, Maier LS. Mechanism of action of the new anti-ischemia drug ranolazine. Clin Res Cardiol 2008;97:222–6.

163. Dipla K, Mattiello JA, Margulies KB, et al. The sarcoplasmic reticulum and the Na+/Ca2+ exchanger both contribute to the Ca2+ transient of failing human ventricular myocytes. Circ Res 1999;84:435–44.

164. Eigel BN, Hadley RW. Antisense inhibition of Na+/Ca2+ exchange during anoxia/reoxygenation in ventricular myocytes. Am J Physiol Heart Circ Physiol 2001;281:H2184–90.

165. Hayashida W, van Eyll C, Rousseau MF, et al. Effects of ranolazine on left ventricular regional diastolic function in patients with ischemic heart disease. Cardiovasc Drugs Ther 1994;8:741–7.

166. Bassand J. Clinical implications of inhibition of the late sodium current: ranolazine. Eur Heart J 2006;8(Suppl A):A14–9.

167. Chaitman BR. Ranolazine for the treatment of chronic angina and potential use in other cardiovascular conditions. Circulation 2006;113:2462–72.

168. Chaitman BR, Pepine CJ, Parker JO, et al. Effects of ranolazine with atenolol, amlodipine, or diltiazem on exercise tolerance and angina frequency in patients with severe chronic angina: a randomized controlled trial. JAMA 2004;291:309–16.

169. Chaitman BR, Skettino SL, Parker JO, et al. Anti-ischemic effects and long-term survival during ranolazine monotherapy in patients with chronic severe angina. J Am Coll Cardiol 2004;43:1375–82.

170. Pepine CJ, Wolff A. A controlled trial with a novel anti-ischemic agent, ranolazine, in chronic stable angina pectoris that is responsive to conventional antianginal agents. Am J Cardiol 1999;84:46–50.

171. Rousseau M, Pouleur H, Cocco G, et al. Comparative efficacy of ranolazine versus atenolol for chronic angina pectoris. Am J Cardiol 2005;95:311–6.

172. Scirica BM. Ranolazine in patients with coronary artery disease. Expert Opin Pharmacother 2007; 8(13):2149–57.

173. Siddiqui AAA, Keam SJ. Ranolazine. A review of its use in chronic stable angina pectoris. Drugs 2006; 66(5):693–710.

174. Stone PH, Gratsiansky NA, Blokhin A, et al. Antianginal efficacy of ranolazine when added to treatment with amlodipine. J Am Coll Cardiol 2006;48:566–75.

175. Timmis AD, Chaitman BR, Crager M. Effects of ranolazine on exercise tolerance and HbA1c in patients with chronic angina and diabetes. Eur Heart J 2006;27:42–8.

176. Wilson SR, Scirica BM, Braunwald E, et al. Efficacy of ranolazine in patients with chronic angina. J Am Coll Cardiol 2009;53:1510–6.

177. Morrow DA, Scirica BM, Prokopczuk E, et al. Effects of ranolazine on recurrent cardiovascular events in patients with non-ST-elevation Acute Coronary Syndromes. JAMA 2007;297:1775–83.

178. Murdock D, Overton N, Kersten M, et al. The effect of ranolazine on maintaining sinus rhythm in patients with resistant atrial fibrillation. Indian Pacing Electrophysiol J 2008;8(3):175–81.

179. Scirica BM, Morrow DA, Hod H, et al. Effect of ranolazine, an antianginal agent with novel electrophysiological properties, on the incidence of arrhythmias in patients with non-ST-segment elevation acute coronary syndrome. Circulation 2007; 116:1647–52.

180. Murdock D, Kaliebe J, Overton N. Ranolazine-induced suppression of ventricular tachycardia in a patient with nonischemic cardiomyopathy: a case report. Pacing Clin Electrophysiol 2008;31:765–8.

181. Eid F, Boden WE. The evolving role of medical therapy for chronic stable angina. Curr Cardiol Rep 2008;10:263–71.

182. Hwang H, Arcidi JM Jr, Hale SL, et al. Ranolazine as an adjunct to cardioplegia: a potential new therapeutic application. J Cardiovasc Pharmacol Ther 2009;14:125–33.

183. Wang P, Fraser H, Lloyd SG, et al. A comparison between ranolazine and CVT-4325, a novel inhibitor of fatty acid oxidation, on cardiac metabolism and left ventricular function in rat isolated perfused heart during ischemia and reperfusion. J Pharmacol Exp Ther 2007;321:213–20.

184. Sharikabad MN, Aronsen JM, Haugen E, et al. Cardiomyocytes from postinfarction failing rat hearts have improved ischemia tolerance. Am J Physiol Heart Circ Physiol 2009;296:H787–95.

185. Tamareille S, Le Grand B, John GW, et al. Anti-ischemic compound KC 12291 prevents diastolic contracture in isolated atria by blockade of voltage-gated sodium channels. J Cardiovasc Pharmacol 2002;40:346–55.

186. Kumar K, Nearing BD, Carvas M, et al. Ranolazine exerts potent effects on atrial electrical properties and abbreviates atrial fibrillation duration in the intact porcine heart. J Cardiovasc Electrophysiol 2009;20:796–802.

187. Maruyama K, Hara A, Hashizume H, et al. Ranolazine attenuates palmitoyl-L-carnitine-induced mechanical and metabolic derangement in the isolated, perfused rat heart. J Pharm Pharmacol 2000;52:709–15.

188. Lu HR, De Clerck F. R 56865, a Na+/Ca(2+)-overload inhibitor, protects against aconitine-induced cardiac arrhythmias in vivo. J Cardiovasc Pharmacol 1993;22:120–5.

189. Sawanobori T, Hirano Y, Hiraoka M. Aconitine-induced delayed afterdepolarization in frog atrium and guinea pig papillary muscles in the presence of low concentrations of Ca2+. Jpn J Physiol 1987;37:59–79.

190. Sawanobori T, Adaniya H, Hirano Y, et al. Effects of antiarrhythmic agents and Mg2+ on aconitine-induced arrhythmias. Jpn Heart J 1996;37:709–18.

191. Leyssens A, Carmeliet E. Block of the transient inward current by R56865 in guinea-pig ventricular myocytes. Eur J Pharmacol 1991;196:43–51.

192. Sheu SS, Lederer WJ. Lidocaine's negative inotropic and antiarrhythmic actions. Dependence on shortening of action potential duration and reduction of intracellular sodium activity. Circ Res 1985;57:578–90.

193. Vollmer B, Meuter C, Janssen PA. R 56865 prevents electrical and mechanical signs of ouabain intoxication in guinea-pig papillary muscle. Eur J Pharmacol 1987;142:137–40.

194. Rastogi S, Sharov VG, Mishra S, et al. Ranolazine combined with enalapril or metoprolol prevents progressive LV dysfunction and remodeling in dogs with moderate heart failure. Am J Physiol Heart Circ Physiol 2008;295:H2149–55.

195. Sabbah HN, Chandler MP, Mishima T, et al. Ranolazine, a partial fatty acid oxidation (pFOX) inhibitor, improves left ventricular function in dogs with chronic heart failure. J Card Fail 2002;8:416–22.

196. Fraser H, Ivey PE, Kato J, et al. Ranolazine reduces ATX-II-induced contracture in rat left atria. The 25th European Section Meeting. International Society for Heart Research. Tromsø, Norway, June 21–25, 2005.

197. Fazekas T, Krassoi I, Lengyel C, et al. Suppression of erythromycin-induced early afterdepolarizations and torsade de pointes ventricular tachycardia by mexiletine. Pacing Clin Electrophysiol 1998;21:147–50.

198. Abrahamsson C, Carlsson L, Duker G. Lidocaine and nisoldipine attenuate almokalant-induced dispersion of repolarization and early afterdepolarizations in vitro. J Cardiovasc Electrophysiol 1996;7:1074–81.

199. Antoons G, Oros A, Beekman JD, et al. Late Na(+) current inhibition by ranolazine reduces torsades de pointes in the chronic atrioventricular block dog model. J Am Coll Cardiol 2010;55:801–9.

200. Burashnikov A, Di Diego JM, Zygmunt AC, et al. Atrium-selective sodium channel block as a strategy for suppression of atrial fibrillation: differences in sodium channel inactivation between atria and ventricles and the role of ranolazine. Circulation 2007;116:1449–57.

201. Carvas M, Nascimento BC, Acar M, et al. Intrapericardial ranolazine prolongs atrial refractory period and markedly reduces atrial fibrillation inducibility in the intact porcine heart. J Cardiovasc Pharmacol 2010;55:286–91.

202. Kumar K, Nearing BD, Bartoli CR, et al. Effect of ranolazine on ventricular vulnerability and defibrillation threshold in the intact porcine heart. J Cardiovasc Electrophysiol 2008;19:1073–9.

203. Burashnikov A, Antzelevitch C. Atrial-selective sodium channel block for the treatment of atrial fibrillation. Expert Opin Emerg Drugs 2009;14:233–49.

204. Ruan Y, Liu N, Bloise R, et al. Gating properties of SCN5A mutations and the response to mexiletine in long-QT syndrome type 3 patients. Circulation 2007;116:1137–44.

205. Moss AJ, Zareba W, Schwarz KQ, et al. Ranolazine shortens repolarization in patients with sustained inward sodium current due to type-3 long-QT syndrome. J Cardiovasc Electrophysiol 2008;19:1289–93.

206. Arakawa J, Hara A, Kokita N. Lidocaine attenuates mechanical and metabolic derangements induced by Palmitoyl-L-Carnitine in the isolated perfused rat heart. Pharmacology 1997;55:259–68.

207. Ravens U, Himmel HM. Drugs preventing Na+ and Ca2+ overload. Pharmacol Res 1999;39:167–74.

Mechanisms Underlying Atrial Fibrillation

David Filgueiras Rama, MD, José Jalife, MD*

KEYWORDS

- Atrial fibrillation • Antiarrhythmic drugs • Reentry
- Rotor dynamics

Atrial fibrillation (AF) is by far the most common sustained arrhythmia seen in clinical practice.[1] AF is associated with a doubling of mortality in both sexes and is a major risk factor for stroke.[1] Specifically, AF is responsible for at least 15% to 20% of all embolic strokes.[2] Overall, AF is thought to be the underlying cause of more than 10,000 deaths per year in the United States. Patients with AF also experience a reduced quality of life compared with controls and the general population.[3] Its prevalence doubles with each advancing decade of age, with a prevalence of 9% in persons 80 years or older.[4] Although it is now clear that AF is already a huge epidemiologic problem, estimates project an increment of 2.5-fold during the next 50 years, and the projected number of persons with AF in the United States may exceed 12 million by 2050.[5] Its importance is also highlighted by the cost of AF management: AF burden has a huge impact on hospitalization costs and on overall health care.[6] It has been suggested that new antiarrhythmic drugs such as dronedarone, which has been shown to decrease hospitalizations,[7] together with implementation of guidelines to reduce the admissions that are not critical for AF care[8] may become essential to support the rapid increase in the prevalence of AF in subsequent years.

However, the authors submit that only a profound and complete understanding of the mechanisms involved in the initiation and maintenance of AF would allow the generation of more specific prevention and/or treatment of new episodes. For many years, various pharmacologic approaches have been tried to convert AF to sinus rhythm, as well as to prevent recurrences. However, many of such drugs, while effective, are associated with substantial side effects and proarrhythmia, and therefore are commonly withdrawn.[9] New, more atrial-selective I_{Kur}, $I_{K,ACh}$, or I_{To} blocking drugs are currently under development. Atrial-selective prolongation of the effective refractory period (ERP) could terminate AF without increasing the risk of ventricular arrhythmias. New variants of older drugs are being tried with the goal of decreasing the incidence of side effects, but concurrently new and often severe adverse effects pop up.[10]

The highly successful catheter-based procedure pioneered by Haïssaguerre and colleagues[11] of ablating ectopic triggers that arise from the pulmonary veins in paroxysmal AF has progressively been extended to a much more heterogeneous population, in which unfortunately the success rate is significantly lower and frequently requires the continuation of antiarrhythmic therapy. Limitations related to the long duration of the procedure, its lack of specificity, and the presence of important side effects[12] make this approach impractical for the AF population at large.

From the foregoing it seems reasonable to conclude that generating insights into AF mechanisms from the use of appropriate experimental and numerical models may have crucial relevance in our attempts to improve patient care and to develop new and more specific therapies. This article focuses on current knowledge about such mechanisms and their translation to real clinical situations.

Supported in part by NHLBI Grants P01-HL039707 and P01-HL087226 and the Leducq Foundation (J.J.) by a Spanish Society of Cardiology Fellowship and Fundación Pedro Barrié de la Maza (D.F.R.).
Department of Internal Medicine, Center for Arrhythmia Research, University of Michigan, 5025 Venture Drive, Ann Arbor, MI 48108, USA
* Corresponding author.
E-mail address: jjalife@umich.edu

Card Electrophysiol Clin 3 (2011) 141–156
doi:10.1016/j.ccep.2010.10.003

CLASSIFICATION OF ATRIAL FIBRILLATION

Several classifications have been proposed for AF, but one based on the temporal pattern of the arrhythmia has been recommended recently. Although such a classification does not account for all aspects of AF, its recommendations are based on its simplicity and clinical relevance.[13]

First, one may distinguish between patients in whom only one AF episode has been detected and patients with 2 or more AF episodes. In such cases with multiple documented episodes, AF is classified as recurrent. In either case, there is no differentiation between symptomatic and asymptomatic episodes, or in terms of the duration or the occurrence of previous, undetected episodes. If the arrhythmia terminates spontaneously it is designated as paroxysmal, but when it is sustained for more than 7 days it is termed persistent. Persistent AF usually requires pharmacologic or electrical cardioversion for termination. The term permanent is used in cases of long-standing AF (>1 year), in which the cardioversion has not been attempted or has failed.

One single patient can be classified into the 3 different categories outlined, depending on the moment.[13] For instance, some patients have episodes of paroxysmal AF for years and never develop persistent AF. Yet others develop persistent or permanent AF. In fact, in a multivariate model, age is the only independent predictor of progression to permanent AF in patients with paroxysmal or persistent AF and no concomitant heart disease or hypertension (lone AF).[14] Furthermore, the presence of premature supraventricular complexes or supraventricular tachycardia on the surface electrocardiogram (ECG) or Holter recording is associated with a decreased risk of progression to permanent AF.[14] The latter highlights the evidence that in some patients rapidly discharging foci, mainly located in the pulmonary veins, initiate the arrhythmia,[11,15] whereas in others a diseased atrial substrate has a dominant role.[16] Therefore, the progression to permanent AF could be explained by the comorbidities associated with the aging process.

In animal models, the stability of AF progressively increases with time in artificially sustained AF by fast atrial pacing.[17,18] After a period of 1 to 2 weeks the AF becomes persistent and the cardioversion success rate decreases until cardioversion is no longer possible in most cases.[19] In humans with paroxysmal and persistent AF it is difficult to know the exact burden and duration of the episodes. Thus, patients with short-lasting episodes and without structural heart disease might not develop permanent AF, because the episodes are usually not long enough to create the remodeling that has been described in animal models.[14]

The clinical relevance of this classification is related to therapeutic implications, specifically related to antithrombotic therapy, because at the present time it is the only therapy that can increase survival in patients with AF.[20] Thus, patients with lone AF who are younger than 60 years would not need antithrombotic therapy to prevent ischemic stroke, because the risk of ischemic stroke is similar to that of the expected risk of the general population.[21] The duration of AF is also important in deciding the cardioversion approach. In those episodes lasting for more than 48 hours or of unknown duration, it is necessary to rule out the possibility of an atrial thrombus by transesophageal echocardiogram or establishing appropriate anticoagulation before the cardioversion. Long-standing AF cases lasting longer than 6 months imply that the likelihood of successful cardioversion is very low, so a strategy focused on rate control and antithrombotic therapy should be pursued.[13]

MECHANISMS OF ARRHYTHMIAS: IMPLICATIONS IN ATRIAL FIBRILLATION
Abnormal Impulse Formation; Abnormal Automaticity

Automaticity is defined as the ability of some excitable cells to produce spontaneous action potentials (AP) in the absence of an external input. In the heart, under normal conditions, sinoatrial (SA) nodal cells, atrioventricular (AV) nodal cells, and His-Purkinje cells possess the property of automaticity. The APs of all 3 cell types have a characteristic ability to gradually undergo spontaneous depolarization during phase 4, which brings the membrane potential to the threshold for activation. The ionic bases of automaticity are complex and controversial. In the SA and AV nodes, it involves a decrease in K^+ conductance and activation of the hyperpolarization-activated current (I_f), as well as of inward Ca^{2+} currents and the current carried by the Na^+/Ca^{2+} exchanger.[22] In Purkinje cells, the I_f current seems to predominate. Under pathologic conditions associated with low intracellular pH, elevated extracellular K^+, and excess catecholamines, abnormal automaticity may arise from either atrial or ventricular cells.[23]

In some cases of AF, it is possible to identify focal discharges from the pulmonary veins (PVs).[11] Although pacemaker cells in the PVs have not been demonstrated as yet in humans,[24] it is generally assumed that discharges in the myocardial venous sleeves[11,25] generated by cells undergoing abnormal automaticity are not only the "triggers" but are also capable of sustaining AF. The fact that in some cases it is possible to restore sinus rhythm after radiofrequency ablation of identifiable foci in the PVs supports the idea that rapid discharges from such foci can maintain AF. However, some cases of AF do not terminate on ablation but are no longer reinducible after cardioversion. The latter supports the "trigger" role of PV foci in the initiation of AF. In either case, arrhythmogenic mechanisms other than automaticity inside the PVs may also be terminated by local ablation.

In isolated PVs from normal dogs it was possible to identify automatic discharges, but the interval between discharges was relatively long (1000 ms).[26] Ischemic conditions may lead to heterogeneous depolarization and depolarization-induced abnormal automaticity, and explain the generation of slow spontaneous discharges. Slow automaticity has been also identified in isolated PVs after catheter ablation in patients with refractory paroxysmal AF (**Fig. 1**).[27] The abnormal automaticity may respond to Ca^{2+} channel blockers, Na channel blockers, and β-blockers.[26] In patients with paroxysmal AF administration of verapamil, propranolol or procainamide decreases the density of ectopic beat bursts that originate in the PVs and initiate AF.[28] Infusion of isoproterenol in cases pretreated with any of these drugs is unable to induce sustained AF.[28] Increasing the inward rectifier potassium channel current I_{K1} should also abolish automaticity, because the resting membrane potential becomes more negative. Nevertheless, the use of adenosine in patients with paroxysmal AF who have undergone an electrophysiological study demonstrated that the maximal dominant frequency (DF_{max}) increases after adenosine at each region compared with baseline.[29] The adenosine effect would be consistent with a reentry mechanism.

Altogether, the evidence does not support the idea that abnormal automaticity maintains AF in the majority of cases. However, this mechanism could be involved in selected cases of paroxysmal AF.[27]

Triggered Activity

Triggered activity arises from membrane potential oscillations that occur during or immediately following an AP. By definition, triggered activity cannot occur in the absence of a previous spontaneous or driven AP, but a triggered AP may itself trigger additional self-sustaining responses. Two different types of triggered activity can be distinguished: early afterdepolarizations (EADs) and delay afterdepolarizations (DADs).

EADs are oscillatory potentials that may occur during phase 2 or 3 of the AP. Increasing the inward currents (eg, $I_{Ca,L}$ or I_{Na}) or decreasing the outward currents during the plateau or phase 3 (eg, I_{Kr} or I_{Ks}) could induce AP prolongation and generate EADs. The L-type Ca^{2+} window current is probably the most likely responsible for the generation of EADs. Situations such as bradycardia and low extracellular K^+ are predisposing factors for EADs. A new type of EADs, called late-phase 3 EADs, has been recently described.[30] Rapid rates of excitation, strong abbreviations of the AP, and intense calcium release from the sarcoplasmic reticulum (SR) were apparently necessary to induce late-phase 3 EADs in the period following rapid pacing and AF termination. Reinitiation of AF was observed after late-phase 3 EADs–induced triggered beats.[25] Although

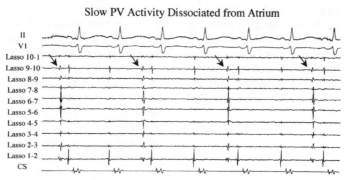

Slow PV Activity Dissociated from Atrium

Fig. 1. Automatic slow pulmonary vein (PV) activity dissociated from the atrium (cycle length 1280 ms) is shown by the arrows. The interval between PV potentials and preceding atrial potentials becomes shorter gradually. II, V1, surface ECG leads II and V1; CS, coronary sinus; Lasso, circular decapolar catheter at the PV ostium. (*Reproduced from* Takahashi Y, Lesaka Y, Takahashi A, et al. Reentrant tachycardia in pulmonary veins of patients with paroxysmal atrial fibrillation. J Cardiovasc Electrophysiol 2003;14:928; with permission.)

EADs may be involved in AF recurrences after termination of paroxysmal AF, their role seems to be very limited in recurrences occurring days or months after AF termination. Likewise, it is difficult to explain their role in AF maintenance.

DADs are the result of intracellular calcium overload. If the cell and the SR are overloaded with Ca^{2+}, then Ca^{2+} waves appear during diastole. These waves activate the electrogenic sodium calcium exchanger and thereby produce DADs. Ischemia, low extracellular K^+, and toxic concentrations of digitalis or catecholamines are all associated with DADs. There is also a rate dependence of the DADs, so it is possible to increase the number of DADs, thus increasing the stimulation rate and burst duration.[31]

Demonstration of triggered activity either initiating or sustaining AF in human electrophysiological studies has been difficult. The few data available come from studies in which the ectopic discharges are confined to their site of initiation after isolation of the PVs or coronary sinus (CS).[32,33] In those cases, pharmacologic and stimulation strategies suggest triggered activity inside the PVs or CS, but it has not been possible to completely rule out microeentrant activity. Induction of EADs was shown to lead to polymorphic atrial tachycardia and AF in anesthetized dogs (**Fig. 2**).[34] In isolated PVs from healthy dogs and dogs with chronic rapid atrial pacing it was possible to identify EADs leading to bursts of high-frequency irregular rhythms.[26] This effect was increased by isoproterenol and was significantly higher in the chronic group.[26]

In stretch-induced AF in Langendorff-perfused sheep hearts, afterdepolarization-induced focal discharges from the PV appear to affect the dynamics by destabilizing the rotors and generating wavebreaks and new rotors. This effect is more evident after adrenergic and cholinergic stimulation with isoproterenol and acetylcholine (ACh), and it is dramatically reduced after reducing intracellular Ca^{2+} overload–related triggered activity with ryanodine or caffeine.[35] The persistence of AF after reducing intracellular calcium overload in almost all cases suggests that the reentrant sources are the main mechanism that sustains the AF.[35]

Reentry

Anatomic reentry, also known as circus movement reentry, may be defined as the circulation of the cardiac impulse around a fixed obstacle, leading to repetitive excitation of the heart at a frequency that depends on the conduction velocity, the duration of the refractory period, and the perimeter of the obstacle. The reentry circuit has an excitable gap, which separates the front of the impulse from its own refractory tail. The basic principles of conditions for anatomic or circus movement reentry are the following: (1) a well-defined anatomic circuit; (2) the wavelength (conduction velocity times refractory period) of the circulating impulse needs to be shorter than the length of the circuit; (3) the initiation of the reentry requires unidirectional block and the presence of slow conduction in part of the circuit; (4) reentrant activity may be stopped by any factor that interrupts the circuit. Similarly, it is possible to reinduce the reentry by means to the application of premature stimuli or by the use of pharmacologic, physiologic, or physical conditions that create unidirectional block.

Although these principles of anatomic reentry may apply to some types of cardiac arrhythmias such as the classic AV nodal reciprocating tachycardias, a different type of reentrant mechanism is responsible for more complex arrhythmias such as polymorphic ventricular tachycardia (PVT),[36] AF,[37,38] and ventricular fibrillation (VF).[39] Understanding reentry in such cases requires a grasp of the concept that the obstacles around which reentrant activity occurs may also be functional, not requiring a fixed circuit.[40] The essential condition for the initiation of functional reentry is that the wavefront should encounter an area of transient refractoriness, which could lead to wavebreak and curling of the wavefront. At the wavebreak point (also known as the "singularity point," SP) the curvature of the wavefront is so steep that the depolarizing wavefront cannot invade the resting excitable tissue ahead of it (source to sink mismatch). Consequently the SP becomes a pivot around which the rest of the wavefront rotates; in other words, the SP becomes the spinning engine (rotor) that organizes the rest of the reentrant activity. Under these conditions, the wavefront acquires the shape of an involute spiral with increasing convex curvature toward the center of rotation (**Fig. 3**).[41]

Functional reentry can occur in 2 dimensions (2D) or 3 dimensions (3D). In 2D, the wave organized by the rotor is called a spiral wave. However, because the atrial and ventricular walls are formed by multiple layers of electrically coupled muscle cells forming a 3D electrical syncytium, spiral waves may stack on top of each other transmurally from epi- to endocardium to result in a scroll wave, which is the 3D equivalent of the spiral wave. In this case the center of rotation becomes a linear, I-shaped filament. However, 3D scroll waves may be more complex than that because their filaments may also

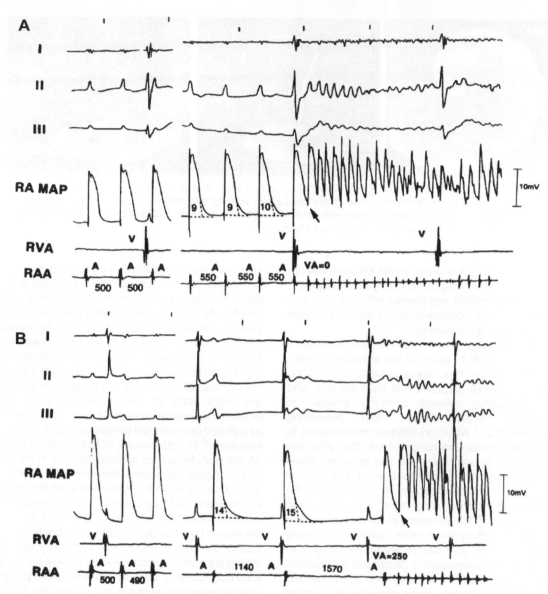

Fig. 2. (*A*) Example of polymorphic atrial tachycardia (P-AT) originating from an early afterdepolarization (EAD: *arrow*) at a normal atrial rate and a ventricular-atrial (VA) interval of zero. (*B*) Example of P-AT initiation in a dog with atrial bradycardia and a VA interval of 250 milliseconds. Numbers in action potentials indicate EAD percentage of total monophasic action potential duration. Control panels are on the left; cesium treatment on the right. RA MAP, right atrial monophasic action potential; RAA, right atrial appendage; RVA, right ventricular apex. (*Reproduced from* Satoh T, Zipes DP. Cesium-induced atrial tachycardia degenerating into atrial fibrillation in dogs: atrial torsades de pointes? J Cardiovasc Electrophysiol 1998;9:973; with permission.)

acquire more complex nonlinear shapes (eg, L-shape, U-shape, O-shape).[42] As such, more often than not the 3D structure of the myocardium makes it very difficult to identify the rotors (scroll waves) responsible for the arrhythmia. In the vast majority of circumstances, one can only observe indirect signs of the complex 3D activity on the epicardial or endocardial surface.[43] Moreover, rotors and scroll waves may be stationary or

they may meander or drift, in which case the pattern of the arrhythmia will be even more complex.

The use of spectral analysis of high-resolution optical mapping data has enabled the identification of discrete sites of high-frequency periodic activity during AF, along with frequency gradients between left and right atria.[44] Spectral analysis has generated strong support for the hypothesis

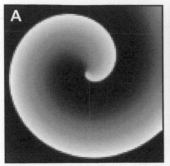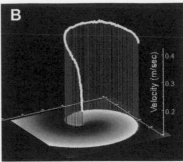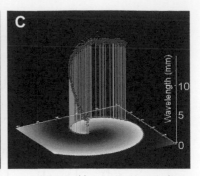

Fig. 3. A rotor and its properties. (*A*) Computational simulation of spiral waves originated by a rotor in a 2-dimensional structure. (*B*) Progressive decrease of the conduction velocity (CV) due to the steeper convex curvature toward the tip of the wave front. (*C*) Progressive decrease of the wavelength (WL) toward the center of rotation (core). The shortest wavelength is localized near the core.

that fast reentrant sources on the left atrial wall are the drivers that support the arrhythmia (**Fig. 4**).[44] The rotors can drift and interact with new anatomic and functional obstacles, giving rise to wavelets and fibrillatory conduction.[45]

An initial step toward understanding the role of reentry in AF is to examine the anatomic characteristics of the PVs. Some patients with paroxysmal AF have ectopic beats from the PVs, and radiofrequency ablation is highly effective in restoring sinus rhythm and preventing recurrences.[11] Although different mechanisms to generate focal discharges from the PVs are described above, reentry is the most accepted mechanism.[27] The architecture of the PVs is complex in that the pattern of orientation of the muscle fiber bundles is highly nonuniform and anisotropic.[46] The presence of fibrosis makes the reentrant activity even more complex and easily inducible.[47] In dog hearts, areas with very slow conduction, progressively decreased conduction, and conduction block have been demonstrated in the PVs. In the same experiments, optical mapping allowed the identification of reentrant activity in the PV samples after extrastimuli and isoproterenol.[48] Data from patients who underwent a PV isolation procedure for AF also support the reentry mechanism in the PVs. Using a rapid stimulation protocol, investigators were able to induce sustained tachycardia inside the isolated PVs in up to 2.6% of cases. Entrainment and termination by burst pacing were also possible. Decremental conduction properties and short refractory periods were observed in all the veins with inducible sustained PV tachycardia in up to 26.4% of patients.[27] Therefore, there is general agreement that a reentrant mechanism inside the PVs is often involved in clinical AF.[27,43]

Experimental studies have demonstrated that high-frequency reentrant sources (rotors) in the

atria manifest as localized areas of organization. The region with the fastest rotors activates at the highest frequency and drives the overall arrhythmia (see **Fig. 4**). The waves emanating from such rotors interact with either functional or anatomic obstacles in their path, resulting in the phenomenon of fibrillatory conduction.[49] As shown by experiments using a model of ACh-induced AF in isolated sheep hearts, the heterogeneous distribution in the left and right atria of ACh-activated potassium (K,ACh) channels results a left to right DF gradient, as well as a dominant left to right propagation of the impulses.[37] In other words, in this model of acute AF the high-frequency sources localize in the left atrium. Additional studies demonstrated that the gradual decrease in AF frequency from the left to the right atria and the pattern of fibrillatory conduction can be easily explained by the breakdown of the waves traveling rightward across Bachmann's bundle and the inferoposterior pathway (CS).[45] In strong support of the above idea, optical mapping data from isolated, coronary-perfused sheep right atrial preparations showed that pacing the Bachmann bundle at rates higher than a critical rate (breakdown frequency) increases the complexity and decreases the organization of wave propagation, in a manner resembling fibrillatory conduction.[45] A different model in which the intraatrial pressure is increased to produce stretch and induce AF in isolated Langendorff-perfused sheep hearts showed that AF is maintained by rapidly activating sources at the junction between the superior PVs and posterior left atrium. In 3 of 9 cases the sources were identified as rotors in the PV junction.[38]

A similar hierarchical organization in the rate of activation of different regions in the atria has also been demonstrated in patients with AF. In paroxysmal AF, DF analysis showed a left to right frequency gradient and demonstrated that the

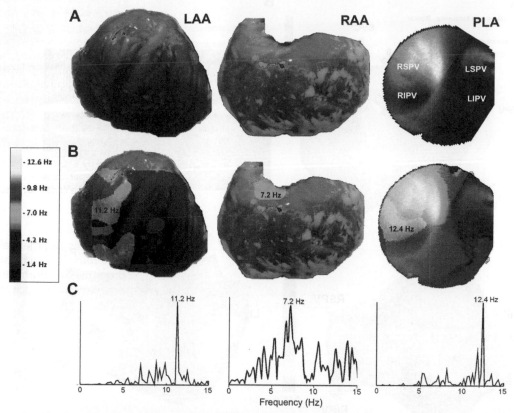

Fig. 4. Identification of the regions with the highest frequency periodic activity during acute stretch–induced atrial fibrillation in a Langendorff-perfused isolated sheep heart. (*A*) Anatomic view of the left atrial appendage (LAA), right atrial appendage (RAA), and posterior left atrium (PLA). PLA shows the endoscopic view of the mapped region with the 4 pulmonary veins (PVs). (*B*) Frequency maps obtained by optical mapping on the LAA and PLA. Frequency value in the RAA was obtained from bipolar electrograms. The highest frequency region is located in the PLA. (*C*) Spectral analysis, in which the maximum dominant frequency corresponds with the PLA region in the right PVs. LIPV, left inferior pulmonary vein; LSPV, left superior pulmonary vein; RIPV, right inferior pulmonary vein; RSPV, right superior pulmonary vein.

PVs and posterior left atrium junction are the most common regions harboring the high-frequency sources.[50,51] Ablation of such sites terminated paroxysmal AF in a high percentage of cases.[52] The arrhythmogenic mechanisms of such high-frequency sources might be focal or automatic. However, the fact that adenosine increases the frequency at sites that activate at the highest rate at baseline supports the reentrant mechanism of AF maintenance.[29]

In persistent and permanent AF, the role of the PVs becomes less prevalent in terms of harboring the highest DF sources (**Fig. 5**).[52] Thus, in patients with persistent and permanent AF many of the so-called high-frequency drivers tend to localize in either or both atria, rather than the PVs.[52] Epicardial mapping of the atria of some patients with chronic AF who underwent open cardiac surgery identified areas of the atria that were activated at

remarkable regular intervals with relatively short cycle lengths (CLs).[53] The electrograms recorded at those sites showed a highly organized and monomorphic beat-to-beat morphology. The rest of the mapped areas showed irregular activation and CLs longer than in the regular area. In most of the cases the most regular and fastest pattern was localized at the left atrium.[53] The limited mapping area might help explain why in some other cases it was not possible to identify the regular and fast area. Although only 9 patients were studied, the results suggested the presence of reentrant sources in patients with chronic AF.

It is interesting that in patients with paroxysmal and persistent AF undergoing an ablation procedure, abolition of the left to right frequency gradient is a long-term predictor of sinus rhythm maintenance.[51] In patients with persistent AF it was necessary to ablate extrapulmonary vein

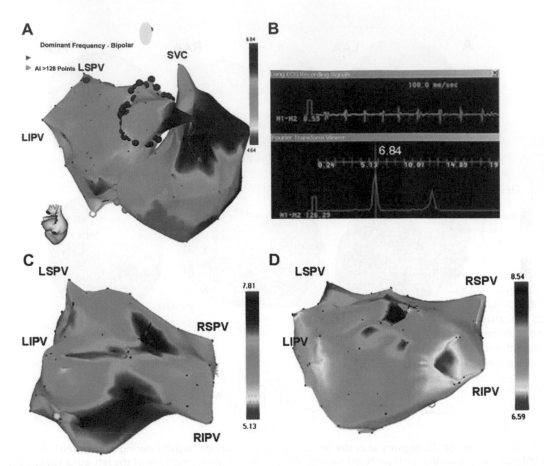

Fig. 5. Dominant frequency (DF) maps in paroxysmal (*A*) and persistent AF (*C, D*). (*A*) Real-time atrial DF map (posterior view; CARTO system) in a paroxysmal AF patient. Purple, primary DF$_{max}$ site (*red arrow*) on right intermediate pulmonary vein (RIPV). Red dots, circumferential ablation line. (*B*) Bipolar recording (*top*) of primary DF$_{max}$ site and its power spectrum (*bottom*) before ablation. (*C, D*) DF maps in a persistent AF patient (left atria [LA] posterior view). (*C*) Before index ablation. (*D*) Before repeat procedure. Purple, primary DF site on the LA posterior wall. Note close correlation between both maps regarding primary DF site location (posterior LA wall) and maximal DF values at primary DF site. (*Modified from* Atienza F, Almendral J, Jalife J, et al. Real-time dominant frequency mapping and ablation of dominant frequency sites in atrial fibrillation with left-to-right frequency gradients predicts long-term maintenance of sinus rhythm. Heart Rhythm 2009;6:34, 37; with permission.)

sites, because half of the DF$_{max}$ locations were outside the PVs[51] (see **Fig. 5**). The data support reentrant activity sustaining AF, and in cases with persistent AF those sources are more often localized outside the PVs.

THEORIES FOR ATRIAL FIBRILLATION. ASSEMBLING THE ATRIAL PUZZLE

AF has been a reason for discussion and continuing investigation since the turn of the twentieth century. The development of the ECG allowed the first striking questions about the origin of new recording rhythms compatible with AF. In the first half of the last century, 2 theories based

on variations of circus movement and ectopic foci were the prevalent scientific explanations for AF.[54] Although initially Sir Thomas Lewis accepted the idea originally proposed by Theodor Engelmann in 1885, and subsequently developed by Heinrich Winterberg (1906) that AF was caused by the synchronous activity of multiple heterotypic foci, it was Carl Rothberger with Winterberg who proposed the idea of "tachysystole," which attributed AF to the extremely rapid discharge rate of an ectopic focus. However, after the theoretical description and experimental demonstration by Mines (1913) and by Garrey (1914) of the circus movement reentry, Lewis adopted such a theory in his description of AF.[55,56] He used it as the basic for his proposal of a single circuit generating fibrillatory activity.

Reentry around an anatomic obstacle could explain either flutter or AF, depending on the size and the refractory period of the circuit. Thus, in the case of a small circuit and a refractory period briefer than in the surrounding atria, the propagation of the waves to the atria would not be uniform, leading to AF in the rest of the atria.[56] According to this theory, elimination of the reentry would terminate the AF.

The focal ectopic focus theory was subsequently revived by Scherf's experiments in the dog in the 1940s.[57] Scherf administered small aconitine crystals to the epicardium of the right atrial appendage, which triggered spontaneous electrical discharges at exceedingly rapid rates. In most cases, the rate of the tachycardia increased to such an extent that it became AF. The isolation of the appendage from the rest of the atria terminated the arrhythmia.[57]

The aforementioned two theories, that is, circus movement and ectopic focal AF, have important limitations, particularly when one attempts to use either one of them to explain persistent or permanent AF. It is difficult to envision any condition in which either mechanism can sustain for months or even years. Thus, by the end of the 1950s, Moe and Abildskov[58] developed a new theory based on the idea that fibrillation can exist as a stable state, which can be self-sustained and independent of its initiating agency. In anesthetized dogs they showed that AF was self-perpetuating as long as the vagus was stimulated. The vagal stimulus would create a nonuniform distribution of the refractory periods. The latter, along with a large enough atrial mass and slow conduction velocity, would favor the perpetuation of the arrhythmia by permitting the coexistence of multiple independent, randomly wandering wavelets.[58] A computer model developed by the same investigators showed that the minimum number of wavelets required to perpetuate the arrhythmia was between 23 and 40.[59] Their studies gave rise to the multiple wavelet hypothesis, which was later on supported by experiments in dogs done by Allessie and coleagues.[60] This group mapped the spread of excitation in the atria during rapid pacing–induced AF in the presence of ACh. The study demonstrated multiple propagating wavelets giving rise to turbulent atrial activity. In those experiments, the number of wavelets required to sustain the arrhythmia was estimated to be between 4 and 6, which was somewhat puzzling given the large number of wavelets previously theorized by Moe and Abildskov. Nevertheless, additional support for the

theory came from animal and human mapping studies, especially after the observation that some cases of chronic AF could be successfully treated with the surgical MAZE procedure, in which the compartmentalization of the atria would create independent regions unable to sustain the multiple wavelets.[61]

In recent years, computer modeling together with the use of voltage-sensitive probes and high-resolution video imaging to record electrical wave propagation on the surface of isolated hearts began to question the validity of the multiple wavelet theory. High spatial (on the order of micrometers) and temporal resolution recordings during fibrillation demonstrated that the turbulent electrical activity in the ECG could be explained by a single or a small number of rapidly spinning rotors.[44,62] The rotor forces the excitation wave to rotate around a pivot point. The spiral waves and scroll waves emitted by the rotor propagate through the cardiac muscle and interact with anatomic and functional obstacles, leading to fragmentation and new wavelet formation. This explanation is incompatible with the multiple wavelet theory, which requires as a condition that the wavelets wander randomly throughout the atria in a manner resembling the Brownian motion of particles in water. Randomness implies that, while at any given point in time the frequency of activation may differ in different parts of the atria, statistically the frequency should be the same everywhere; this is not what happens in AF, in which frequency of activation is hierarchical in both experimental animals and humans. Unfortunately, it is currently not possible to observe the filaments or the scroll waves propagating through the 3D atrial muscle, due to technical limitations. However, high-resolution spectral analysis makes it possible to identify the regions of periodic activity. The highest frequency sites suggest the presence of organized reentrant sources (rotors), and in many cases the domains harboring the higher frequencies are localized in the left atrium (see **Figs. 4** and **5**), and occasionally it is possible to identify a long-persistent rotor in the highest frequency domain.[35,38,44] Indeed, rotors and spiral waves, whether electrical or chemical, have the tendency to be remarkably stable.[42]

In the left atrium, the posterior wall harbors the fastest spatiotemporally organized activity[49] (see **Figs. 4** and **5**). Further analysis also demonstrates that waves generated by stable rotors in the left atrium undergo complex, spatially distributed conduction block patterns as they head toward the right atrium, manifesting as fibrillatory conduction.[45] The outer limit of the DF_{max} domain is the area where the most fractionated activity surrounds the most regular activity.[49] Therefore, left to right dominant frequency gradients during AF may not be explained by the multiple wavelet theory. In fact, given the new evidence, the authors are almost certain that should Gordon Moe be alive today he would agree.

Recently, data published in patients with long persistent AF who underwent a stepwise ablation procedure support the role of high-frequency sources in long-lasting persistent AF.[63] Ablation was performed in the right atrium after all left atrial AF sources had been ablated and a right to left atrial gradient existed. In 55% of cases with persistent right to left frequency gradient the AF terminated on right atrial ablation. Of note, those patients with right to left frequency gradient after left atrial ablation had a longer AF history and a larger right atrial diameter.[63] It is reasonable to speculate that continuous high frequency and heterogeneous bombardment with fibrillatory waves during long-lasting AF produced electrical remodeling substantial enough to spread the likelihood of new sources and rotors to appear in either atria outside the PVs. This proposal would also explain the lower success rate after ablation of the left atrial sources, raising secondary rotors in the right atrium.

Computer simulations also support the rotor theory[39]; however, the computational model by Moe and colleagues[59] was based on random distribution of the refractory periods, in such a way that closely apposed cardiac cells could have widely different refractory periods. Such an assumption is not compatible with current knowledge in cardiac cellular electrophysiology, whereby electrical intercellular connections tend to minimize any difference at the microscopic level and to create gradients of refractory period across tissues.[64]

IONIC MECHANISMS INVOLVED IN THE MODULATION OF ROTOR DYNAMICS

Although not universally accepted, rotor theory has become an important mechanistic explanation for AF. The authors submit that understanding the dynamics of rotors will allow more specific strategies to stop them and prevent their de novo formation, and thus prevent AF. The initial step in the initiation of a rotor is a wavebreak after the interaction of a wavefront with a functional or anatomic obstacle. This process may occur in a totally homogeneous medium with the only condition of a transient heterogeneity in the system, which can be simulated with an S1-S2 protocol. The S1 wave is followed by a second wave (S2) perpendicular to S1. If S2 is initiated before the repolarizing tail of S1 has disappeared, S1 acts as a barrier for S2 propagation at the intersection point, resulting in a rotating spiral wave.[65] Under certain conditions of excitability, the presence of an anatomic or functional obstacle with sharp edges may destabilize the propagation of electrical waves, giving rise to the formation of self-sustained vortices and turbulent cardiac electrical activity.[66,67] Both situations may initiate high-frequency reentrant sources in the heart and give rise to new reentrant sources and wave fragmentation.

The propagation velocity of a wavefront depends on its curvature, in such a way that waves whose fronts are concave propagate faster than planar waves, and the latter move faster than convex waves.[68] As illustrated in **Fig. 3**A and B, the wavefronts of the spiral waves emitted by a rotor have an increasingly steeper convex curvature, which results in a progressive decrease of the conduction velocity (CV) toward the center of rotation (ie, the core). At the perimeter of the core the curvature reaches a critical value, leading to a mismatch between the depolarizing current supplied by the wavefront and the electrotonic current required to depolarize the resting cells inside the core. Thus, the powerful electrotonic effect exerted by the core shortens the AP duration (APD) in its vicinity.[69] Consequently, the shortest wavelength (WL = CV × APD) will be near the core (see **Fig. 3**C).

Whereas I_{Na} is the main component of the depolarizing current at the wavefront, I_{K1} is crucial for control of the cardiac excitability and the frequency and stability of rotors.[39] I_{K1} plays an important role controlling the electrotonic gradient between the resting cells in the core and the active cells at its immediate periphery. The crucial role of the interplay between I_{k1} and I_{Na} in controlling rotor frequency and stability became evident in experiments conducted by Noujaim and colleagues[70] using an I_{K1} overexpressing mouse model. I_{K1} up-regulation accelerated the final phase of the AP repolarization and induced membrane hyperpolarization during diastole. During reentry the overexpression translated into a shorter WL and greater Na channel availability, increasing the excitability ahead of the rotating wavefront. I_{k1} overexpression increased the voltage gradient in between the active cells surrounding the core and the resting cells inside the core. The latter contributed to enhancement of the electrotonic currents flowing between the resting and active cells, which further accelerated the repolarization of the active cells and reduced the CV in the vicinity of the core.[70] Likewise, the nonexcited cells in the center of the core provided a larger outward conductance than normal, which further decreased the probability of the cells being excited by the surrounding actively depolarized cells, helping to reduce both the core size and meandering. Finally, during fibrillation, faster and more stable ventricular rotors were present in the I_{K1} overexpressing mouse heart.[70]

The ACh-sensitive potassium current ($I_{K,ACh}$) plays an important role in experimental AF as well as in some patients.[29] $I_{K,ACh}$ hyperpolarizes the cell membrane, and abbreviates the APD and refractory period, increasing the frequency of the reentrant sources and the resting membrane conductance.[29] ACh produces a dose-dependent increase in AF frequency (**Fig. 6**). The higher the ACh concentration, the higher is the rotor frequency and the more complex the fibrillatory patterns.[71] The current displays larger density in the left atrium than in the right atrium, which is related to heterogeneous distribution of both vagal innervation and muscarinic receptors, as well as K,ACh channels. Both muscarinic receptors and

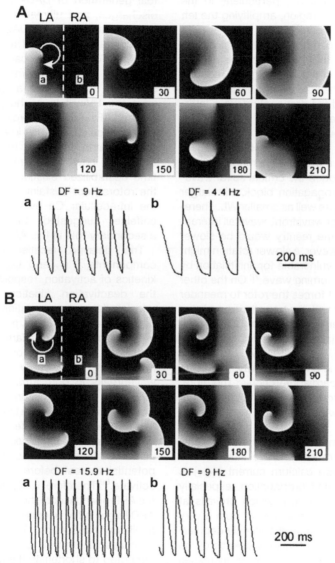

Fig. 6. Computer simulations in a 2-dimensional sheet of paroxysmal AF at baseline (*A*) and peak $I_{K,ACh}$ effect (*B*). For each snapshot, stable reentry in the left half of the sheet acted as the high-frequency source of fibrillatory waves in the LA (*a*) that propagated toward the RA (*b*) in the right part of the sheet. At baseline (*A*), LA DF (*a*; 9 Hz) is higher than RA DF (*b*; 4.4 Hz); left-to right gradient is 4.6 Hz. At peak adenosine effect (*B*), DFs in the LA (*a*) is 15.9 Hz and in the RA (*b*) is 9 Hz; the left-to-right gradient is 6.9 Hz. Numbers in frames indicate relative time in milliseconds. (*Reproduced from* Atienza F, Almendral J, Moreno J, et al. Activation of inward rectifier potassium channels accelerates atrial fibrillation in humans: evidence for a reentrant mechanism. Circulation 2006;114:2439; with permission.)

K,ACh channels are more abundant in the left atrium than the right atrium.[71] Progressively increasing the ACh concentration in isolated Langendorff-perfused hearts increases progressively the frequency of the rotors and the number of rotations, with a greater effect in the left than the right atrium. In addition, the augmented heterogeneity in activation frequency increases the likelihood for wavebreak and the complexity of the fibrillatory patterns.[71] In humans with paroxysmal AF, activation of $I_{K,ACh}$ ($I_{K,Ado}$) channels by adenosine increases the local DF, particularly in the PVs-left atrium junction region, amplifying the left to right frequency gradient.[29]

In a simpler scenario, reducing the excitability by decreasing I_{Na} leads to smaller upstroke velocity (dVdt) and amplitude of the AP along with reduced APD, CV, and WL. When the excitability is reduced to a critical point and the propagating wave interacts with a functional or anatomic obstacle, the wavefront may break, curl, and initiate self-sustained reentry.[66] Na channel blockade will affect reentry in such a way that the reduced excitability will tend to reduce the critical spiral wavefront curvature for propagation block, with larger path length and core, as well as smaller WL. Therefore, the probability for wavefront-wavetail interaction decreases and the reentry would be slower and more stable. However, a slower rotation might make the rotor more vulnerable for annihilation by interacting with an incoming wave.[72] On the other hand, a substrate that forces the rotor to meander may favor interaction with the boundaries and also lead to eventual termination.[72] In this regard, although class IC antiarrhythmics effectively terminate recent-onset AF, their well-known proarrhythmic action leads to increased mortality in patients with a history of myocardial infarction.[73] Therefore, the ventricular substrate after an infarction might increase the risk of wavebreak and reentry on Na channel blockade.

The duration and morphology of the AP is highly dependent on the transmembrane influx of the Ca^{2+} ions. The L-type calcium current (I_{Ca-L}) is necessary for sustained propagation, especially during very slow conduction, which prevails at the core of a spiral wave because of both a very steep wavefront curvature and a slightly depolarized resting membrane potential. Blockade of the L-type calcium channel by verapamil increases the size of the core, and decreases the rotor frequency and the degree of fragmentation of the excitation wavefronts.[74] In one clinical study, patients with persistent AF and at least 7 days under treatment with verapamil were assessed by frequency analysis from surface ECG recordings. The fibrillatory frequency was significantly lower in those patients treated with the drug as compared with controls.[75] Although the study was not randomized, the known electrophysiological effects of I_{Ca-L} blockade along with other small published series[76] support the results.

Alterations in intracellular Ca^{2+} kinetics are intimately related to the development of DADs. For example, during high-frequency pacing or during treatment with digoxin, the intracellular Ca^{2+} increases, leading to a higher propensity for spontaneous calcium release from the SR and to eventual generation of DADs that trigger premature discharges, and ultimately result in wavebreaks and fibrillation.[77] In VF, DADs are thought to play a secondary role behind reentry.[77] On the other hand, in AF a few clinical cases have been reported in which the most likely mechanism sustaining the arrhythmia was triggered activity from the PVs.[28] In a sheep model of stretch-induced AF under adrenergic and cholinergic stimulation, focal discharges identified in the optically mapped atria enhanced the likelihood of wavebreak and new rotor formation, but at the same time destabilized existing rotors.[35] The fact that the rotors kept sustaining the AF after reducing the intracellular Ca overload with ryanodine or caffeine suggested that DADs also play a secondary role in this AF model.[35]

The delayed rectifier current (I_K) has 2 components,[78] I_{Kr} and I_{Ks}, with fast and slow kinetics of activation, respectively. In both cases, the deactivation kinetics show considerable species-dependent variation.[79] The combination of slow deactivation of I_{Kr} and I_{Ks} helps explain the mechanism of post-repolarization refractoriness.[80] Therefore, the presence of spatial heterogeneities in I_K density would easily explain the formation of wavebreaks in both atria and ventricles. During functional reentry, uniform I_K reduction should increase the APD more in the periphery than closer to the center of rotation. Near the center, repolarization occurs prematurely because of the electrotonic influence of the core, which returns the membrane potential to rest before I_K has enough time to activate.[69] Therefore, I_K blockade should not affect the APD near the core; however, it should make the APD larger in the periphery of the rotor, resulting in fibrillatory conduction. Of note, gain of function of I_{Ks} is associated with familial AF, which has been attributed to shortening the atrial APD and ERP.[81] In well-controlled optically mapping experiment, adenovirally mediated upregulation of I_{Ks} in neonatal rat ventricular monolayers showed rotors with higher rotation frequencies, lower CV, and shorter APD than controls. However, despite the shorter APD, multiple wavebreaks leading to fibrillatory conduction occurred in 46% of the reentry episodes in the I_{Ks}-overexpressing monolayers but in none of the controls.[80] Computer simulations demonstrated that spatially inhomogeneous I_{Ks} recovery kinetics during diastole may be sufficient to allow the formation of wavebreaks leading to reentry.[80] It is noteworthy that although the monolayer data cannot be directly extrapolated to the human situation, the results do allow the speculation that the most likely mechanism leading to fibrillation in the familial cases of I_{Ks} gain of function[81] is post-repolarization refractoriness, leading to multiple wavebreaks and fibrillatory conduction.

The ultra-rapid delayed rectifier current (I_{Kur}) is an important player in atrial repolarization.[82] The current is absent in the ventricles, which makes it a target for new antiarrhythmic therapy in AF.[83] In isolated human atrial myocytes, I_{Kur} shows relatively slow recovery from inactivation at diastolic potentials, as well as significant frequency dependence at physiologic temperatures.[84] The rate-dependence decrease in I_{Kur} may tend to result in longer APD during tachycardia than if I_{Kur} was rate-independent. Thus, the I_{Kur} properties might be protective against reentrant arrhythmia. However, the results are controversial with regard to the use of I_{Kur} blockade to terminate AF, with some data suggesting proarrhythmic effects due to abbreviation of the ventricular APD_{90} and ERP in healthy dogs.[85]

In human atrial cells, the transient outward current (I_{To}) activates in the plateau range of membrane potential and is responsible for the transient repolarization during phase 1 of the AP. I_{To} recovery from inactivation is slow, leading to smaller amplitude at fast rates and AP prolongation. In isolated rabbit ventricular cells, I_{To} plays a key role in the mechanism of Wenckebach rhythms.[86] The latter might play an important role in the boundaries between frequency domains, favoring fibrillatory conduction. Studies in goats 48 hours after AF-induced electrical remodeling have shown that AF terminates in a dose-dependent manner after I_{Kur}/I_{To} blockade, as a result of prolongation of the atrial ERP and WL.[87] The effect was stronger than that produced by I_{Kr} blockade with dofetilide, which could be explained by a larger contribution of I_{Kur} and I_{To} to atrial repolarization in the electrically remodeled atria. Although AF leads to downregulation of I_{Kur}, I_{To}, and I_{Ca-L}, a greater reduction of I_{Ca-L} might explain the postulated larger contribution of I_{Kur} and I_{To}.

SUMMARY

This article presents a brief and necessarily incomplete discussion on various clinically relevant aspects of AF. The first part addresses the epidemiology of the arrhythmia, its importance in the general population, and the limitations of currently available pharmacologic and invasive therapeutic strategies. Such interventions often cause side effects, due to lack of specificity and mechanical complications. Attention is also paid to the current classification of AF and how its duration and temporal pattern influences the therapeutic strategy in terms of cardioversion and anticoagulation. The second part focuses on the arrhythmogenic mechanisms that have been proposed to underlie AF, including variants of reentry and focal discharge. Each mechanism is discussed individually and is linked to the current evidence in experimental and human AF, in an effort to provide hypotheses covering the wide range between paroxysmal and permanent AF. Finally, the third part briefly reviews the ionic bases underlying rotor dynamics, which nowadays is gaining support as a relevant mechanistic theory for AF and may be helpful in the development of new, safer, and more effective antiarrhythmic strategies.

In short, we may conclude that AF is still a huge challenge for basic scientists and clinicians alike. Achieving an understanding of AF mechanisms and being able to translate basic science findings to human AF will allow us to generate more specific therapies designed to prevent and/or terminate this most interesting, yet difficult to treat arrhythmia. It is likely that new drugs capable of blocking specific atrial ion channels that are essential for the sustainment of rotors will decrease the need for invasive, highly destructive procedures. The hope is that AF prevention/termination and long-term maintenance of sinus rhythm using conservative next-generation pharmacologic approaches will significantly improve the quality of life of patients and even decrease the need for anticoagulation.

ACKNOWLEDGMENTS

The authors thank Dr Sergey Mironov for his help in the illustration of conduction velocity and wavelength (see **Fig. 3**) and Dr Steven R. Ennis for his help in some of the experiments (see **Fig. 4**).

REFERENCES

1. Kannel WB, Wolf PA, Benjamin EJ, et al. Prevalence, incidence, prognosis, and predisposing conditions for atrial fibrillation: population-based estimates. Am J Cardiol 1998;82:2N–9N.

2. Wolf PA, Abbott RD, Kannel WB. Atrial fibrillation as an independent risk factor for stroke: the Framingham Study. Stroke 1991;22:983–8.

3. Thrall G, Lane D, Carroll D, et al. Quality of life in patients with atrial fibrillation: a systematic review. Am J Med 2006;119:448.e1–448.e19.

4. Go AS, Hylek EM, Phillips KA, et al. Prevalence of diagnosed atrial fibrillation in adults: national implications for rhythm management and stroke prevention: the AnTicoagulation and Risk Factors in Atrial Fibrillation (ATRIA) Study. JAMA 2001;285:2370–5.

5. Miyasaka Y, Barnes ME, Gersh BJ, et al. Secular trends in incidence of atrial fibrillation in Olmsted County, Minnesota, 1980 to 2000, and implications on the projections for future prevalence. Circulation 2006;114:119–25.

6. Coyne KS, Paramore C, Grandy S, et al. Assessing the direct costs of treating nonvalvular atrial fibrillation in the United States. Value Health 2006;9:348–56.

7. Hohnloser SH, Crijns HJ, van Eickels M, et al. Effect of dronedarone on cardiovascular events in atrial fibrillation. N Engl J Med 2009;360:668–78.

8. Zimetbaum P, Reynolds MR, Ho KK, et al. Impact of a practice guideline for patients with atrial fibrillation on medical resource utilization and costs. Am J Cardiol 2003;92:677–81.

9. Lafuente-Lafuente C, Mouly S, Longas-Tejero MA, et al. Antiarrhythmic drugs for maintaining sinus rhythm after cardioversion of atrial fibrillation: a systematic review of randomized controlled trials. Arch Intern Med 2006;166:719–28.

10. Kober L, Torp-Pedersen C, McMurray JJ, et al. Increased mortality after dronedarone therapy for severe heart failure. N Engl J Med 2008;358:2678–87.

11. Haissaguerre M, Jais P, Shah DC, et al. Spontaneous initiation of atrial fibrillation by ectopic beats originating in the pulmonary veins. N Engl J Med 1998;339:659–66.

12. Cappato R, Calkins H, Chen SA, et al. Worldwide survey on the methods, efficacy, and safety of catheter ablation for human atrial fibrillation. Circulation 2005;111:1100–5.

13. Fuster V, Ryden LE, Cannom DS, et al. ACC/AHA/ESC 2006 guidelines for the management of patients with atrial fibrillation: full text: a report of the American College of Cardiology/American Heart Association Task Force on practice guidelines and the European Society of Cardiology Committee for Practice Guidelines (Writing Committee to Revise the 2001 guidelines for the management of patients with atrial fibrillation) developed in collaboration with the European Heart Rhythm Association and the Heart Rhythm Society. Europace 2006;8:651–745.

14. Jahangir A, Lee V, Friedman PA, et al. Long-term progression and outcomes with aging in patients with lone atrial fibrillation: a 30-year follow-up study. Circulation 2007;115:3050–6.

15. Waktare JE, Hnatkova K, Sopher SM, et al. The role of atrial ectopics in initiating paroxysmal atrial fibrillation. Eur Heart J 2001;22:333–9.

16. Allessie M, Ausma J, Schotten U. Electrical, contractile and structural remodeling during atrial fibrillation. Cardiovasc Res 2002;54:230–46.

17. Morillo CA, Klein GJ, Jones DL, et al. Chronic rapid atrial pacing. Structural, functional, and electrophysiological characteristics of a new model of sustained atrial fibrillation. Circulation 1995;91:1588–95.

18. Wijffels MC, Kirchhof CJ, Dorland R, et al. Atrial fibrillation begets atrial fibrillation. A study in awake chronically instrumented goats. Circulation 1995;92:1954–68.

19. Eijsbouts S, Ausma J, Blaauw Y, et al. Serial cardioversion by class IC Drugs during 4 months of persistent atrial fibrillation in the goat. J Cardiovasc Electrophysiol 2006;17:648–54.

20. Singer DE, Albers GW, Dalen JE, et al. Antithrombotic therapy in atrial fibrillation: the Seventh ACCP Conference on Antithrombotic and Thrombolytic Therapy. Chest 2004;126:429S–56S.

21. Kopecky SL, Gersh BJ, McGoon MD, et al. The natural history of lone atrial fibrillation. A population-based study over three decades. N Engl J Med 1987;317:669–74.

22. Anumonwo J, Jalife J. Cardiac electrophysiology and arrhythmias. In: Fisch C, Surawicz B, editors. Cardiac electrophysiology and arrhythmias. New York: Elsevier; 1991. p. 35–50.

23. Katzung BG, Morgenstern JA. Effects of extracellular potassium on ventricular automaticity and evidence for a pacemaker current in mammalian ventricular myocardium. Circ Res 1977;40:105–11.

24. Ho SY, Cabrera JA, Tran VH, et al. Architecture of the pulmonary veins: relevance to radiofrequency ablation. Heart 2001;86:265–70.

25. Anderson KP, Stinson EB, Mason JW. Surgical exclusion of focal paroxysmal atrial tachycardia. Am J Cardiol 1982;49:869–74.

26. Chen YJ, Chen SA, Chang MS, et al. Arrhythmogenic activity of cardiac muscle in pulmonary veins of the dog: implication for the genesis of atrial fibrillation. Cardiovasc Res 2000;48:265–73.

27. Takahashi Y, Iesaka Y, Takahashi A, et al. Reentrant tachycardia in pulmonary veins of patients with paroxysmal atrial fibrillation. J Cardiovasc Electrophysiol 2003;14:927–32.

28. Chen SA, Hsieh MH, Tai CT, et al. Initiation of atrial fibrillation by ectopic beats originating from the pulmonary veins: electrophysiological characteristics, pharmacological responses, and effects of radiofrequency ablation. Circulation 1999;100:1879–86.

29. Atienza F, Almendral J, Moreno J, et al. Activation of inward rectifier potassium channels accelerates atrial fibrillation in humans: evidence for a reentrant mechanism. Circulation 2006;114:2434–42.

30. Burashnikov A, Antzelevitch C. Reinduction of atrial fibrillation immediately after termination of the

arrhythmia is mediated by late phase 3 early afterdepolarization-induced triggered activity. Circulation 2003;107:2355–60.

31. Fujiwara K, Tanaka H, Mani H, et al. Burst emergence of intracellular Ca^{2+} waves evokes arrhythmogenic oscillatory depolarization via the Na^+-Ca^{2+} exchanger: simultaneous confocal recording of membrane potential and intracellular Ca^{2+} in the heart. Circ Res 2008;103:509–18.

32. Rostock T, O'Neill MD, Takahashi Y, et al. Interactions between two simultaneous tachycardias within an electrically isolated pulmonary vein. J Cardiovasc Electrophysiol 2007;18:441–5.

33. Knecht S, O'Neill MD, Matsuo S, et al. Focal arrhythmia confined within the coronary sinus and maintaining atrial fibrillation. J Cardiovasc Electrophysiol 2007;18:1140–6.

34. Satoh T, Zipes DP. Cesium-induced atrial tachycardia degenerating into atrial fibrillation in dogs: atrial torsades de pointes? J Cardiovasc Electrophysiol 1998;9:970–5.

35. Yamazaki M, Vaquero LM, Hou L, et al. Mechanisms of stretch-induced atrial fibrillation in the presence and the absence of adrenocholinergic stimulation: interplay between rotors and focal discharges. Heart Rhythm 2009;6:1009–17.

36. Cerrone M, Noujaim SF, Tolkacheva EG, et al. Arrhythmogenic mechanisms in a mouse model of catecholaminergic polymorphic ventricular tachycardia. Circ Res 2007;101:1039–48.

37. Mansour M, Mandapati R, Berenfeld O, et al. Left-to-right gradient of atrial frequencies during acute atrial fibrillation in the isolated sheep heart. Circulation 2001;103:2631–6.

38. Kalifa J, Jalife J, Zaitsev AV, et al. Intra-atrial pressure increases rate and organization of waves emanating from the superior pulmonary veins during atrial fibrillation. Circulation 2003;108:668–71.

39. Samie FH, Berenfeld O, Anumonwo J, et al. Rectification of the background potassium current: a determinant of rotor dynamics in ventricular fibrillation. Circ Res 2001;89:1216–23.

40. Allessie MA, Bonke FI, Schopman FJ. Circus movement in rabbit atrial muscle as a mechanism of tachycardia. Circ Res 1973;33:54–62.

41. Jalife J, Berenfeld O. Molecular mechanisms and global dynamics of fibrillation: an integrative approach to the underlying basis of vortex-like reentry. J Theor Biol 2004;230:475–87.

42. Wellner M, Berenfeld O, Jalife J, et al. Minimal principle for rotor filaments. Proc Natl Acad Sci U S A 2002;99:8015–8.

43. Berenfeld O, Mandapati R, Dixit S, et al. Spatially distributed dominant excitation frequencies reveal hidden organization in atrial fibrillation in the Langendorff-perfused sheep heart. J Cardiovasc Electrophysiol 2000;11:869–79.

44. Mandapati R, Skanes A, Chen J, et al. Stable microreentrant sources as a mechanism of atrial fibrillation in the isolated sheep heart. Circulation 2000;101:194–9.

45. Berenfeld O, Zaitsev AV, Mironov SF, et al. Frequency-dependent breakdown of wave propagation into fibrillatory conduction across the pectinate muscle network in the isolated sheep right atrium. Circ Res 2002;90:1173–80.

46. Saito T, Waki K, Becker AE. Left atrial myocardial extension onto pulmonary veins in humans: anatomic observations relevant for atrial arrhythmias. J Cardiovasc Electrophysiol 2000;11:888–94.

47. Spach MS, Josephson ME. Initiating reentry: the role of nonuniform anisotropy in small circuits. J Cardiovasc Electrophysiol 1994;5:182–209.

48. Arora R, Verheule S, Scott L, et al. Arrhythmogenic substrate of the pulmonary veins assessed by high-resolution optical mapping. Circulation 2003;107:1816–21.

49. Kalifa J, Tanaka K, Zaitsev AV, et al. Mechanisms of wave fractionation at boundaries of high-frequency excitation in the posterior left atrium of the isolated sheep heart during atrial fibrillation. Circulation 2006;113:626–33.

50. Lazar S, Dixit S, Marchlinski FE, et al. Presence of left-to-right atrial frequency gradient in paroxysmal but not persistent atrial fibrillation in humans. Circulation 2004;110:3181–6.

51. Atienza F, Almendral J, Jalife J, et al. Real-time dominant frequency mapping and ablation of dominant frequency sites in atrial fibrillation with left-to-right frequency gradients predicts long-term maintenance of sinus rhythm. Heart Rhythm 2009;6:33–40.

52. Sanders P, Berenfeld O, Hocini M, et al. Spectral analysis identifies sites of high-frequency activity maintaining atrial fibrillation in humans. Circulation 2005;112:789–97.

53. Sahadevan J, Ryu K, Peltz L, et al. Epicardial mapping of chronic atrial fibrillation in patients: preliminary observations. Circulation 2004;110:3293–9.

54. Lewis T. The mechanism and graphic registration of the heart beat. 3rd edition. London: Shaw; 1925. p. 319–74.

55. Garrey WE. Auricular fibrillation. Physiol Rev 1924;4:215.

56. Lewis T, Fell HS, Stroud WD. Observations upon flutter and fibrillation. II. The nature of auricular flutter. Heart 1920;7:191–233.

57. Scherf D. Studies on auricular tachycardia caused by aconitine administration. Proc Soc Exp Biol Med 1947;64:233–9.

58. Moe GK, Abildskov JA. Atrial fibrillation as a self-sustaining arrhythmia independent of focal discharge. Am Heart J 1959;58:59–70.

59. Moe GK, Rheinboldt WC, Abildskov JA. A computer model of atrial fibrillation. Am Heart J 1964;67:200–20.

60. Allessie MA, Lammers WE, Bonke FI, et al. Experimental evaluation of Moe's multiple wavelet hypothesis of atrial fibrillation. In: Zipes DP, Jalife J, editors. Cardiac electrophysiology and arrhythmias. Orlando: Grune & Stratton; 1985. p. 265–75.

61. Cox JL. The surgical treatment of atrial fibrillation. IV. Surgical technique. J Thorac Cardiovasc Surg 1991; 101:584–92.

62. Gray RA, Jalife J, Panfilov AV, et al. Mechanisms of cardiac fibrillation. Science 1995;270:1222–3 [author reply: 4–5].

63. Hocini M, Nault I, Wright M, et al. Disparate evolution of right and left atrial rate during ablation of long-lasting persistent atrial fibrillation. J Am Coll Cardiol 2010;55:1007–16.

64. Delmar M, Duffy HS, Soren PL, et al. Molecular organization and regulation of the cardiac gap junction channel connexin43. In: Zipes DP, Jalife J, editors. Cardiac electrophysiology: from cell to bedside. 4th edition. Philadelphia: Saunders; 2004. p. 66–76.

65. Keldermann RH, ten Tusscher KH, Nash MP, et al. A computational study of mother rotor VF in the human ventricles. Am J Physiol Heart Circ Physiol 2009;296:H370–9.

66. Cabo C, Pertsov AM, Davidenko JM, et al. Vortex shedding as a precursor of turbulent electrical activity in cardiac muscle. Biophys J 1996;70: 1105–11.

67. Jalife J, Pandit SV. Ionic mechanisms of wavebreak in fibrillation. Heart Rhythm 2005;2:660–3.

68. Fast VG, Kleber AG. Role of wavefront curvature in propagation of cardiac impulse. Cardiovasc Res 1997;33:258–71.

69. Beaumont J, Davidenko N, Davidenko JM, et al. Spiral waves in two-dimensional models of ventricular muscle: formation of a stationary core. Biophys J 1998;75:1–14.

70. Noujaim SF, Pandit SV, Berenfeld O, et al. Up-regulation of the inward rectifier K^+ current (I K1) in the mouse heart accelerates and stabilizes rotors. J Physiol 2007;578:315–26.

71. Sarmast F, Kolli A, Zaitsev A, et al. Cholinergic atrial fibrillation: I(K, ACh) gradients determine unequal left/right atrial frequencies and rotor dynamics. Cardiovasc Res 2003;59:863–73.

72. Kneller J, Kalifa J, Zou R, et al. Mechanisms of atrial fibrillation termination by pure sodium channel blockade in an ionically-realistic mathematical model. Circ Res 2005;96:e35–47.

73. Preliminary report: effect of encainide and flecainide on mortality in a randomized trial of arrhythmia suppression after myocardial infarction. The Cardiac Arrhythmia Suppression Trial (CAST) Investigators. N Engl J Med 1989;321:406–12.

74. Samie FH, Mandapati R, Gray RA, et al. A mechanism of transition from ventricular fibrillation to tachycardia: effect of calcium channel blockade on the dynamics of rotating waves. Circ Res 2000; 86:684–91.

75. Bollmann A, Sonne K, Esperer HD, et al. Patients with persistent atrial fibrillation taking oral verapamil exhibit a lower atrial frequency on the ECG. Ann Noninvasive Electrocardiol 2002;7:92–7.

76. Meurling CJ, Ingemansson MP, Roijer A, et al. Attenuation of electrical remodelling in chronic atrial fibrillation following oral treatment with verapamil. Europace 1999;1:234–41.

77. Lakireddy V, Bub G, Baweja P, et al. The kinetics of spontaneous calcium oscillations and arrhythmogenesis in the in vivo heart during ischemia/reperfusion. Heart Rhythm 2006;3:58–66.

78. Wang Z, Fermini B, Nattel S. Delayed rectifier outward current and repolarization in human atrial myocytes. Circ Res 1993;73:276–85.

79. Cheng JH, Kodama I. Two components of delayed rectifier K^+ current in heart: molecular basis, functional diversity, and contribution to repolarization. Acta Pharmacol Sin 2004;25:137–45.

80. Munoz V, Grzeda KR, Desplantez T, et al. Adenoviral expression of IKs contributes to wavebreak and fibrillatory conduction in neonatal rat ventricular cardiomyocyte monolayers. Circ Res 2007;101:475–83.

81. Chen YH, Xu SJ, Bendahhou S, et al. KCNQ1 gain-of-function mutation in familial atrial fibrillation. Science 2003;299:251–4.

82. Firek L, Giles WR. Outward currents underlying repolarization in human atrial myocytes. Cardiovasc Res 1995;30:31–8.

83. Ehrlich JR, Nattel S. Novel approaches for pharmacological management of atrial fibrillation. Drugs 2009;69:757–74.

84. Feng J, Xu D, Wang Z, et al. Ultrarapid delayed rectifier current inactivation in human atrial myocytes: properties and consequences. Am J Physiol 1998;275:H1717–25.

85. Burashnikov A, Antzelevitch C. Can inhibition of IKur promote atrial fibrillation? Heart Rhythm 2008;5: 1304–9.

86. Yehia AR, Shrier A, Lo KC, et al. Transient outward current contributes to Wenckebach-like rhythms in isolated rabbit ventricular cells. Am J Physiol 1997; 273:H1–11.

87. Blaauw Y, Gogelein H, Tieleman RG, et al. "Early" class III drugs for the treatment of atrial fibrillation: efficacy and atrial selectivity of AVE0118 in remodeled atria of the goat. Circulation 2004;110:1717–24.

Advances in the Pharmacologic Management of Atrial Fibrillation

Alexander Burashnikov, PhD, FHRS,
Charles Antzelevitch, PhD, FHRS*

KEYWORDS
- Atrial fibrillation • Antiarrhythmic drugs • Cardiac arrhythmia
- Electrophysiology • Pharmacology

Atrial fibrillation (AF) is a growing clinical problem associated with increased morbidity and mortality. The rising prevalence of AF is largely due to the increase in the aging sector of the population. AF is expected to reach epidemic proportions, increasing from about 2.66 million to 15 million affected people by 2050 in the United States alone.[1] Currently available tools for the treatment of patients with AF remain far from ideal. The development of safe and effective treatments for AF is one of the greatest unmet medical needs. There is an emerging paradigm shift in the management of patients with AF from electric end points (rate and rhythm control) to more general end points (such as mortality and morbidity).[2] This review describes current strategies and novel developments in the pharmacologic management of AF (**Fig. 1**).

RHYTHM CONTROL

Rhythm control strategies are focused on the maintenance of sinus rhythm, with its restoration when required. Rhythm control can be achieved with antiarrhythmic agents (AADs), catheter ablation, electric cardioversion, or, rarely, by using surgical techniques. AADs are also used to maintain sinus rhythm after catheter ablation or cardioversion. Although the use and efficacy of catheter ablation–based approaches in AF rhythm control treatment have increased significantly over the past decade, AADs remain the first line therapy for rhythm management of most patients with AF.[3,4] The recent European Society of Cardiology (ESC) guidelines indicate that left atrial ablation may be considered as the frontline therapy in select patients with paroxysmal symptomatic AF (ie, relatively young individuals with minimal to no heart disease).[4]

Modulation of Ion Channel Activity

Most AADs in current clinical use, and those under development, exert their anti-AF actions exclusively or primarily via modulation of cardiac ion channel activity. Agents that inhibit the early sodium channel current (I_{Na}), such as flecainide and propafenone, have proven to be effective in terminating paroxysmal episodes of AF but far less effective in dealing with persistent AF. Because of a proclivity for arrhythmogenesis, these agents are contraindicated in patients with acute coronary syndrome and structural heart disease, which account for more than 70% of patients with AF.[3] Agents that as a primary action inhibit the rapidly activating delayed rectified

Financial support: Supported by grant HL47678 from NHLBI (CA) and the Masons of New York State and Florida.
Conflict of interest statement: Dr Antzelevitch is a consultant to Gilead Sciences and AstraZeneca and received grant support from Gilead Sciences, AstraZeneca, and Merck and Cardiome.
Masonic Medical Research Laboratory, 2150 Bleecker Street, Utica, NY 13501, USA
* Corresponding author.
E-mail address: ca@mmrl.edu

Card Electrophysiol Clin 3 (2011) 157–167
doi:10.1016/j.ccep.2010.10.006

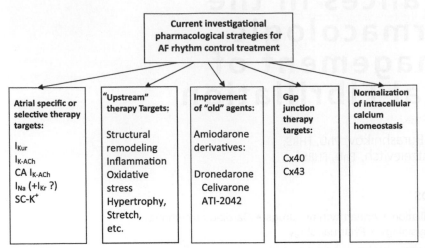

Fig. 1. Current prominent investigational strategies for rhythm control of AF. CA, constitutively active; Cx, connexin; I_{K-ACh}, acetylcholine-regulated inward rectifying potassium current; I_{Kr}, rapidly activating delayed rectified potassium current; I_{Kur}, ultrarapid delayed rectifier potassium current; I_{Na}, early sodium current; SC-K$^+$, small conductance calcium-activated potassium channels. (*From* Burashnikov A, Antzelevitch C. New pharmacological strategies for the treatment of atrial fibrillation. Ann Noninvasive Electrocardiol 2009;14:291; with permission.)

potassium current (I_{Kr}), such as dofetilide, also effectively terminate paroxysmal AF and less effectively persistent AF but these drugs also cause acquired long QT syndrome and may be associated with the development of torsades de pointes arrhythmias. The success rate for terminating persistent AF is greater for I_{Kr} blockers than for I_{Na} blockers.[3] The efficacy of long-term maintenance of sinus rhythm with I_{Na} and I_{Kr} blockers (at 1 year) does not exceed 50%.[5] Amiodarone, a mixed ion channel blocker, is widely used for the long-term maintenance of sinus rhythm and is effective in 65% of cases at 1 year.[6] Advantages of amiodarone are that it can be safely used in most patients with structural heart disease and its application is rarely associated with ventricular proarrhythmia. A major disadvantage of the long-term use of amiodarone is the relatively high rate of multiorgan toxicity. Dronedarone, a derivative of amiodarone, was approved by the Food and Drug Administration (FDA) in 2009 for the treatment of patients with AF, with the indication that it reduces cardiovascular hospitalization. Anti-AF efficacy of dronedarone is superior to placebo but significantly inferior to that of amiodarone.[7–9] Although dronedarone is generally safer than amiodarone, its major drawback is its apparent action to aggravate congestive heart failure (CHF) in patients with preexisting severe CHF (New York Heart Association [NYHA] class IV).[10] Amiodarone has also been reported to increase mortality in NYHA class IV patients.[11]

It is speculated that rhythm control with AADs would be preferable for most patients with AF if safer and more effective anti-AF drugs were available.[12,13] Thus, development of safe and effective AADs for rhythm control management of AF is highly desirable. The search for new anti-AF AADs focuses largely on the delineation of atria-specific or atria-selective targets/agents, as well as on "an improvement of existing AADs" (see **Fig. 1**). Atria-selective strategies[14] are designed to avoid or reduce the risk of induction of ventricular proarrhythmia. Atria-specific targets for AF treatment are those that are present exclusively or almost exclusively in the atria and include the ultrarapid delayed rectified potassium current (I_{Kur}), the acetylcholine-activated inward rectifying potassium current (I_{K-ACh}), and the constitutively active (CA) I_{K-ACh}, which does not require acetylcholine or muscarinic receptors for activation.[15]

I_{Kur} is among the most investigated ion current and until recently, it was widely considered to be the most promising target for the treatment of AF.[15] However, it is becoming increasingly evident that I_{Kur} block alone is unlikely to be sufficient to effectively suppress AF.[16,17] In fact, inhibition of I_{Kur} may promote AF in nonremodeled atria.[18] The contribution of I_{Kur} in AF may be relatively small because I_{Kur} density is reduced with the acceleration of activation rate.[19] I_{Kur} density is also reduced in cells isolated from atria of patients with chronic AF.[20] Although block of I_{Kur} alone may not be effective, when combined with I_{Kr} and/or

I_{Na} inhibition, the role of I_{Kur} in anti-AF actions may be substantial.[16,21]

Block of I_{K-ACh} may be a useful target in clinical cases of vagally mediated AF. CA I_{K-ACh} can be an atria-specific and pathology-specific target for AF treatment. Indeed, CA I_{K-ACh} is only marginally present in healthy nonfibrillating atria and is significantly increased in persistent or chronically fibrillating atria.[15,22] CA I_{K-ACh} could be a valuable target for safe AF treatment, provided it can be inhibited independent of the conventional I_{K-ACh} channels present in many organs other than the heart (eg, in the central nervous system). However, no selective CA I_{K-ACh} blocker is available now.

Recent studies have focused on the small conductance calcium–activated potassium channels (SK channels) present in the hearts of mice, rats, rabbits, and humans.[23,24] There are 3 SK channel isoforms in the heart (ie, SK1, SK2, and SK3); SK1 and SK2 are selectively expressed in atria versus ventricles. Inhibition of the SK channels or genetic ablation of SK2 causes electrophysiological changes selectively in atria.[24,25] Block of SK channels can effectively terminate AF and prevent the recurrence of arrhythmia in experimental rat, guinea pig, and rabbit models of AF.[24] Thus, pilot experimental data suggest that SK channels could be an atria-selective pharmacologic target for AF suppression. However, the role of SK channels in large animals and humans remains poorly defined, as are the functional consequences of modulation of SK channels, including the proarrhythmic potential. For instance, it has been reported that genetic ablation of SK2 channels is associated with the induction of AF in mice.[25]

Atria-selective ionic channel targets are those that are present in both the chambers of the heart but their inhibition produces greater effects in atria than ventricles. These targets include I_{Na} and I_{Kr} channels (see **Fig. 1**). I_{Na} blockers (such as ranolazine, AZD7009, AZD1305, and long-term amiodarone) produce atria-selective depression of I_{Na} and I_{Na}-dependent parameters and effectively suppress AF in the canine heart at concentrations causing little to no electrophysiological changes in the ventricles.[16,17,26–28] A selective I_{Kr} block produces a greater prolongation of action potential duration (APD) and effective refractory period in atria versus ventricles at normal activation rates.[16,27,29] All atria-selective identified I_{Na} blockers also inhibit I_{Kr} and preferentially prolong APD in atria. APD prolongation in atria has been shown to potentiate the development of use-dependent block of I_{Na} (**Fig. 2**).[16,26,27] Atria-selective I_{Na} blockers, including ranolazine, amiodarone, AZD7009, and AZD1305, effectively suppress AF in the clinic.[30–33]

With the exception of I_{Kr} blockers, such as dofetilide, currently available drugs showing anti-AF efficacy (such as amiodarone, dronedarone, flecainide, propafenone, vernakalant, quinidine) as well as promising investigational AADs (such as ranolazine) inhibit multiple ion channels. Among these multiple ion channel blockers, those that inhibit I_{Na} and exhibit rapid dissociation kinetics (such as amiodarone, dronedarone, vernakalant, and ranolazine) rarely, if ever, produce ventricular proarrhythmia. In contrast, AADs (eg, propafenone and flecainide) that inhibit I_{Na} and exhibit slow dissociation kinetics are capable of inducing ventricular proarrhythmia and are contraindicated in structurally compromised hearts as well as in acute coronary syndrome. Another important side effect of AF therapy with slowly dissociating I_{Na} blockers is an induction of atrial flutter with 1:1 conduction to the ventricles. Of note, rapidly dissociating I_{Na} blockers tend to be atrial selective, whereas slowly dissociating blockers are not.[16] Vernakalant recently received FDA approval for its intravenous administration for acute cardioversion of paroxysmal AF and rapid termination of postoperative AF.[34,35]

Recent experimental studies conducted in canine atrial and ventricular preparations demonstrate that the combinations of long-term amiodarone and short-term ranolazine as well as short-term dronedarone and ranolazine (at a relatively low ranolazine concentration; 5 μM) cause a potent synergistic atria-selective depression of sodium channel–mediated parameters (**Fig. 3**).[36,37] These combinations were shown to effectively suppress and prevent the induction of AF, while exerting little to no electrophysiological influence in the ventricles.[36,37] The combination of dronedarone and ranolazine is likely to be associated with little to no adverse effects or organ toxicity because each has a safe clinical record.[38,39] Available data indicate that dronedarone alone is not an atria-selective agent.[37,40,41]

The long-term adverse effects of AADs, both arrhythmic and nonarrhythmic, remain difficult to predict.[10,42] Clinical experience indicates that an optimal long-term risk-benefit ratio is best achieved with multiple ion channel blockers, which inhibit I_{Na} with rapid dissociation kinetics, as well as late I_{Na} and I_{Kr}.[16,17]

Upstream Therapy

AF is commonly associated with both electric and structural atrial abnormalities as well as with a number of other conditions such as oxidation injury, inflammation, stretch, ischemia. Many of these AF-associated abnormalities are caused by

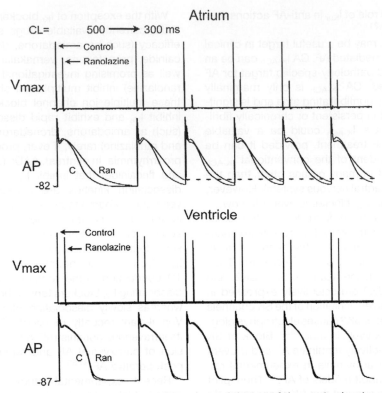

Fig. 2. Ranolazine produces a much greater rate-dependent inhibition of the maximal action potential upstroke velocity (V_{max}) in atria than in ventricles. Shown are V_{max} and action potential (AP) recordings obtained from coronary-perfused canine right atrium and left ventricle before (C) and after ranolazine (10 μM) administration. Ranolazine prolongs late repolarization in atria but not ventricles (due to IKr inhibition[27]). Acceleration of rate then leads to elimination of the diastolic interval, during which much of the recovery from sodium channel block occurs, thus contributing to the atrial selectivity of the drug. CL, cycle length; Ran, ranolazine. (*From* Antzelevitch C, Burashnikov A. Atrial-selective sodium channel block as a novel strategy for the management of atrial fibrillation. J Electrocardiol 2009;42:545; with permission.)

intracardiac and extracardiac diseases, including heart failure, hypertension, coronary artery diseases, myocardial infarction. Oxidative stress may induce inflammation, and both of these factors may promote atrial structural remodeling (ie, interstitial fibrosis, fibroblast proliferation, accumulation of collagen, dilatation, hypertrophy). Atrial structural remodeling can be principally involved in the development and maintenance of AF and may play a greater role in AF maintenance than electric atrial abnormalities.[43] Amelioration of diseases and/or conditions/factors promoting atrial structural remodeling (such as hypertension, heart failure, infarction, oxidative stress, inflammation, stretch) may reduce AF occurrence. A relatively novel investigational approach for AF rhythm control management is upstream therapy, which targets structural remodeling in the atria, factors/diseases that promote such remodeling, or both.[44]

The precise contribution of structural remodeling, inflammation, oxidative injury, ischemia, and stretch (and numerous mediating factors/signaling pathways) in the development of AF remains poorly understood and is likely to vary significantly among different AF pathologies.[45] Experimental and clinical evidence indicate that angiotensin-converting enzyme inhibitors, angiotensin receptor blockers, statins, aldosterone antagonists, and ω-3 polyunsaturated fatty acids may or may not be beneficial in the management of AF.[44,46,47] The anti-AF mechanisms of these interventions are not well established and are presumed to be largely because of their antihypertensive, antiinflammatory, and antioxidative stress actions, reducing structural remodeling.

Several factors have been identified to mediate the generation of atrial fibrosis/inflammation/oxidative stress, including angiotensin II, angiotensin II receptors, transforming growth factor β1, mitogen-activated protein kinase, platelet-derived growth factor, peroxisome proliferator-activated receptor λ, Janus kinase, Rac1, NADPH oxidase, signal transducers and activators of

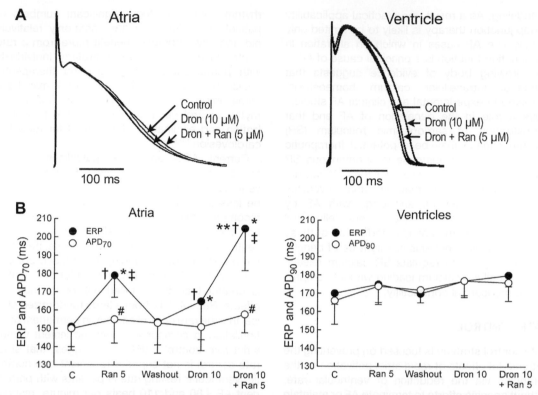

Fig. 3. Atria-selective induction of postrepolarization refractoriness (PRR) by ranolazine (Ran), dronedarone (Dron), and a combination of both (PRR) was approximated by the difference between effective refractory period (ERP) and action potential duration (APD) measured at 70% repolarization (APD_{70}) in atria and by the difference between ERP and APD measured at 90% repolarization (APD_{90}) in ventricles; ERP corresponds to APD_{70-75} in atria and APD_{90} in ventricles. (*A*) Shown are superimposed action potentials demonstrating relatively small changes with Dron, Ran, and their combination. (*B*) Summary of atria-selective induction of PRR. Ventricular data were obtained from epicardium and atrial data from endocardial pectinate muscle. n = 7–8. *, $P<.05$ versus respective control (C); †, $P<.05$ versus washout; ‡, $P<.05$ versus Dron 10; #, $P<.05$ versus respective ERP; **, $P<.05$, change in ERP induced by combination of Ran and Dron (from washout) versus the sum of changes caused by Ran and Dron independently (both from washout). CL = 500 ms. (*From* Burashnikov A, Sicouri S, Di Diego JM, et al. Synergistic effect of the combination of dronedarone and ranolazine to suppress atrial fibrillation. J Am Coll Cardiol 2010;56:1216–24; with permission.)

transcription, and calcineurin.[45,48] The precise cause-effect relationship of the changes observed in all these factors/cascades with AF is difficult to establish, so some of these changes could be the consequences of AF. Most of the current clinical data on upstream AF therapy are derived from observational studies that were not sufficiently powered, and hence, practical clinical applicability of the upstream therapies remains to be determined.[46,47]

Other Preclinical Rate Control Strategies

Several investigational approaches for the pharmacologic treatment of AF have some supporting experimental evidence but remain far from clinical testing (such as modulation of gap junctions or

intracellular calcium activity).[17] It is well recognized that conduction disturbances may have a pivotal role in the generation of AF. Gap junctions, composed of proteins called connexins, are complexes that connect myocardial cells through low-resistance pathways and affect the propagation of excitation in the myocardium. Improving gap junction conductance using the gap junction modulator rotigaptide suppresses AF in a canine chronic mitral regurgitation AF model[49] and canine acute ischemia AF model.[50] Rotigaptide, however, did not affect AF development in AF models associated with heart failure or atrial tachypacing.[49,50] An apparent limitation of gap junction therapy for the treatment of AF is that atrial conduction slowing in most patients with AF occurs largely due to structural remodeling. As a result, the practical applicability of gap junction therapy is likely to be limited only to selective AF cases in which an alteration in gap junction function is a principal cause of AF.

A growing body of evidence suggests that abnormal intracellular calcium homeostasis, observed in experimental and clinical AF studies, plays a role in the generation of AF and that normalization of sarcoplasmic reticulum (SR) calcium release may be a potential therapeutic approach.[51–54] An increase in spontaneous SR calcium release as well as a significant SR calcium leak have been observed in atrial myocytes isolated from humans and dogs with AF by tachypacing-induced atrial remodeling.[52,53] Although the pharmacologic modulation of these arrhythmogenic mechanisms might be of benefit, the challenge is to regulate SR calcium release and intracellular calcium loading without compromising myocardial contractility.

RATE CONTROL

Rate control strategy is focused on preventing the detrimental effects of rapid atrial activation on the ventricles via the reduction of ventricular rate, without specific efforts to terminate AF or maintain sinus rhythm. Major harmful consequences of sustained nontreated AF on ventricles are the development of cardiomyopathy and heart failure. Rate control is most often achieved with the use of pharmacologic agents such as β-blockers, calcium channel blockers, and digoxin. These drugs reduce the excitability of the atrioventricular node, decreasing the number of activations conducted to the ventricles from the fibrillating atria.

It is commonly believed that normality (ie, sinus rhythm) is better than abnormality (ie, AF and related rate control). Indeed, patients with AF who are maintained in sinus rhythm (with or without AADs) have a better survival rate and quality of life than those in whom AF persists,[55–57] although this is not always the case.[58] Currently available AADs do not reliably maintain sinus rhythm over the long term without the substantial risk of adverse effects in many patients with AF. Results from a number of multicenter, randomized, and prospective clinical trials suggest that rhythm control strategies with currently available AADs are not superior to rate control in terms of morbidity and mortality.[59–62] It likely that the adverse effects of using available AADs for rhythm control, secondary to extracardiac toxicity and ventricular proarrhythmia, balances or exceeds the benefit derived from a limited capability of these AADs to maintain sinus rhythm. Due to the limitations and shortcomings of the AAD-based

rhythm control strategy, significant numbers of patients with AF, who are commonly relatively old and asymptomatic, benefit more from a rate control than a rhythm control strategy. Individuals with permanent AF may have no therapeutic choice but rate control. Rate control may have some important advantages over AAD-based rhythm control, such as a reduced rate of hospitalization and elimination of the need for repeated cardiovesion.[59,60]

Current ACC and AHA guidelines for the management of patients with AF suggest that ventricular rate in the rate control approach should be less than 80 beats per minute at rest.[3] This recommendation is largely based on the assumption that in patients with AF, (1) the closer the ventricular rate is to the normal sinus rate, the lower the probability of developing AF-induced complications and (2) the benefit from strict rate control is greater than the entailed risk of the adverse effects. Recent data from a large randomized clinical trial the rate control efficacy in permanent atrial fibrillation: a comparison between lenient versus strict rate control II (RACE-II) suggest that strict rate control is not superior to lenient rate control (ie, ventricular resting rate in patients with permanent AF ≤80 and 110 beats per minute, respectively) for preventing cardiovascular morbidity and mortality.[63] Previous retrospective analysis of the Atrial Fibrillation Follow-up Investigation of Rhythm Management (AFFIRM) trial also did not find differences in morbidity and mortality or quality of life in strict versus mild rate controls.[64] Considering the results of RACE-II, as well as the practical convenience and advantages of lenient versus strict rate controls (easier to achieve with fewer outpatient visits), the new ESC guidelines suggest that lenient rate control may be preferable in select patients with permanent AF.[4]

Aspirin, a less effective but safer agent than warfarin, is often prescribed to low-risk patients with AF (risk of stroke ≤2% per year).[65] Rate and rhythm control with AADs are not mutually exclusive, that is, many AADs used for rhythm control (such as amiodarone, dronedarone, sotalol) possess rate control abilities as well, which may contribute to their total therapeutic positive actions.

ANTICOAGULATION

Stroke is a major detrimental consequence of AF. The incidence of stroke is increased 5-fold in patients with AF compared with those without AF.[66] Most patients with AF, regardless of the choice of rhythm or rate control strategies, require anticoagulation therapy to reduce the risk of stroke. The decision is commonly made with the aid of the CHADS2 score that counts the following risk factors: CHF, hypertension, age greater than 75 years, diabetes mellitus (each scored as 1), and prior stroke or transient ischemic attack (each scored as 2). Patients with AF with a score of 2 or more are considered to have a high risk for stroke (>4% annually). The most commonly used anticoagulants include vitamin K antagonists; among them, warfarin is most widely prescribed for patients at intermediate to high risk for stroke.[67] Aspirin, a less effective but safer agent than warfarin, is often prescribed to low-risk patients with AF (risk of stroke = 2% per year).[65] Antiplatelet agents are also anticoagulants. Randomized clinical trials have consistently shown that in high-risk AF patients, warfarin therapy results in reduction of about 65% in the incidence of stroke whereas antiplatelet agents (clopidogrel and aspirin) reduce it by approximately 20%.[68]

A major complication of anticoagulant therapy is bleeding, and so before the initiation of antithrombotic therapy, a risk-benefit ratio needs to be evaluated. The risk of bleeding is increased with age and diabetes.[65,68]

Warfarin, despite its limitations, remains the best available anticoagulant for high-risk patients with AF.[67] Several novel anticoagulants (such as dabigatran, rivaroxaban, edoxaban, apixaban) are currently in their late stages of clinical development for providing an alternative to warfarin, which is capable of providing safe and effective anticoagulation. Notably, in the Randomized Evaluation of Long-Term Anticoagulation (RE-LY) trial, which includes 18,113 patients with AF and at risk of stroke, a dosage of 150 mg/d of dabigatran was associated with a lower rate of stroke and systemic embolism than warfarin; both agents were associated with a similar rate of major hemorrhage.[69] With a lower dose, dabigatran (110 mg/d) reduced stroke and systemic embolism similar to warfarin but caused a lower incidence of major bleeding.[69]

COMPREHENSIVE MANAGEMENT OF PATIENTS WITH AF

A recent trend in the management of AF involves a shift from electric end points such as rate or rhythm control to hard end points such as morbidity and mortality.[2] Indeed, improving morbidity and mortality should be the prime focus of any therapy. Many patients with AF have coexisting ailments (such as hypertension, heart failure, coronary artery diseases, myocardial ischemia, diabetes) that are often more serious than AF. These diseases often develop independent of AF but may promote AF or may be aggravated by AF. A comprehensive approach to therapy addressing these comorbidities is therefore the key to reducing morbidity and mortality in patients with AF. Dronedarone has been promoted as such an agent owing to its ability to reduce stroke, blood pressure, and ventricular rate during AF, as well as reduce the incidence of AF.[8,38,70] This ability of dronedarone may explain the significant reduction of cardiovascular-related hospitalization and mortality in patients with AF treated with dronedarone in the Placebo-Controlled, Double Blind, Parallel Arm Trial to asses the efficacy of dronedarone 400 mg bid for the prevention of cardiovascular hospitalization and death from any cause in patients with atrial fibrillation/flutter (ATHENA) trial.[38] The anti-AF efficacy of dronedarone seems to be relatively poor.[7-9] It is possible that a significant reduction in hospitalization (and, thus, morbidity) can be achieved without substantial AF suppression. All-cause mortality was not significantly reduced by dronedarone in ATHENA,[38] as is the case for all large clinical trials of anti-AF agents conducted to date.[3,38,60,71,72]

The authors' recent experimental data demonstrating a potent synergistic effect of a combination of dronedarone and ranolazine to atrial-selectively suppress sodium channel–mediated parameters and effectively suppress AF (see **Fig. 3**),[37] which may represent another comprehensive approach to the management of patients with AF. Ranolazine, in addition to its potent antiarrhythmic actions,[26,30,73,74] is capable of ameliorating ischemia-related and heart failure–related symptoms,[75-77] suggesting that it may suppress AF both directly (ie, electrically) and indirectly via its actions to counter AF-promoting conditions (heart failure and ischemia). Both drugs have an excellent clinically-proven safety profile.

SUMMARY

Development of safe and effective pharmacologic therapy for AF is one of the greatest unmet medical needs. Although rhythm control strategies are preferable to those of rate control, pharmacologic therapy capable of widely applicable, safe, and effective AF suppression is not available. Ion channel inhibition remains the principal strategy for suppression of AF. Practical clinical experience indicates that multiple ion channel blockers are generally more optimally effective for rhythm control of AF than ion channel–selective blockers. Concurrent inhibition of sodium and potassium ion channels is more likely to produce atria-selective suppression of sodium channel–mediated parameters, so long as dissociation of the drug from the sodium channel is rapid. Such drugs can effectively suppress AF with a relatively low or no risk of induction of ventricular arrhythmias. Upstream therapy targeting nonelectric factors such as structural remodeling may be required for optimally effective pharmacologic management. Pharmacologic strategies that aim to ameliorate both electric and structural substrates and triggers in the atrium as well as to treat AF-associated extracardiac diseases and AF-induced adverse consequences (primarily stroke and heart failure) are likely to be most successful in reducing morbidity and mortality in patients with AF.

REFERENCES

1. Miyasaka Y, Barnes ME, Gersh BJ, et al. Secular trends in incidence of atrial fibrillation in Olmsted County, Minnesota, 1980 to 2000, and implications on the projections for future prevalence. Circulation 2006;114:119–25.
2. Prystowsky EN, Camm J, Lip GY, et al. The impact of new and emerging clinical data on treatment strategies for atrial fibrillation. J Cardiovasc Electrophysiol 2010;21:946–58.
3. Fuster V, Ryden LE, Cannom DS, et al. ACC/AHA/ESC 2006 guidelines for the management of patients with atrial fibrillation—executive summary: a report of the American College of Cardiology/American Heart Association Task Force on Practice Guidelines and the European Society of Cardiology Committee for Practice Guidelines (Writing Committee to Revise the 2001 Guidelines for the Management of Patients With Atrial Fibrillation). J Am Coll Cardiol 2006;48:854–906.
4. Camm AJ, Kirchhof P, Lip GY, et al. Guidelines for the management of atrial fibrillation: the Task Force for the Management of Atrial Fibrillation of the European Society of Cardiology (ESC). Eur Heart J 2010; 31(19):2369–429.
5. Naccarelli GV, Gonzalez MD. Atrial fibrillation and the expanding role of catheter ablation: do antiarrhythmic drugs have a future? J Cardiovasc Pharmacol 2008;52:203–9.
6. Zimetbaum P. Amiodarone for atrial fibrillation. N Engl J Med 2007;356:935–41.
7. Piccini JP, Hasselblad V, Peterson ED, et al. Comparative efficacy of dronedarone and amiodarone for the maintenance of sinus rhythm in patients with atrial fibrillation. J Am Coll Cardiol 2009;54:1089–95.
8. Singh D, Cingolani E, Diamond GA, et al. Dronedarone for atrial fibrillation: have we expanded the antiarrhythmic armamentarium? J Am Coll Cardiol 2010; 55:1569–76.
9. Burashnikov A, Belardinelli L, Antzelevitch C. Acute dronedarone is inferior to amiodarone in terminating

and preventing atrial fibrillation in canine atria. Heart Rhythm 2010;7:1273–9.
10. Kober L, Torp-Pedersen C, McMurray JJ, et al. Increased mortality after dronedarone therapy for severe heart failure. N Engl J Med 2008;358:2678–87.
11. Bardy GH, Lee KL, Mark DB, et al. Amiodarone or an implantable cardioverter-defibrillator for congestive heart failure. N Engl J Med 2005;352:225–37.
12. Savelieva I, Camm J. Anti-arrhythmic drug therapy for atrial fibrillation: current anti-arrhythmic drugs, investigational agents, and innovative approaches. Europace 2008;10:647–65.
13. Reiffel JA. Rate versus rhythm control pharmacotherapy for atrial fibrillation: where are we in 2008? J Atr Fibrillation 2008;1:31–47.
14. Wang ZG, Fermini B, Nattel S. Sustained depolarization-induced outward current in human atrial myocytes: evidence for a novel delayed rectifier K^+ current similar to Kv1.5 cloned channel currents. Circ Res 1993;73:1061–76.
15. Nattel S, Carlsson L. Innovative approaches to antiarrhythmic drug therapy. Nat Rev Drug Discov 2006; 5:1034–49.
16. Burashnikov A, Antzelevitch C. Atrial-selective sodium channel block for the treatment of atrial fibrillation. Expert Opin Emerg Drugs 2009;14: 233–49.
17. Burashnikov A, Antzelevitch C. New development in atrial antiarrhythmic drug therapy. Nat Rev Cardiol 2010;7:139–48.
18. Burashnikov A, Antzelevitch C. Can inhibition of I_{Kur} promote atrial fibrillation? Heart Rhythm 2008;5: 1304–9.
19. Feng J, Xu D, Wang Z, et al. Ultrarapid delayed rectifier current inactivation in human atrial myocytes: properties and consequences. Am J Physiol 1998;275:H1717–25.
20. Van Wagoner DR, Pond AL, McCarthy PM, et al. Outward K^+ current densities and Kv1.5 expression are reduced in chronic human atrial fibrillation. Circ Res 1997;80:772–81.
21. Blaauw Y, Schotten U, van HA, et al. Cardioversion of persistent atrial fibrillation by a combination of atrial specific and non-specific class III drugs in the goat. Cardiovasc Res 2007;75:89–98.
22. Ravens U. Potassium channels in atrial fibrillation: targets for atrial and pathology-specific therapy? Heart Rhythm 2008;5:758–9.
23. Tuteja D, Xu D, Timofeyev V, et al. Differential expression of small-conductance Ca2+ -activated K+ channels SK1, SK2, and SK3 in mouse atrial and ventricular myocytes. Am J Physiol Heart Circ Physiol 2005;289:H2714–23.
24. Diness JG, Sorensen US, Nissen JD, et al. Inhibition of small conductance Ca2+ -activated potassium channels terminates and protects against atrial fibrillation. Circ Arrhythm Electrophysiol 2010;3:380–90.

25. Li N, Timofeyev V, Tuteja D, et al. Ablation of a Ca^{2+} - activated K^+ channel (SK2 channel) results in action potential prolongation in atrial myocytes and atrial fibrillation. J Physiol 2009;587:1087–100.

26. Burashnikov A, Di Diego JM, Zygmunt AC, et al. Atrium-selective sodium channel block as a strategy for suppression of atrial fibrillation: differences in sodium channel inactivation between atria and ventricles and the role of ranolazine. Circulation 2007;116:1449–57.

27. Burashnikov A, Di Diego JM, Sicouri S, et al. Atrial-selective effects of chronic amiodarone in the management of atrial fibrillation. Heart Rhythm 2008;5:1735–42.

28. Goldstein RN, Khrestian C, Carlsson L, et al. Azd7009: a new antiarrhythmic drug with predominant effects on the atria effectively terminates and prevents reinduction of atrial fibrillation and flutter in the sterile pericarditis model. J Cardiovasc Electrophysiol 2004;15:1444–50.

29. Spinelli W, Parsons RW, Colatsky TJ. Effects of WAY-123,398, a new class III antiarrhythmic agent, on cardiac refractoriness and ventricular fibrillation threshold in anesthetized dogs: a comparison with UK-68798, E-4031, and dl-sotalol. J Cardiovasc Pharmacol 1992;20:913–22.

30. Murdock DK, Overton N, Kersten M, et al. The effect of ranolazine on maintaining sinus rhythm in patients with resistant atrial fibrillation. Indian Pacing Electrophysiol J 2008;8:175–81.

31. Geller JC, Egstrup K, Kulakowski P, et al. Rapid conversion of persistent atrial fibrillation to sinus rhythm by intravenous AZD7009. J Clin Pharmacol 2009;49:312–22.

32. Toivonen L, Raatikainen P, Walfridsson H, et al. A randomized, invasive cardiac electrophysiology study of the combined ion channel blocker AZD1305 in patients after catheter ablation of atrial flutter. J Cardiovasc Pharmacol 2010; 56:300–8.

33. Murdock DK, Reiffel JA, Kaliebe J, et al. The conversion of paroxysmal or initial onset atrial fibrillation with oral ranolazine: implications for a new "pill-in-pocket" approach in structural heart disease. J Atr Fibrillation 2010;2:705–10.

34. Roy D, Pratt CM, Torp-Pedersen C, et al. Vernakalant hydrochloride for rapid conversion of atrial fibrillation. A phase 3, randomized, placebo-controlled trial. Circulation 2008;117:1518–25.

35. Kowey PR, Dorian P, Mitchell LB, et al. Vernakalant hydrochloride for the rapid conversion of atrial fibrillation after cardiac surgery: a randomized, double-blind, placebo-controlled trial. Circ Arrhythm Electrophysiol 2009;2:652–9.

36. Sicouri S, Burashnikov A, Belardinelli L, et al. Synergistic electrophysiologic and antiarrhythmic effects of the combination of ranolazine and chronic amiodarone in canine atria. Circ Arrhythm Electrophysiol 2010;3:88–95.

37. Burashnikov A, Sicouri S, Di Diego JM, et al. Synergistic effect of the combination of dronedarone and ranolazine to suppress atrial fibrillation. J Am Coll Cardiol 2010;56:1216–24.

38. Hohnloser SH, Crijns HJ, van EM, et al. Effect of dronedarone on cardiovascular events in atrial fibrillation. N Engl J Med 2009;360:668–78.

39. Koren MJ, Crager MR, Sweeney M. Long-term safety of a novel antianginal agent in patients with severe chronic stable angina: the Ranolazine Open Label Experience (ROLE). J Am Coll Cardiol 2007; 49:1027–34.

40. Manning A, Thisse V, Hodeige D, et al. SR 33589, a new amiodarone-like antiarrhythmic agent: electrophysiological effects in anesthetized dogs. J Cardiovasc Pharmacol 1995;25:252–61.

41. Varro A, Takacs J, Nemeth M, et al. Electrophysiological effects of dronedarone (SR 33589), a noniodinated amiodarone derivative in the canine heart: comparison with amiodarone. Br J Pharmacol 2001;133:625–34.

42. Preliminary report: Effect of encainide and flecainide on mortality in a randomized trial of arrhythmia suppression after myocardial infarction. The Cardiac Arrhythmia Suppression Trial (CAST) Investigators. N Engl J Med 1989;321:406–12.

43. Cha TJ, Ehrlich JR, Zhang L, et al. Atrial ionic remodeling induced by atrial tachycardia in the presence of congestive heart failure. Circulation 2004;110: 1520–6.

44. Goette A, Bukowska A, Lendeckel U. Non-ion channel blockers as anti-arrhythmic drugs (reversal of structural remodeling). Curr Opin Pharmacol 2007;7:219–24.

45. Nattel S, Burstein B, Dobrev D. Atrial remodeling and atrial fibrillation: mechanisms and implications. Circ Arrhythm Electrophysiol 2008;1:62–73.

46. Savelieva I, Camm J. Statins and polyunsaturated fatty acids for treatment of atrial fibrillation. Nat Clin Pract Cardiovasc Med 2008;5:30–41.

47. Dawe DE, Ariyarajah V, Khadem A. Is there a role for statins in atrial fibrillation? Pacing Clin Electrophysiol 2009;32:1063–72.

48. Burashnikov A. Are there atrial selective/predominant targets for "upstream" atrial fibrillation therapy? Heart Rhythm 2008;5:1294–5.

49. Guerra JM, Everett TH, Lee KW, et al. Effects of the gap junction modifier rotigaptide (ZP123) on atrial conduction and vulnerability to atrial fibrillation. Circulation 2006;114:110–8.

50. Shiroshita-Takeshita A, Sakabe M, Haugan K, et al. Model-dependent effects of the gap junction conduction-enhancing antiarrhythmic peptide rotigaptide (ZP123) on experimental atrial fibrillation in dogs. Circulation 2007;115:310–8.

51. Burashnikov A, Antzelevitch C. Reinduction of atrial fibrillation immediately after termination of the arrhythmia is mediated by late phase 3 early after depolarization-induced triggered activity. Circulation 2003;107:2355–60.

52. Hove-Madsen L, Llach A, Bayes-Genis A, et al. Atrial fibrillation is associated with increased spontaneous calcium release from the sarcoplasmic reticulum in human atrial myocytes. Circulation 2004;110: 1358–63.

53. Vest JA, Wehrens XH, Reiken SR, et al. Defective cardiac ryanodine receptor regulation during atrial fibrillation. Circulation 2005;111:2025–32.

54. Burashnikov A, Antzelevitch C. Late-phase 3 EAD. A unique mechanism contributing to initiation of atrial fibrillation. PACE 2006;29:290–5.

55. Corley SD, Epstein AE, DiMarco JP, et al. Relationships between sinus rhythm, treatment, and survival in the Atrial Fibrillation Follow-Up Investigation of Rhythm Management (AFFIRM) Study. Circulation 2004;109:1509–13.

56. Pedersen OD, Bagger H, Keller N, et al. Efficacy of dofetilide in the treatment of atrial fibrillation-flutter in patients with reduced left ventricular function: a Danish investigations of arrhythmia and mortality on dofetilide (diamond) substudy. Circulation 2001; 104:292–6.

57. Guglin M, Chen R, Curtis AB. Sinus rhythm is associated with fewer heart failure symptoms: insights from the AFFIRM trial. Heart Rhythm 2010;7: 596–601.

58. Talajic M, Khairy P, Levesque S, et al. Maintenance of sinus rhythm and survival in patients with heart failure and atrial fibrillation. J Am Coll Cardiol 2010; 55:1796–802.

59. Wyse DG, Waldo AL, DiMarco JP, et al. A comparison of rate control and rhythm control in patients with atrial fibrillation. N Engl J Med 2002; 347:1825–33.

60. Roy D, Talajic M, Nattel S, et al. Rhythm control versus rate control for atrial fibrillation and heart failure. N Engl J Med 2008;358:2667–77.

61. Van Gelder I, Hagens VE, Bosker HA, et al. A comparison of rate control and rhythm control in patients with recurrent persistent atrial fibrillation. N Engl J Med 2002;347:1834–40.

62. Hohnloser SH, Kuck KH, Lilienthal J. Rhythm or rate control in atrial fibrillation—Pharmacological Intervention in Atrial Fibrillation (PIAF): a randomised trial. Lancet 2000;356:1789–94.

63. Van GI, Groenveld HF, et al. Lenient versus strict rate control in patients with atrial fibrillation. N Engl J Med 2010;362:1363–73.

64. Cooper HA, Bloomfield DA, Bush DE, et al. Relation between achieved heart rate and outcomes in patients with atrial fibrillation (from the Atrial Fibrillation Follow-up Investigation of Rhythm

Management [AFFIRM] study). Am J Cardiol 2004;93:1247–53.

65. Padanilam BJ, Prystowsky EN. Atrial fibrillation: goals of therapy and management strategies to achieve the goals. Med Clin North Am 2008;92: 217, xiii.

66. Wolf PA, D'Agostino RB, Belanger AJ, et al. Probability of stroke: a risk profile from the Framingham study. Stroke 1991;22:312–8.

67. Gopinathannair R, Sullivan RM, Olshansky B. Update on medical management of atrial fibrillation in the modern era. Heart Rhythm 2009;6: S17–22.

68. Hart RG, Pearce LA, Aguilar MI. Meta-analysis: antithrombotic therapy to prevent stroke in patients who have nonvalvular atrial fibrillation. Ann Intern Med 2007;146:857–67.

69. Connolly SJ, Ezekowitz MD, Yusuf S, et al. Dabigatran versus warfarin in patients with atrial fibrillation. N Engl J Med 2009;361:1139–51.

70. Connolly SJ, Crijns HJ, Torp-Pedersen C, et al. Analysis of stroke in ATHENA: a placebo-controlled, double-blind, parallel-arm trial to assess the efficacy of dronedarone 400 mg BID for the prevention of cardiovascular hospitalization or death from any cause in patients with atrial fibrillation/atrial flutter. Circulation 2009;120:1174–80.

71. Lafuente-Lafuente C, Mouly S, Longas-Tejero MA, et al. Antiarrhythmics for maintaining sinus rhythm after cardioversion of atrial fibrillation. Cochrane Database Syst Rev 2007;4:CD005049.

72. Torp-Pedersen C, Moller M, Bloch-Thomsen PE, et al. Dofetilide in patients with congestive heart failure and left ventricular dysfunction. Danish Investigations of Arrhythmia and Mortality on Dofetilide Study Group. N Engl J Med 1999;341: 857–65.

73. Scirica BM, Morrow DA, Hod H, et al. Effect of ranolazine, an antianginal agent with novel electrophysiological properties, on the incidence of arrhythmias in patients with non ST-segment elevation acute coronary syndrome: results from the Metabolic Efficiency With Ranolazine for Less Ischemia in Non ST-Elevation Acute Coronary Syndrome Thrombolysis in Myocardial Infarction 36 (MERLIN-TIMI 36) randomized controlled trial. Circulation 2007;116: 1647–52.

74. Murdock DK, Reiffel JA, Kaliebe JW, et al. The conversion of paroxysmal or initial onset atrial fibrillation with oral ranolazine: implications for "pill in the pocket" approach in structural heart disease. J Am Coll Cardiol 2010;55:A6.E58.

75. Chaitman BR. Ranolazine for the treatment of chronic angina and potential use in other cardiovascular conditions. Circulation 2006;113:2462–72.

76. Wilson SR, Scirica BM, Braunwald E, et al. Efficacy of ranolazine in patients with chronic angina

observations from the randomized, double-blind, placebo-controlled MERLIN-TIMI (Metabolic Efficiency With Ranolazine for Less Ischemia in Non-ST-Segment Elevation Acute Coronary Syndromes) 36 Trial. J Am Coll Cardiol 2009;53:1510–6.

77. Undrovinas AI, Belardinelli L, Undrovinas NA, et al. Ranolazine improves abnormal repolarization and contraction in left ventricular myocytes of dogs with heart failure by inhibiting late sodium current. J Cardiovasc Electrophysiol 2006;17:S161–77.

From Cell to Bedside—Why Make the Journey?

John C. Lopshire, MD, PhD*, Douglas P. Zipes, MD

KEYWORDS

- Cardiac electrophysiology • Translational research
- Arrhythmias • Conduction system disease

It is 1 am, and the physician is called by the emergency department to see a 52 year-old man who presented with a complaint that his heart was pounding with associated shortness of breath. The patient, Mr Y, reveals these symptoms became apparent at approximately 10 p.m. while walking his dog. He denies prior similar symptoms or other active complaints, although he claims that his heart often seems to skip beats. He has no past medical history of illnesses or medical conditions, although he admits to an active 60 pack per year tobacco smoking habit. On examination, Mr Y is a thin man who appears moderately distressed. The patient's blood pressure is 124/76; the respiratory rate is 22 breaths per minute, and oxygen saturation is 92% on 2 L of oxygen via nasal cannula. A focused bedside physical examination is remarkable only for audible chest wheezing and an irregularly—irregular tachycardia with no audible murmurs or rubs. An electrocardiogram reveals atrial fibrillation with a rapid ventricular rate averaging 145 beats per minute (bpm). The QRS duration is 88 milliseconds. There is no evidence of active ischemia. Prior to the physician's arrival, a spiral chest computed tomography (CT) scan had ruled out pulmonary embolism, and the patient's serum tests, including cardiac enzymes, were unremarkable. The emergency department physician placed orders to start the patient on therapeutic anticoagulation and a beta agonist nebulizer for his wheezing. After initiation of the nebulizer, Mr Y's ventricular rate accelerated to 160 bpm. He remained in atrial fibrillation. His other vital signs were: blood pressure 130/82, respiratory rate 20, and oxygen saturation of 97% on 2 L nasal cannula.

The physician rapidly considers the best treatment options for Mr Y's atrial fibrillation. Although he is experiencing some measure of distress, the physician deems him clinically stable and rules out the need for urgent direct current cardioversion to restore sinus rhythm. The physician considers the relative pros and cons of rate versus rhythm control strategies. The physician suspects that the patient's rapid ventricular rate likely began when his symptoms started, but has some concerns over the possibility that his atrial fibrillation has been present for an indeterminate duration given his history of skipped beats. Thus, the physician decides against rhythm control to decrease the possibility of thromboembolic complications. That leaves rate control using atrioventricular nodal blockade as the treatment option. Beta-adrenergic antagonists would effectively slow atrioventricular conduction but likely worsen the patient's respiratory status. Therefore, the physician decides to use an intravenous calcium channel blocking agent, namely diltiazem, to attempt to slow Mr Y's ventricular rate and alleviate his symptoms. Approximately 5 minutes after receiving 10 mg intravenous diltiazem followed with slow intravenous continuous infusion, Mr Y's

Disclosures: JCL receives research funding from Medtronic, Incorporated. DPZ receives research funding and serves as a consultant for Medtronic, Incorporated.
Division of Cardiology, Department of Medicine, Krannert Institute of Cardiology, Indiana University School of Medicine, 1800 North Capitol Avenue, Suite E310, Indianapolis, IN 46202, USA
* Corresponding author.
E-mail address: jlopshir@iupui.edu

Card Electrophysiol Clin 3 (2011) 169–172
doi:10.1016/j.ccep.2010.10.011
1877-9182/11/$ — see front matter © 2011 Elsevier Inc. All rights reserved.

ventricular rate had slowed to the 70 bpm. Importantly, although he remained in atrial fibrillation, his symptoms abated; his blood pressure remained stable, and his respiratory status improved. The physician then is called to see another patient who is in complete heart block. As the physician makes his or her way towards this next clinical encounter, he or she briefly marvels at the number of time-tested treatment options that are readily available for patients like Mr Y and this next patient—and feel gratitude for the legion of prior investigators whose fundamental basic science discoveries provide the foundation for much of today's clinical practice.

This clinical vignette highlights a scene repeated an untold number of times daily where a practicing cardiac electrophysiologist uses a commonplace therapy born from a benchtop basic science observation in cardiac cells or tissues that finds its way to bedside practice. In this case, the use of selective calcium channel blocking agents to specifically target the cells of the atrioventricular node (AVN) was suggested by early work of Zipes and colleagues in isolated rabbit heart preparations.[1] In this work, they demonstrated that manganese (which has calcium channel blocking properties) could slow or block AVN propagation, whereby the toxin tetrodotoxin (which blocks sodium ion channels) had no effect. This basic science observation led to further investigation and eventual widespread clinical use of calcium channel blockade therapy to control rapid ventricular rates in atrial fibrillation, atrial flutter, and other supraventricular arrhythmias involving the AVN.

In their daily clinical practice, cardiac electrophysiologists routinely utilize what are now commonplace diagnostic and therapeutic interventions to treat arrhythmias and cardiac conduction system disease. Most of these interventions went through a lengthy process of basic science discovery, followed by early developmental and validation studies to prepare for human application. Most then underwent further refinement and improvements prior to becoming the standard of care for patients in the form now recognized. Many then evolve further into advanced research or diagnostic or therapeutic tools. One notable example of this evolutionary process is the modern 12 lead electrocardiogram (ECG). At the core of this seemingly routine, everyday test is the phenomenon of cardiac electrical activity. In the late 1800s, British physiologist John Sanderson used primitive techniques to be among the first to directly record and visualize cardiac electrical activity from the frog heart using a Lippmann capillary electrometer.[2] In 1878, Augustus Waller assembled a Lippmann capillary

electrometer connected to a projector to be one of the first to record cardiac electrical activity from a person in real time.[3] In the early 1900s, Einthoven developed the string galvanometer, which allowed for higher resolution recordings, to systematically record human cardiac activity in normal and abnormal conditions.[4] His descriptions of the important features of the ECG endure to this day and earned him the Nobel prize in medicine. Subsequently, Lewis and others made important refinements to the ECG and its clinical applications to produce the modern instrument utilized today. Interestingly, the evolution of the ECG continues, as Yoram Rudy and others are developing new noninvasive techniques that allow for much higher resolution imaging of real-time cardiac electrical activity.[5]

In considering this example of the evolution of the ECG, the major point to be made is that as basic science discoveries in cardiac electrophysiology are made, these eventually get translated into clinical practice, are refined through clinical use, and become part of standardized practice. This is a truly translational, bench-to-bedside process. Moreover, as basic science discoveries are translated into clinical applications, they often prompt the creation of spin-off technologies and techniques, and sometimes even drive bedside-to-bench research. In this instance, a clinical observation is made. A deficiency in knowledge is identified; a hypothesis is generated, and that hypothesis is tested in the basic research laboratory. The results of this testing then may reveal new knowledge that subsequently returns to the clinical venue. The key difference seen in modern basic science research, as compared to the 20th century, is often the difference in speed in which these findings can be disseminated to the scientific and clinical communities. The successful clinician and researcher in this modern era will be able to rapidly assimilate these findings into their knowledge base and leverage them to adapt his or her research or practice efforts for the synergistic benefit of the scientific and clinical communities.

For the practicing cardiac electrophysiologist, one might ask why in-depth knowledge of basic cardiac electrophysiology is necessary. Short of helping with the board certification examination questions that deal with basic science principles and phenomenon, what benefit can the practicing electrophysiologist hope to realize from this effort? To put it another way, why make the journey? There are several compelling reasons to make this journey. The first and most notable is that a strong scientific knowledge base is the foundation of successful clinical practice. That is the reason that most medical schools around the globe initiate training of medical students with 2 or more years of basic medical science education. Most post-graduate clinical cardiac electrophysiology training programs now have a significant didactic lecture component dedicated to teaching essential basic science cardiac electrophysiology principles to trainees. The electrophysiologist who possesses at least a basic understanding of the cellular-, tissue-, and organ-level anatomy and physiology of the cardiovascular system will be in a position to appreciate the finer, deeper issues associated with the diagnostic and therapeutic modalities they may employ on a routine basis. Thus, when such a routine tool produces an unexpected result, they may be able to form a plausible explanation for this aberrant result, and formulate an appropriate course of action. Furthermore, with this knowledge base, they will be able to independently evaluate the merits and pitfalls of new therapies and treatments as they become available. Ideally, this knowledge should include a reasonable familiarity with the important determinants of excitability (ionic gradients, ion channels, and gap junctions) in different cardiac tissues, from the sino-atrial node to ventricular muscle, in both health and disease.

The second reason that the practicing cardiac electrophysiologist should acquire and maintain a solid understanding of basic science cardiac electrophysiology principles is to simply keep up with the pace of new discoveries that will impact the care of their patients. Scientific understanding of electrophysiological disease processes at the molecular level is increasing exponentially. An illustrative example is in the area of genetics. The human genome project mapped the human genome. The area of functional genomics is now being explored. There is now an understanding of the way various genes influence or even cause cardiac disease. In the 1990s, there were fewer than 10 genes identified that were known to be associated with arrhythmias or conduction system disease; that number now runs into the hundreds. If one factors in molecules identified that can interact with or alter gene expression and promote arrhythmias, that number grows much higher. Commercial and private laboratory tests are now available to screen for some of these genetic defects. On the therapeutic side, scientists and clinicians are actively developing genetic therapies to ameliorate or even reverse arrhythmic disease. An innumerable number of new, targeted, molecular-based diagnostic and therapeutic treatments for arrhythmias and conduction system disease are on the horizon, and increasingly-informed patients will demand their physicians be able to utilize these novel technologies to enhance their care. By securing and maintaining a basic science knowledge base, the clinician will be able to effectively deliver care to the arrhythmia patient in this rapidly changing clinical arena.

The final, and most compelling reason that practicing cardiac electrophysiologists should make the effort to understand and appreciate the basic science underpinnings of cardiac electrophysiology is that this knowledge may allow them to identify and appreciate deficits in the broader basic and clinical knowledge base and possibly contribute to increasing understanding in these areas. In this way, the practicing clinician could exert a huge impact on arrhythmia patient care. Maybe a clinician will not conduct basic research himself or herself, but he or she may be able to share personal experiences or provide unbiased insight that prompts other investigators to pursue novel avenues of scientific inquiry. Alternatively, a clinician could refer patients for participation in trials and registries whose outcome goals are to better understand arrhythmias and conduction system disease. There are many unanswered questions or areas of serious deficits in knowledge related to the maintenance and control of cardiac electrical activity. For instance, a fundamental understanding of sinus node regulation in patients with other arrhythmias is lacking. Atrial fibrillation is occurring at alarmingly increasing rates in patients, but there are serious deficits in understanding of the etiologies, natural history, or progression of this increasingly common arrhythmia. It remains unknown why patients with atrial fibrillation have an increased risk of sudden cardiac arrest. In patients with a prior history of sudden cardiac arrest, it is known that they are at elevated risk of recurrent arrest, but clinicians cannot tell them when, where, or why this may occur. The same holds for patients with compromised left ventricular function and no prior history of sudden cardiac arrest; clinicians know they have a heightened risk of sudden cardiac arrest, but they cannot tell them when, or even if, this will occur. This can certainly be frustrating for the patient and clinician when determining treatment options that involve invasive procedures and large expense such as implantable defibrillators. On the pharmacological arena, the development of new antiarrhythmic medications needs to be fostered. This listing could continue. Although there has been significant progress in understanding the biological basis of arrhythmic and conduction system diseases, there remain serious knowledge deficits that the practicing clinician can help eliminate by maintaining a personal knowledge base of basic science principles, sharing observations and theories of arrhythmia mechanisms with other clinicians and basic scientists, and encouraging patient participation in basic science and biomarker trials and registries.

In summary, the modern clinical environment for the cardiac electrophysiology clinician is rapidly changing. As the basic science knowledge base in this area grows, the clinician must endeavor to assimilate the essential basic science principles into his or her knowledge base that will allow him or her to deliver competent and cutting edge care to patients. Other chapters within this issue will discuss the clinical relevance of basic science electrophysiology in greater detail and will provide a solid foundation for the clinician's ongoing journey to master the science behind the clinical care of patients with complex arrhythmia and conduction system disorders.

REFERENCES

1. Zipes DP, Mendez C. Action of manganese ions and tetrodotoxin on atrioventricular nodal transmembrane potentials in isolated rabbit hearts. Circ Res 1973;32:447–54.
2. Sanderson J. Experimental results relating to the rhythmical and excitatory motions of the ventricle of the frog heart. Proc Roy Soc Lond 1878;27:410–4.
3. Waller AD. A demonstration on man of electromotive changes accompanying the heart's beat. J Physiol 1887;8:229–34.
4. Einthoven W. Le telecardiogramme. Arch Int Physiol 1906;4:132–64 [in French].
5. Ramanathan C, Ghanem RN, Jia P, et al. Noninvasive electrocardiographic imaging for cardiac electrophysiology and arrhythmias. Nat Med 2004;10:422–8.

Index

Note: Page numbers of articles titles are in **boldface** type.

A

Action potential (AP), 58–61
  ventricular, prolongation of, 58–61
Acute myocardial ischemia
  phase 2 reentry in, 54
  ST segment elevation in, 54
Afterdepolarization(s), 26–27
  early. See *Early afterdepolarizations (EADs)*.
Afterpotentials, delayed, history of, 6
Altered currents, in heart failure, 61
Altered repolarization
  acquired long QT syndrome due to, 13–14
  heart failure due to, 11–12
Anderson-Tawill syndrome (ATS), loss-of-function
  of potassium channels and, 118–119
Anticoagulation, pharmacologic management of
  atrial fibrillation in, 162–163
AP. See *Action potential (AP)*.
Arrhythmia(s)
  defined, 23
  electrophysiologic basis of, history of, 6–7
  gender differences in, calcium and, 16–17
  in heart failure, cellular mechanisms of, 58–61
  mechanisms of, **23–45,** 142–148
    abnormal impulse formation, 23–24
    afterdepolarization, 26–27
    altered repolarization and acquired long QT
      syndrome, 13–14
    altered repolarization and heart failure,
      11–12
    apex-base gradients of repolarization, 14
    automaticity, 24–26
    Brugada syndrome, 33–34
    calcium in, 15–17
    channelopathy-related, 33–39
    circus movement reentry without anatomic
      obstacle, 29–30
    deciphering of, **11–21**
    delayed afterdepolarization–induced triggered
      activity, 27
    early repolarization syndrome, 35–36
    J wave syndromes, 33–36
    long QT syndrome, 36–38
    reentrant arrhythmias, 27–32. See also
      Reentrant arrhythmias.
    repolarization and congenital long QT
      syndrome, 14–15
    short QT syndrome, 38

spatial dispersion of repolarization in
  channelopathy-mediated sudden death,
  38–39
transmural repolarization gradients in heart
  failure, 12–13
triggered activity, 26–27
Arrhythmogenesis
  heart failure and, mechanisms underlying, **57–68**
    described, 57–58
  in heart failure, altered metabolism in, 61–62
  late I_{Na} in, **125–140.** See also *Late sodium channel
    current (I_{Na}).*
  of J wave, 48–51
Arrhythmogenic right ventricular cardiomyopathy,
  sodium channel effects on, 105
Atrial fibrillation
  classification of, 142
  described, 141
  familial
    gain-of-function of potassium channels and,
      121–122
    sodium channel effects on, 102
  management of
    comprehensive, 163
    pharmacologic
      advances in, **157–167**
      in anticoagulation, 162–163
      in rate control, 162
      in rhythm control, 157–162
        modulation of ion channel activity,
          157–159
        preclinical rate control strategies,
          161–162
        upstream therapy, 159–161
  mechanisms underlying, **141–156**
    abnormal automaticity, 142–143
    abnormal impulse formation, 142–143
    reentry, 144–148
    rotor dynamics modulation, ionic mechanisms
      in, 150–153
    triggered activity, 143–144
    theories for, 148–150
Atrial standstill, sodium channel effects on, 102
ATS. See *Anderson-Tawill syndrome (ATS)*.
Automaticity
  abnormal, in atrial fibrillation, 142–143
  defined, 23
  enhanced, 25

Card Electrophysiol Clin 3 (2011) 173–177
doi:10.1016/S1877-9182(10)00181-4

Printed and bound by CPI Group (UK) Ltd, Croydon, CR0 4YY

03/10/2024

01040351-0020